Clinical Advances in MRI of Kidney

Clinical Advances in MRI of Kidney

Editor: Eliza Harris

MURPHY & MOORE
www.murphy-moorepublishing.com

www.murphy-moorepublishing.com

MURPHY & MOORE

Cataloging-in-Publication Data

Clinical advances in MRI of kidney / edited by Eliza Harris.
p. cm.
Includes bibliographical references and index.
ISBN 978-1-63987-110-0
1. Kidneys--Magnetic resonance imaging. 2. Kidneys--Imaging. 3. Kidneys--Radiography.
4. Kidneys--Diseases--Diagnosis. I. Harris, Eliza.
RC904.5.I42 C55 2022
616.610 757--dc23

Murphy & Moore Publishing,
1 Rockefeller Plaza,
New York City, NY 10020, USA

ISBN 978-1-63987-110-0 (Hardback)

Contents

Preface VII

Chapter 1 **Renal pH Imaging Using Chemical Exchange Saturation Transfer (CEST) MRI: Basic Concept** 1
Dario Livio Longo, Pietro Irrera, Lorena Consolino, Phillip Zhe Sun and Michael T. McMahon

Chapter 2 **Preparation and Monitoring of Small Animals in Renal MRI** 17
Tamas Kaucsar, Adam Hosszu, Erdmann Seeliger, Henning M. Reimann and Andrea Fekete

Chapter 3 **Dynamic Contrast Enhancement (DCE) MRI-Derived Renal Perfusion and Filtration: Basic Concepts** 28
Michael Pedersen, Pietro Irrera, Walter Dastrù, Frank G. Zö llner, Kevin M. Bennett, Scott C. Beeman, G. Larry Bretthorst, Joel R. Garbow and Dario Livio Longo

Chapter 4 **Preparation of Ex Vivo Rodent Phantoms for Developing, Testing, and Training MR Imaging of the Kidney and Other Organs** 51
Jason M. Millward, João S. Periquito, Paula Ramos Delgado, Christian Prinz, Thoralf Niendorf and Sonia Waiczies

Chapter 5 **MRI Mapping of Renal T_1: Basic Concept** 62
Stefanie J. Hectors, Philippe Garteiser, Sabrina Doblas, Gwenaël Pagé, Bernard E. Van Beers, John C. Waterton and Octavia Bane

Chapter 6 **Noninvasive Renal Perfusion Measurement Using Arterial Spin Labeling (ASL) MRI: Basic Concept** 75
Min-Chi Ku, María A. Fernández-Seara, Frank Kober and Thoralf Niendorf

Chapter 7 **Hardware Considerations for Preclinical Magnetic Resonance of the Kidney** 86
Paula Ramos Delgado, Ekkehard Küstermann, André Kühne, Jason M. Millward, Thoralf Niendorf, Andreas Pohlmann and Martin Meier

Chapter 8 **Recommendations for Preclinical Renal MRI: A Comprehensive Open-Access Protocol Collection to Improve Training, Reproducibility, and Comparability of Studies** 111
Andreas Pohlmann, Susan J. Back, Andrea Fekete, Iris Friedli, Stefanie Hectors, Neil Peter Jerome, Min-Chi Ku, Dario Livio Longo, Martin Meier, Jason M. Millward, Joa˜o S . Periquito, Erdmann Seeliger, Suraj D. Serai, Sonia Waiczies, Steven Sourbron, Christoffer Laustsen and Thoralf Niendorf

Chapter 9 **Animal Models of Renal Pathophysiology and Disease....132**
Adam Hosszu, Tamas Kaucsar, Erdmann Seeliger and Andrea Fekete

Chapter 10 **Ultrasound and Photoacoustic Imaging of the Kidney: Basic Concepts and Protocols....150**
Sandra Meyer, Dieter Fuchs and Martin Meier

Chapter 11 **MRI Mapping of the Blood Oxygenation Sensitive Parameter T_2* in the Kidney: Basic Concept....172**
Lu-Ping Li, Bradley Hack, Erdmann Seeliger and Pottumarthi V. Prasad

Chapter 12 **Reversible (Patho)Physiologically Relevant Test Interventions: Rationale and Examples....187**
Kathleen Cantow, Mechthild Ladwig-Wiegard, Bert Flemming, Andrea Fekete, Adam Hosszu and Erdmann Seeliger

Chapter 13 **Renal Diffusion-Weighted Imaging (DWI) for Apparent Diffusion Coefficient (ADC), Intravoxel Incoherent Motion (IVIM), and Diffusion Tensor Imaging (DTI): Basic Concepts....204**
Neil Peter Jerome, Anna Caroli and Alexandra Ljimani

Chapter 14 **Quantitative Assessment of Renal Perfusion and Oxygenation by Invasive Probes: Basic Concepts....222**
Kathleen Cantow, Roger G. Evans, Dirk Grosenick, Thomas Gladytz, Thoralf Niendorf, Bert Flemming and Erdmann Seeliger

Permissions

List of Contributors

Index

Preface

The world is advancing at a fast pace like never before. Therefore, the need is to keep up with the latest developments. This book was an idea that came to fruition when the specialists in the area realized the need to coordinate together and document essential themes in the subject. That's when I was requested to be the editor. Editing this book has been an honour as it brings together diverse authors researching on different streams of the field. The book collates essential materials contributed by veterans in the area which can be utilized by students and researchers alike.

MRI stands for magnetic resonance imaging and it is used to take pictures of the internal organs and soft tissues of the body without using X-rays. It uses magnets and radio waves to produce detailed pictures of the body's soft tissues and internal organs. During the process of magnetic resonance imaging, a dye known as contrast medium is injected into the person's blood via a vein in the forearm or hand. A type of MRI, known as magnetic resonance angiography (MRA) is used to provide a detailed view of blood vessels that supply blood to the kidneys. Another type of MRI known as magnetic resonance urography (MRU) is used to evaluate patients with hematuria. The ever growing need of advanced technology is the reason that has fueled the research in the field of MRI in recent times. This book traces the progress of this field and highlights some of its key concepts and applications. It will help the readers in keeping pace with the clinical advances in this field.

Each chapter is a sole-standing publication that reflects each author's interpretation. Thus, the book displays a multi-facetted picture of our current understanding of application, resources and aspects of the field. I would like to thank the contributors of this book and my family for their endless support.

Editor

1

Renal pH Imaging Using Chemical Exchange Saturation Transfer (CEST) MRI: Basic Concept

Dario Livio Longo, Pietro Irrera, Lorena Consolino, Phillip Zhe Sun, and Michael T. McMahon

Abstract

Magnetic Resonance Imaging (MRI) has been actively explored in the last several decades for assessing renal function by providing several physiological information, including glomerular filtration rate, renal plasma flow, tissue oxygenation and water diffusion. Within MRI, the developing field of chemical exchange saturation transfer (CEST) has potential to provide further functional information for diagnosing kidney diseases. Both endogenous produced molecules as well as exogenously administered CEST agents have been exploited for providing functional information related to kidney diseases in preclinical studies. In particular, CEST MRI has been exploited for assessing the acid-base homeostasis in the kidney and for monitoring pH changes in several disease models. This review summarizes several CEST MRI procedures for assessing kidney functionality and pH, for monitoring renal pH changes in different kidney injury models and for evaluating renal allograft rejection.

This chapter is based upon work from the COST Action PARENCHIMA, a community-driven network funded by the European Cooperation in Science and Technology (COST) program of the European Union, which aims to improve the reproducibility and standardization of renal MRI biomarkers. This introduction chapter is complemented by two separate chapters describing the experimental procedure and data analysis.

Key words Magnetic resonance imaging (MRI), Kidney, Mice, Rats, pH, Iopamidol, Chemical exchange saturation transfer (CEST), Acute kidney injury, Ischemia–reperfusion injury, Renal damage

1 Introduction

Renal dysfunction is recognized as a significant health problem originating from a variety of causes leading to acute or chronic kidney diseases. Predisposition to acute kidney injury and premature mortality are frequent outcomes for chronic kidney diseases [1]. Moreover, according to the Global Burden of Disease 2013 study, the age-standardized death rates for chronic kidney diseases showed one of the highest increases in the last two decades [2]. Therefore, reliable and early diagnosis of acute and chronic kidney diseases is needed to preserve renal functionality and

Andreas Pohlmann and Thoralf Niendorf (eds.), *Preclinical MRI of the Kidney: Methods and Protocols*, Methods in Molecular Biology, vol. 2216, https://doi.org/10.1007/978-1-0716-0978-1_14,

improve patients' outcome. Despite these premises, current clinical evaluation of renal function is still based on measurement of serum creatinine, which is well known to have several limitations. In fact, an elevated serum creatinine concentration is only discovered at late stages of the disease when renal functionality is already compromised. Therefore, novel noninvasive imaging approaches are needed for a more accurate and early diagnosis of renal physiology. Magnetic resonance imaging (MRI) has been exploited for tissue anatomic imaging, owing to the high spatial resolution and lack of ionizing radiation. In research, novel MRI techniques have been investigated for assessing multiple functional parameters of the kidneys, including perfusion, filtration, oxygenation and tissue elasticity [3–11]. Several reviews covering the role of these MRI approaches for assessing renal functionality have been published [12–15]. This additional information should enable a better characterization of acute and chronic kidney diseases in comparison to standard urine and serum-based assays.

Recently, Chemical Exchange Saturation Transfer (CEST) MRI has emerged as a novel approach for functional and molecular imaging with great promise for clinical translation [16–18]. In addition, CEST MRI pH imaging has emerged as a valuable approach for assessing extracellular pH values in several tissues, including kidneys and tumors, providing the highest accuracy and spatial resolution achievable so far [19]. Owing to the key role of the kidneys in maintaining the acid-base homeostasis, CEST MRI pH mapping has emerged as a novel and promising approach in monitoring kidney functionality.

In this chapter, we will address the basic concept and the developments of renal CEST pH imaging with the emphasis on kidney disease models in rodents.

This introduction chapter is complemented by two separate chapters describing the experimental procedure and data analysis, which are part of this book.

This chapter is part of the book Pohlmann A, Niendorf T (eds) (2020) Preclinical MRI of the Kidney—Methods and Protocols. Springer, New York.

2 Measurement Concept

2.1 Basic Concept of Chemical Exchange Saturation Transfer (CEST) Imaging

CEST is a new technique that enables the indirect detection of molecules possessing mobile protons in exchange with water [20]. Because of this, CEST makes MRI sensitive to endogenous or exogenous molecules that possess suitable protons [21–32]. The generation of contrast is based on a selective irradiation with a radiofrequency pulse at the specific absorption frequency of the exchanging proton, followed by a subsequent transfer, due to chemical exchange with bulk water, of the saturated signal. Upon the application of a long saturation RF (radiofrequency) pulse, the water signal decreases, allowing the amplification of the labeled protons from the molecule to water. As a consequence, low concentration molecules can be specifically and indirectly detected, owing to the frequency selective irradiation of their mobile proton pool(s) [33–38].

2.2 CEST Contrast Agents for Imaging Kidneys and Mapping pH

Several classes of CEST contrast agents can be used as pH responsive agents and exploited for in vivo experiments.

2.2.1 Diamagnetic CEST Agents

Several molecules, including natural occurring molecules, possess exchangeable protons that can be indirectly detected within the CEST approach [39]. Most of these labile protons have chemical exchange rates that show a strong pH dependence. Hence differences in CEST contrast can be exploited for assessing the pH of the solution where they are dissolved. Due to the concomitant contribution of concentration and exchange rate to the observed CEST contrast, several approaches have been proposed to rule out the concentration term, based on the ratiometric method, that is, taking the ratio of the observed contrast, providing accurate pH readouts [40, 41]. Most of the pH responsive diamagnetic molecules investigated so far in vivo are iodinated contrast agents used for radiographic procedures, since they have been used in the last 40 years in clinical examinations owing to their high safety profiles [42, 43]. The presence of amide groups in their chemical structure allow them to be exploited as CEST MRI contrast agents, upon selective irradiation of the mobile proton pool [44].

Among the radiographic contrast media, Iopamidol (Isovue®, Bracco Imaging, Italy) (Fig. 1) was the first agent exploited for mapping pH thanks to the presence of two amide groups with different resonance frequencies, at 4.2 ppm and at 5.5 ppm, respectively, that can be selectively irradiated [45–47]. This chemical peculiarity led to the development of a ratiometric approach based on the ratio of the CEST effects at these two frequencies to provide accurate pH measurements. In vitro experiments showed a high pH responsiveness within the physiological range and accurate pH measurements (Fig. 2a, b). Following intravenous administration, it can provide selective contrast at specific frequency offsets and from the ratio of these two parametric maps it is possible to measure renal pH map (Fig. 2c–f). To validate the approach and test the pH-responsiveness of the agent, induced alkalinisation or acidification of urine was obtained in mice upon providing acidic or alkaline drinking water for a week. For control mice, mean pH values calculated for cortex, medulla and calyx regions were: 7.0 ± 0.11; 6.85 ± 0.15 and 6.6 ± 0.20, respectively. In mice drinking acidic water a significant acidification of renal pH values was obtained. Conversely, a marked increase of renal pH values was

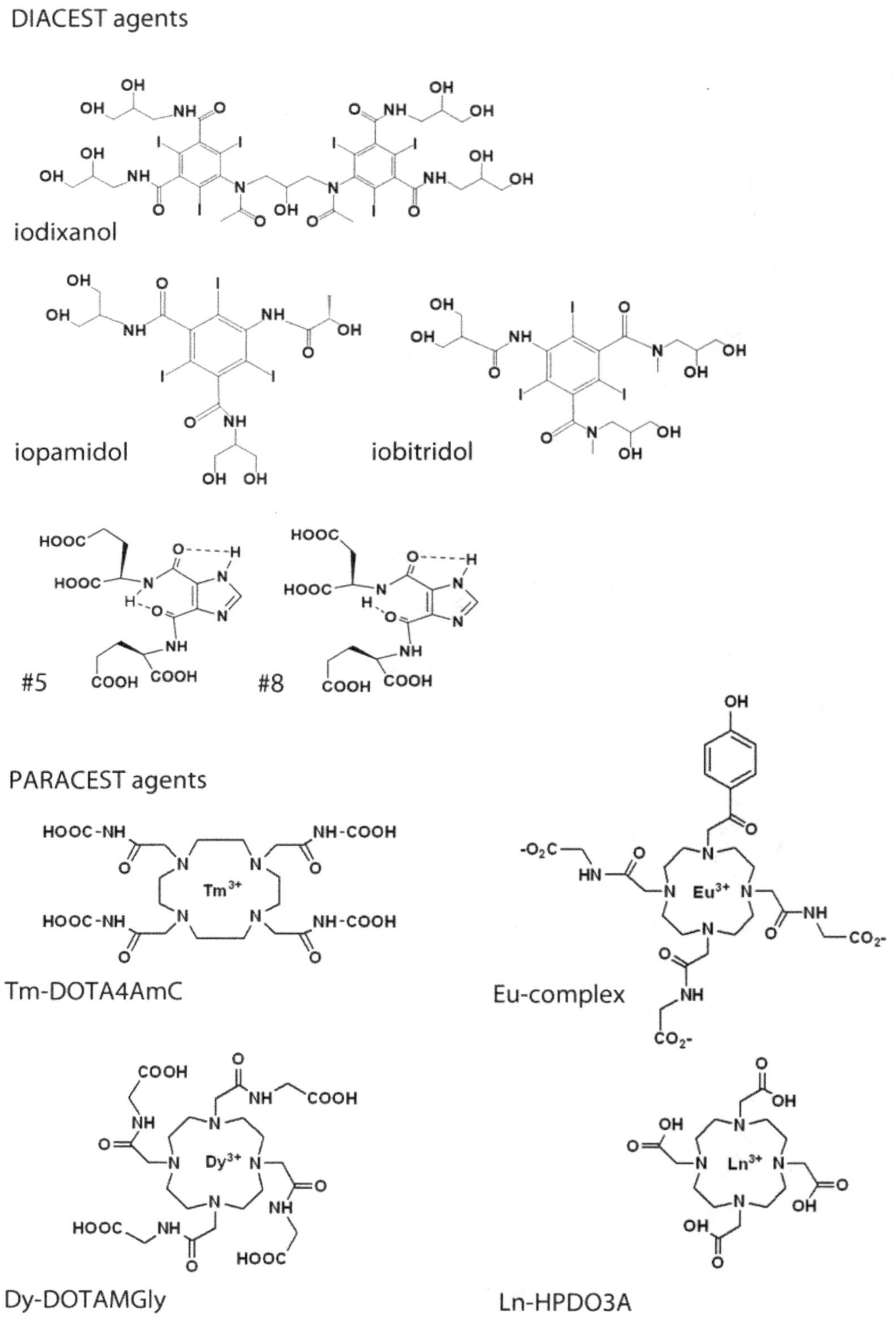

Fig. 1 Chemical structures of the reported pH-responsive CEST agents investigated for renal pH mapping

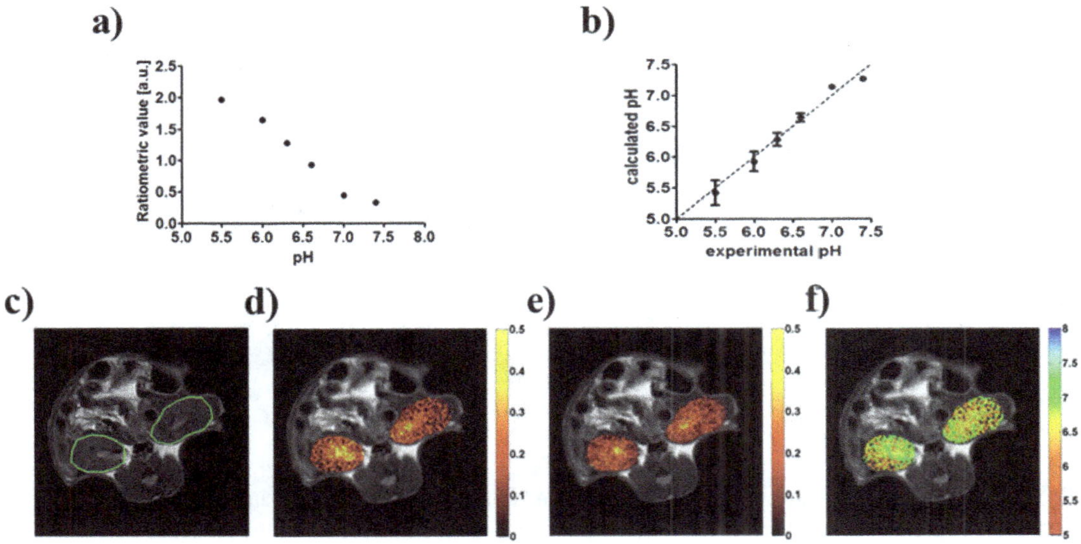

Fig. 2 Iopamidol ratiometric curve obtained from the rations of the CEST contrast upon irradiating at 4.2 and 5.5 ppm, respectively, showing the high pH responsiveness of Iopamidol. Irradiation power levels of 3 μT, Iopamidol 30 mM, 7.05 T, 310 K, irradiation time 5 s (**a**). Calculated pH values obtained by the ratiometric method (Iopamidol 30 mM, 7.05 T, 310 K, irradiation time 5 s, B_1 3 μT) are compared with the values read on the pH-meter (**b**). Representative images of in vivo renal pH mapping showing the anatomical image (**c**) and the CEST contrast parametric maps overlaid to the anatomical image at 4.2 ppm (**d**) and 5.5 ppm (**e**) and the observed pH map (**f**) obtained by ratioing maps (**d**) and (**e**) and using the calibration curve in (**a**) for calculating the pH values. (Adapted with permission from *Magnetic Resonance in Medicine* 2011 (Iopamidol as a responsive MRI-chemical exchange saturation transfer contrast agent for pH mapping of kidneys: in vivo studies in mice at 7 T. Volume: 65, Issue: 1, Pages: 202–211, DOI: https:/doi.org/10.1002/mrm.22608))

observed upon alkaline water administration. Both observations demonstrate the capability to measure in vivo renal pH changes with CEST MRI.

Since the accuracy in measuring pH depends on several factors, including chemical exchange rate, irradiation conditions (saturation power and duration), and main magnetic field, quantification of multisite pH-dependent chemical exchange properties is needed to improve pH accuracy [48]. This characterization of chemical exchange rates and optimal irradiation RF pulses led to the development of an optimized saturation for each single amide proton pools, hence resulting in a higher pH sensitivity. As a result, the capability to measure pH was demonstrated also at magnetic field strengths of 4.7 T, where amide resonances partially overlap. In the study of Wu and coworkers, they demonstrated an improved pH sensitivity, extending the pH detection range from 5.5 to 7.5, with high resolution pH maps of the kidneys in healthy rats (Fig. 3) [49]. More recently, the exploitation of the same ratiometric approach for measuring in vivo pH was also demonstrated at magnetic fields as low as 3 T, which still preserved good pH accuracy [50].

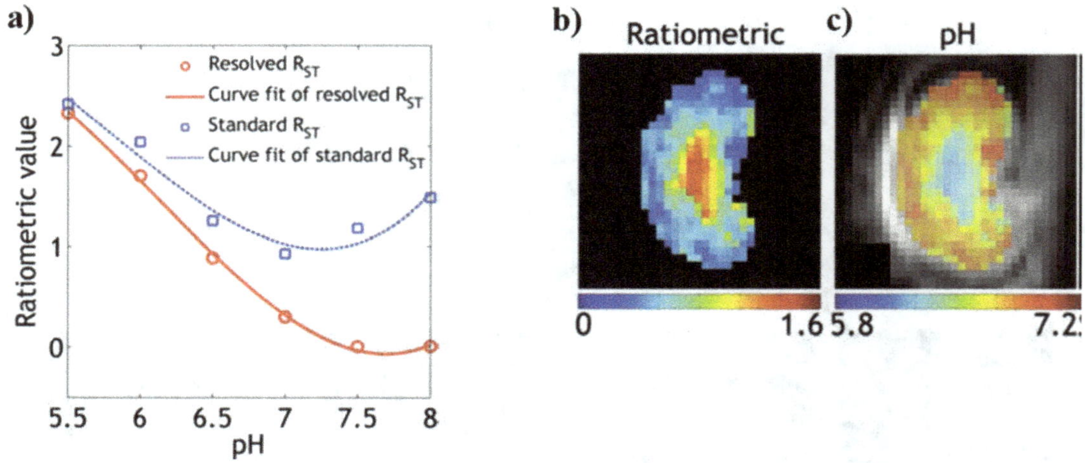

Fig. 3 Extension of pH detection range using the modified ratiometric analysis (red circles) versus the standard ratiometric approach (blue squares) (**a**). Representative in vivo ratiometric map for the proposed approach (**b**). pH map shows the renal pH gradually decreasing from the cortex, medulla to calyx (**c**). Maps are overlaid on the corresponding T_2-weighted image. (Adapted with permission from *Magnetic Resonance in Medicine* 2018 (A generalized ratiometric chemical exchange saturation transfer (CEST) MRI approach for mapping renal pH using Iopamidol, Volume: 79, Issue: 3, Pages: 1553–1558, DOI: https:/doi.org/10.1002/mrm.26817))

Another similar iodinated contrast media, Iopromide (Ultravist®, Bayer Healthcare, Germany), was also demonstrated and compared to Iopamidol for measuring pH, with a pH sensitivity that was not substantially different, although Iopamidol allows for more precise pH measurements [51].

The exploitation of the ratiometric approach requires two distinguishable protons pools on the same molecule, therefore it is limited to a select group of compounds possessing this feature. To overcome this limitation, Longo and Sun proposed a novel approach based on the irradiation of a single pool under different radiofrequency powers [52]. The proposed approach, called ratio of RF power mismatch or RPM, was demonstrated by using Iobitridol (Omnipaque®, GE Healthcare, USA), a radiographic contrast medium possessing only one amide proton pool resonating at 5.5 ppm (Fig. 1). Since the measured CEST contrast is dependent on both pH and irradiation power (B_1), a strong pH dependence was demonstrated by calculating the ratio of the CEST contrast at two different B_1 power levels. In comparison to the conventional ratiometric approach, a good pH accuracy and an even higher pH sensitivity were demonstrated. When investigated in healthy kidneys, the measured pH values upon iobitridol injection strongly correlated with the pH values obtained following iopamidol injection. Recently, to overcome the specific absorption rate (SAR) limitations when using a continuous wave (CW) irradiation of the mobile proton pools, a pulsed ratiometric approach has been exploited and tested on the Iodixanol (Visipaque®, GE Healthcare, USA) X-ray contrast medium for CEST pH imaging [53].

Diamagnetic contrast agents possess resonances that are close in frequency to the bulk water signal resulting in a reduction of sensitivity (due to an inefficient labeling selectivity) when moving from high to low magnetic fields. Following previous investigations, McMahon and colleagues developed new diamagnetic systems based on the imidazole, salicylate or anthranilate moieties which possess mobile protons shifted very far from the bulk water peak [54–56]. In particular, candidate compounds derived from imidazole-4,5-dicarboxamides (#5 and #8, Fig. 1) show a CEST signal shifted up to 7.8 ppm upfield by exploiting the presence of intramolecular bond shifted hydrogens. Besides the large chemical shift, a good pH sensitivity and a high-water solubility made compound **#5** suitable as a pH sensor and so it has been tested in vivo [57]. pH imaging of the kidneys at 11.7 T resulted in average pH values for the whole kidneys of 6.5 ± 0.1, consistent with renal pH values reported by radiographic contrast agents (Fig. 4).

2.2.2 Paramagnetic CEST Agents

Paramagnetic chemical exchange saturation transfer (paraCEST) agents typically consist of a paramagnetic metal ion and an organic chelate based on a macrocyclic cage due to the high kinetic stability of these metal chelates to prevent the release of the toxic free lanthanide cation [58]. The CEST signal is therefore generated by selective irradiation of the bound water molecule, or of the slowly exchanging ligand protons, such as hydroxyl, amine, or amide groups [59–62]. The main advantage of paraCEST agents in comparison to diamagnetic ones relies in the exceptionally large chemical shifts (MR frequency relative to the water frequency) due to the hypershift contribution of the lanthanide metal ion. This large range of chemical shifts increases the specificity of the exchanging proton pools, hence reducing the adverse contributions of direct saturation and of the endogenous semisolid macromolecular effects [63]. Since the chemical exchange rate of the paraCEST agent can be altered by environmental factors such as pH, changes in CEST amplitudes can be used as well for deriving pH values.

The first demonstration of CEST detection in kidneys using a paraCEST agent (TmDOTA-4AmC, Fig. 1) was provided by Vinogradov et al., showing good detectability in the whole kidney regions [64]. Later on, a Europium paraCEST pH responsive agent (europium(III) DO3A-tris(amide) complex, Fig. 1) was exploited to measure pH in mouse kidneys [65]. Owing to its chemical structure, a quite large frequency shift of the ion-bound water molecule due to the delocalization of negative charge coming from deprotonation of phenolic residue was observed. This shift is pH dependent, therefore an alkalinisation from 6.0 to 7.6 at 298 K leads to a 4 ppm shift in frequencies, from 50.5 to

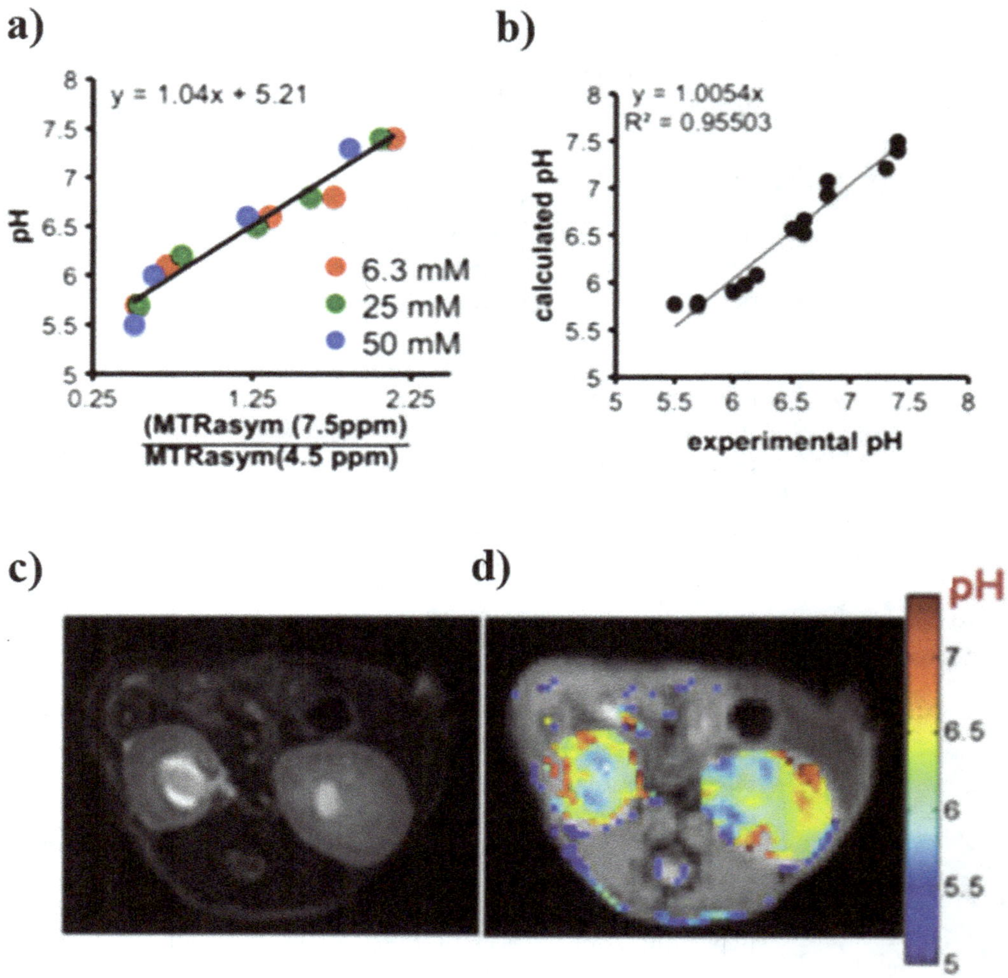

Fig. 4 pH calibration curve of compound #5 (**a**) and calibration plot using all tubes in the phantom showing experimental versus calculated pH (**b**). Experimental conditions: CEST data were obtained at 6.25 mM, 25 mM, or 50 mM concentration, saturation time = 3 s, saturation power = 5.9 μT and 37 °C. pH measurements were made with a precision of ±0.1 unit. T_2-weighted image (**c**) and pH map (**d**) following administration of compound #5. (Adapted with permission from *Contrast Media Molecular Imaging* 2016 (Developing imidazoles as CEST MRI pH sensors, Volume: 11, Issue: 4, Pages: 304–312, DOI: https:/doi.org/10.1002/cmmi.1693))

54.5 ppm, respectively, that can be exploited for assessing pH. By exploiting a 9.4 T MR scanner and ensuring stable temperature homogeneity, in vivo pH measurements were feasible in kidneys upon the administration of a dose of 0.4 mmol/kg [66].

2.3 Imaging Readout

CEST MRI techniques includes continuous wave (CW) or pulsed train RF saturation to prepare the magnetization followed by a fast image readout such as echo planar imaging (EPI), Rapid Imaging with Refocused Echoes (RARE) and/or fast imaging with steady-state precession (FISP) [45, 67, 68]. More advanced methods now provide more sophisticated sampling schemes, such as 3D radial or spiral acquisitions, but those are currently available only on clinical scanners and not on preclinical scanners, thus limiting CEST acquisition in mice and rats to single slice based approaches [69, 70]. However, recent studies have utilized multislice acquisition schemes on preclinical scanners as well [67, 71, 72].

2.3.1 Rapid Imaging with Refocused Echoes (RARE)

Fast spin echo (FSE) or rapid imaging with refocused echoes (RARE) are commonly used because of the strong SNR (signal-to-noise ratio), high tolerance to B_0 inhomogeneities and moderate to short acquisition times. These methods allow acquisitions of several lines for full sampling the k-space for a single slice within a single TR, which greatly reduces the acquisition time and still preserves SNR. With single shot acquisitions, usually centric encoding is exploited to maximize the SNR. Further reductions in acquisition time can be achieved by adjusting the bandwidth (hence reducing the echo times or the distance between each refocused echo time) or by partial Fourier approaches (i.e., by acquiring only a portion of the k-space).

2.3.2 Fast Imaging with Steady-State Precession (FISP)

FISP readout has been used with CEST MRI that provides robust image readout with little distortion, although more sensitive to B_0 inhomogeneity than RARE. B_0 inhomogeneity might be an important issue particularly for body applications like the kidneys.

2.3.3 Spin-Echo Echo Planar Imaging (EPI)

CEST MRI is often combined with EPI acquisition, which provides fast image readout after a relatively long RF saturation. Whereas both gradient echo and spin echo EPI have been used, SE EPI is often preferred for body application because it is less susceptible to mild magnetic field inhomogeneity distortions that are common in body applications. The use of an EPI readout also enables multislice acquisitions in reasonable times.

3 Overview of Applications

CEST imaging has been exploited for assessing renal pH values in healthy and in several models of renal damage, including either bilateral or unilateral acute kidney injury models. Both endogenous CEST approaches and exogenous CEST approaches have been proposed and validated in vivo.

3.1 Endogenous CEST Methods for Assessing Renal Diseases

Since diabetic nephropathies (DNs) are associated with changes in renal metabolites, the utility of CEST MRI to detect changes in glucose/glycogen hydroxylic protons was investigated in murine models of diabetic nephropathies. The study was conducted longitudinally from 8 to 24 weeks on two groups of diabetic mice and on nondiabetic mice as control. Based on the variation of glucose/

glycogen composition and the consequent CEST effects measured in kidney regions, a significantly increased CEST of hydroxyl metabolites was observed in diabetic mice during the progression of DN [73].

3.2 CEST pH Imaging for Assessing Renal Diseases

Most of the studies reported so far have exploited the pH-responsiveness of Iopamidol for investigating the changes in pH homeostasis following renal injuries. In one of these studies, the pH evolution in an acute kidney injury model induced by intramuscular glycerol injection and consequent rhabdomyolysis was monitored [74]. Renal pH maps acquired at 1, 3, 7, 14, 21 days after the injury reported a marked increase of pH values during the damage evolution up to 3–7 days, followed by recovery of pH toward baseline values at 14 and 21 days. These results were in good agreement with morphological and Blood Urean Nitrogen (BUN) quantification supporting this CEST MRI pH mapping approach for investigating renal function. Furthermore, along with the progression of the damage, a reduction of pixels where Iopamidol was detectable was observed, suggesting that also the percentage of CEST-detected pixels can be used as an imaging biomarker of renal injury.

In another study, Longo and coworkers investigated a unilateral kidney ischemia reperfusion injury (KIRI) model to validate MRI-CEST pH mapping for assessing single kidney functionality [75]. Two different times of ischemia duration, 20 and 40 min, were applied to model moderate or severe KIRI, respectively. Following the damage evolution at days 0, 1, 2, 7, a significant increase in renal pH values was observed even at day 1 in both cases. Furthermore, in the following MRI acquisitions a clear distinction between moderate and severe AKI is possible since a recovery of normal acid-base balance was observed only in the moderate KIRI mice whereas in severe KIRI mice the increased pH values did not restore to baseline values (Fig. 5a, b). In additions, as in the previous study, the percentage of CEST detected pixels, representing a marker of the filtration fraction, showed significant differences between the injured kidneys and the contralateral ones, reflecting the different evolution of moderate-to-severe damage (Fig. 5c, d).

3.3 GlucoCEST Imaging for Assessing Renal Diseases

Since the capability of CEST imaging to detect hydroxyl protons, native glucose has also been proposed as a tracer for MRI GlucoCEST imaging [76–78]. Besides its exploitation in oncological applications, it has been applied for monitoring allograft rejection [79]. In this study, Brown Norway rat kidneys were transplanted into Lewis rats and imaged 4 days following the surgery, before and after glucose administration. By calculating the cortex-to-medulla CEST ratio (CESTR), dependent on the accumulation of the administered glucose, rats that underwent allogeneic transplant showed the highest CESTR values compared to syngeneic transplant group and to control mice.

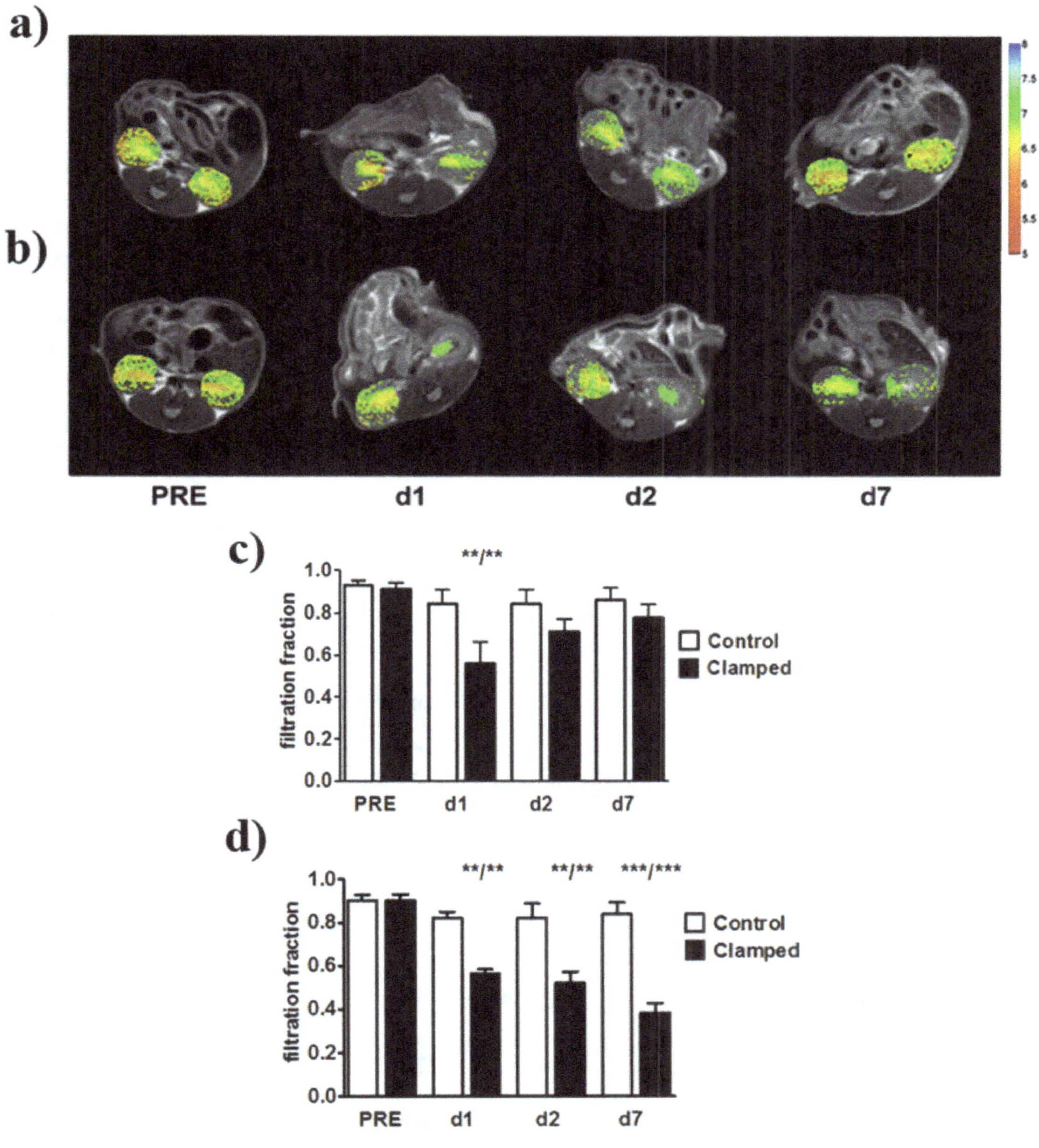

Fig. 5 MRI-CEST pH mapping detects renal pH changes and regional distribution of damage after moderate and severe unilateral kidney ischemia reperfusion injury (KIRI) showing clamped (right) and contralateral normal kidney (left). Representative MRI-CEST pH maps overimposed onto anatomical images before and after moderate (**a**) and severe (**b**) KIRI at different time points (day 1, day 2, and day 7) showing pronounced alkalinization and reduced filtration (noncolored pixels within the renal region, **c**, **d**) of the pH-responsive contrast agent in clamped kidney in comparison to contralateral kidney. (Adapted with permission from: *NMR in Biomedicine* 2017 (Noninvasive evaluation of renal pH homeostasis after ischemia reperfusion injury by CEST-MRI, Volume: 30, Issue: 7, DOI: https:/doi.org/10.1002/nbm.3720))

Acknowledgments

The Italian Ministry for Education and Research (MIUR) is gratefully acknowledged for yearly FOE funding to the Euro-BioImaging Multi-Modal Molecular Imaging Italian Node (MMMI).

This chapter is based upon work from COST Action PARENCHIMA, supported by European Cooperation in Science and Technology (COST). COST (www.cost.eu) is a funding agency for research and innovation networks. COST Actions help connect research initiatives across Europe and enable scientists to enrich their ideas by sharing them with their peers. This boosts their research, career, and innovation.

PARENCHIMA (renalmri.org) is a community-driven Action in the COST program of the European Union, which unites more than 200 experts in renal MRI from 30 countries with the aim to improve the reproducibility and standardization of renal MRI biomarkers.

References

1. Al Malla M, Varghese NV, AlAbdullatif M, Narchi H, Khassawneh M (2017) Prevalence and outcome of acute kidney injury, as defined by the new kidney disease improving global outcomes guideline, in very low birth weight infants. World J Nephrol 6(5):229–235. https://doi.org/10.5527/wjn.v6.i5.229
2. Kassebaum NJ, Lopez AD, Murray CJ, Lozano R (2014) A comparison of maternal mortality estimates from GBD 2013 and WHO. Lancet 384(9961):2209–2210. https://doi.org/10.1016/S0140-6736(14)62421-1
3. Zollner FG, Kalayciyan R, Chacon-Caldera J, Zimmer F, Schad LR (2014) Pre-clinical functional magnetic resonance imaging part I: the kidney. Z Med Phys 24(4):286–306. https://doi.org/10.1016/j.zemedi.2014.05.002
4. Neugarten J, Golestaneh L (2014) Blood oxygenation level-dependent MRI for assessment of renal oxygenation. Int J Nephrol Renovasc Dis 7:421–435. https://doi.org/10.2147/IJNRD.S42924
5. Zimmer F, Zollner FG, Hoeger S, Klotz S, Tsagogiorgas C, Kramer BK, Schad LR (2013) Quantitative renal perfusion measurements in a rat model of acute kidney injury at 3T: testing inter- and intramethodical significance of ASL and DCE-MRI. PLoS One 8(1): e53849. https://doi.org/10.1371/journal.pone.0053849
6. Ichikawa S, Motosugi U, Ichikawa T, Sano K, Morisaka H, Araki T (2013) Intravoxel incoherent motion imaging of the kidney: alterations in diffusion and perfusion in patients with renal dysfunction. Magn Reson Imaging 31 (3):414–417. https://doi.org/10.1016/j.mri.2012.08.004
7. Clatworthy MR, Kettunen MI, Hu DE, Mathews RJ, Witney TH, Kennedy BW, Bohndiek SE, Gallagher FA, Jarvis LB, Smith KG, Brindle KM (2012) Magnetic resonance imaging with hyperpolarized [1,4-(13)C2]fumarate allows detection of early renal acute tubular necrosis. Proc Natl Acad Sci U S A 109 (33):13374–13379. https://doi.org/10.1073/pnas.1205539109
8. Warner L, Yin M, Glaser KJ, Woollard JA, Carrascal CA, Korsmo MJ, Crane JA, Ehman RL, Lerman LO (2011) Noninvasive in vivo assessment of renal tissue elasticity during graded renal ischemia using MR elastography. Investig Radiol 46(8):509–514. https://doi.org/10.1097/RLI.0b013e3182183a95
9. Oostendorp M, de Vries EE, Slenter JM, Peutz-Kootstra CJ, Snoeijs MG, Post MJ, van Heurn LW, Backes WH (2011) MRI of renal oxygenation and function after normothermic ischemia-reperfusion injury. NMR Biomed 24 (2):194–200. https://doi.org/10.1002/nbm.1572

10. Notohamiprodjo M, Reiser MF, Sourbron SP (2010) Diffusion and perfusion of the kidney. Eur J Radiol 76(3):337–347. https://doi.org/10.1016/j.ejrad.2010.05.033
11. Prasad PV (2006) Evaluation of intra-renal oxygenation by BOLD MRI. Nephron Clin Pract 103(2):c58–c65. https://doi.org/10.1159/000090610
12. Kline TL, Edwards ME, Garg I, Irazabal MV, Korfiatis P, Harris PC, King BF, Torres VE, Venkatesh SK, Erickson BJ (2018) Quantitative MRI of kidneys in renal disease. Abdom Radiol (NY) 43(3):629–638. https://doi.org/10.1007/s00261-017-1236-y
13. Zhang JL, Morrell G, Rusinek H, Sigmund EE, Chandarana H, Lerman LO, Prasad PV, Niles D, Artz N, Fain S, Vivier PH, Cheung AK, Lee VS (2014) New magnetic resonance imaging methods in nephrology. Kidney Int 85 (4):768–778. https://doi.org/10.1038/ki.2013.361
14. Zhang JL, Rusinek H, Chandarana H, Lee VS (2013) Functional MRI of the kidneys. J Magn Reson Imaging 37(2):282–293. https://doi.org/10.1002/jmri.23717
15. Grenier N, Pedersen M, Hauger O (2006) Contrast agents for functional and cellular MRI of the kidney. Eur J Radiol 60 (3):341–352. https://doi.org/10.1016/j.ejrad.2006.06.024
16. Liu G, Song X, Chan KW, McMahon MT (2013) Nuts and bolts of chemical exchange saturation transfer MRI. NMR Biomed 26 (7):810–828. https://doi.org/10.1002/nbm.2899
17. Kogan F, Hariharan H, Reddy R (2013) Chemical exchange saturation transfer (CEST) imaging: description of technique and potential clinical applications. Curr Radiol Rep 1(2):102–114. https://doi.org/10.1007/s40134-013-0010-3
18. Jones KM, Pollard AC, Pagel MD (2018) Clinical applications of chemical exchange saturation transfer (CEST) MRI. J Magn Reson Imaging 47(1):11–27. https://doi.org/10.1002/jmri.25838
19. Anemone A, Consolino L, Arena F, Capozza M, Longo DL (2019) Imaging tumor acidosis: a survey of the available techniques for mapping in vivo tumor pH. Cancer Metastasis Rev 38(1-2):25–49. https://doi.org/10.1007/s10555-019-09782-9
20. Ward KM, Aletras AH, Balaban RS (2000) A new class of contrast agents for MRI based on proton chemical exchange dependent saturation transfer (CEST). J Magn Reson 143 (1):79–87. https://doi.org/10.1006/jmre.1999.1956
21. Sun PZ, Benner T, Copen WA, Sorensen AG (2010) Early experience of translating pH-weighted MRI to image human subjects at 3 Tesla. Stroke 41(10 Suppl):S147–S151. https://doi.org/10.1161/STROKEAHA.110.595777
22. Aime S, Castelli DD, Crich SG, Gianolio E, Terreno E (2009) Pushing the sensitivity envelope of lanthanide-based magnetic resonance imaging (MRI) contrast agents for molecular imaging applications. Acc Chem Res 42 (7):822–831. https://doi.org/10.1021/ar800192p
23. McMahon MT, Gilad AA, DeLiso MA, Berman SM, Bulte JW, van Zijl PC (2008) New "multicolor" polypeptide diamagnetic chemical exchange saturation transfer (DIACEST) contrast agents for MRI. Magn Reson Med 60(4):803–812. https://doi.org/10.1002/mrm.21683
24. Sun PZ, Zhou J, Huang J, van Zijl P (2007) Simplified quantitative description of amide proton transfer (APT) imaging during acute ischemia. Magn Reson Med 57(2):405–410. https://doi.org/10.1002/mrm.21151
25. McMahon MT, Gilad AA, Zhou J, Sun PZ, Bulte JW, van Zijl PC (2006) Quantifying exchange rates in chemical exchange saturation transfer agents using the saturation time and saturation power dependencies of the magnetization transfer effect on the magnetic resonance imaging signal (QUEST and QUESP): Ph calibration for poly-L-lysine and a starburst dendrimer. Magn Reson Med 55(4):836–847. https://doi.org/10.1002/mrm.20818
26. Jones CK, Schlosser MJ, van Zijl PC, Pomper MG, Golay X, Zhou J (2006) Amide proton transfer imaging of human brain tumors at 3T. Magn Reson Med 56(3):585–592. https://doi.org/10.1002/mrm.20989
27. Sun PZ, Wang E, Cheung JS (2012) Imaging acute ischemic tissue acidosis with pH-sensitive endogenous amide proton transfer (APT) MRI--correction of tissue relaxation and concomitant RF irradiation effects toward mapping quantitative cerebral tissue pH. NeuroImage 60(1):1–6. https://doi.org/10.1016/j.neuroimage.2011.11.091
28. Haris M, Nath K, Cai K, Singh A, Crescenzi R, Kogan F, Verma G, Reddy S, Hariharan H, Melhem ER, Reddy R (2013) Imaging of glutamate neurotransmitter alterations in Alzheimer's disease. NMR Biomed 26(4):386–391. https://doi.org/10.1002/nbm.2875
29. Longo DL, Di Gregorio E, Abategiovanni R, Ceccon A, Assfalg M, Molinari H, Aime S

(2014) Chemical exchange saturation transfer (CEST): an efficient tool for detecting molecular information on proteins' behaviour. Analyst 139(11):2687–2690. https://doi.org/10.1039/c4an00346b

30. Ceccon A, D'Onofrio M, Zanzoni S, Longo DL, Aime S, Molinari H, Assfalg M (2013) NMR investigation of the equilibrium partitioning of a water-soluble bile salt protein carrier to phospholipid vesicles. Proteins 81 (10):1776–1791. https://doi.org/10.1002/prot.24329
31. Castelli DD, Terreno E, Longo D, Aime S (2013) Nanoparticle-based chemical exchange saturation transfer (CEST) agents. NMR Biomed 26(7):839–849. https://doi.org/10.1002/nbm.2974
32. Dastru W, Longo D, Aime S (2011) Contrast agents and mechanisms. Drug Discov Today 8 (2–4):e109–e115. https://doi.org/10.1016/j.ddtec.2011.11.013
33. Sherry AD, Woods M (2008) Chemical exchange saturation transfer contrast agents for magnetic resonance imaging. Annu Rev Biomed Eng 10:391–411. https://doi.org/10.1146/annurev.bioeng.9.060906.151929
34. Zaiss M, Windschuh J, Goerke S, Paech D, Meissner JE, Burth S, Kickingereder P, Wick W, Bendszus M, Schlemmer HP, Ladd ME, Bachert P, Radbruch A (2016) Downfield-NOE-suppressed amide-CEST-MRI at 7 Tesla provides a unique contrast in human glioblastoma. Magn Reson Med 77 (1):196–208. https://doi.org/10.1002/mrm.26100
35. Rivlin M, Navon G (2016) Glucosamine and N-acetyl glucosamine as new CEST MRI agents for molecular imaging of tumors. Sci Rep 6:32648. https://doi.org/10.1038/srep32648
36. Li Y, Chen H, Xu J, Yadav NN, Chan KW, Luo L, McMahon MT, Vogelstein B, van Zijl PC, Zhou S, Liu G (2016) CEST theranostics: label-free MR imaging of anticancer drugs. Oncotarget 7(6):6369–6378. https://doi.org/10.18632/oncotarget.7141
37. Desmond KL, Mehrabian H, Chavez S, Sahgal A, Soliman H, Rola R, Stanisz GJ (2017) Chemical exchange saturation transfer for predicting response to stereotactic radiosurgery in human brain metastasis. Magn Reson Med 78(3):1110–1120. https://doi.org/10.1002/mrm.26470
38. Goerke S, Breitling J, Zaiss M, Windschuh J, Kunz P, Schuenke P, Paech D, Longo DL, Klika KD, Ladd ME, Bachert P (2018) Dual-frequency irradiation CEST-MRI of endogenous bulk mobile proteins. NMR Biomed 31 (6):e3920. https://doi.org/10.1002/nbm.3920
39. Longo DL, Moustaghfir FZ, Zerbo A, Consolino L, Anemone A, Bracesco M, Aime S (2017) EXCI-CEST: exploiting pharmaceutical excipients as MRI-CEST contrast agents for tumor imaging. Int J Pharm 525 (1):275–281. https://doi.org/10.1016/j.ijpharm.2017.04.040
40. Ward KM, Balaban RS (2000) Determination of pH using water protons and chemical exchange dependent saturation transfer (CEST). Magn Reson Med 44(5):799–802. https://doi.org/10.1002/1522-2594
41. Longo D, Aime S (2017) Iodinated contrast media as pH-responsive CEST agents. In: McMahon MT, Gilad AA, Bulte JBM, Van Zijl PCM (eds) Chemical exchange saturation transfer imaging, Advances and applications. Pan Stanford Publishing, Singapore, pp 447–466. https://doi.org/10.1201/9781315364421-20
42. McDonald RJ, McDonald JS, Bida JP, Carter RE, Fleming CJ, Misra S, Williamson EE, Kallmes DF (2013) Intravenous contrast material-induced nephropathy: causal or coincident phenomenon? Radiology 267 (1):106–118. https://doi.org/10.1148/radiol.12121823
43. McDonald JS, McDonald RJ, Comin J, Williamson EE, Katzberg RW, Murad MH, Kallmes DF (2013) Frequency of acute kidney injury following intravenous contrast medium administration: a systematic review and meta-analysis. Radiology 267(1):119–128. https://doi.org/10.1148/radiol.12121460
44. Aime S, Calabi L, Biondi L, De Miranda M, Ghelli S, Paleari L, Rebaudengo C, Terreno E (2005) Iopamidol: exploring the potential use of a well-established x-ray contrast agent for MRI. Magn Reson Med 53(4):830–834. https://doi.org/10.1002/mrm.20441
45. Longo DL, Dastru W, Digilio G, Keupp J, Langereis S, Lanzardo S, Prestigio S, Steinbach O, Terreno E, Uggeri F, Aime S (2011) Iopamidol as a responsive MRI-chemical exchange saturation transfer contrast agent for pH mapping of kidneys: in vivo studies in mice at 7 T. Magn Reson Med 65(1):202–211. https://doi.org/10.1002/mrm.22608
46. Anemone A, Consolino L, Longo DL (2017) MRI-CEST assessment of tumour perfusion using X-ray iodinated agents: comparison with a conventional Gd-based agent. Eur Radiol 27 (5):2170–2179. https://doi.org/10.1007/s00330-016-4552-7
47. Longo DL, Michelotti F, Consolino L, Bardini P, Digilio G, Xiao G, Sun PZ, Aime S

(2016) In vitro and in vivo assessment of non-ionic iodinated radiographic molecules as chemical exchange saturation transfer magnetic resonance imaging tumor perfusion agents. Investig Radiol 51(3):155–162. https://doi.org/10.1097/RLI.0000000000000217

48. Sun PZ, Longo DL, Hu W, Xiao G, Wu R (2014) Quantification of iopamidol multi-site chemical exchange properties for ratiometric chemical exchange saturation transfer (CEST) imaging of pH. Phys Med Biol 59 (16):4493–4504. https://doi.org/10.1088/0031-9155/59/16/4493
49. Wu Y, Zhou IY, Igarashi T, Longo DL, Aime S, Sun PZ (2018) A generalized ratiometric chemical exchange saturation transfer (CEST) MRI approach for mapping renal pH using iopamidol. Magn Reson Med 79 (3):1553–1558. https://doi.org/10.1002/mrm.26817
50. Longo DL, Bartoli A, Consolino L, Bardini P, Arena F, Schwaiger M, Aime S (2016) In vivo imaging of tumor metabolism and acidosis by combining PET and MRI-CEST pH imaging. Cancer Res 76(22):6463–6470. https://doi.org/10.1158/0008-5472.CAN-16-0825
51. Moon BF, Jones KM, Chen LQ, Liu P, Randtke EA, Howison CM, Pagel MD (2015) A comparison of iopromide and iopamidol, two acidoCEST MRI contrast media that measure tumor extracellular pH. Contrast Media Mol Imaging 10(6):446–455. https://doi.org/10.1002/cmmi.1647
52. Longo DL, Sun PZ, Consolino L, Michelotti FC, Uggeri F, Aime S (2014) A general MRI-CEST ratiometric approach for pH imaging: demonstration of in vivo pH mapping with iobitridol. J Am Chem Soc 136 (41):14333–14336. https://doi.org/10.1021/ja5059313
53. Arena F, Irrera P, Consolino L, Colombo Serra S, Zaiss M, Longo DL (2018) Flip-angle based ratiometric approach for pulsed CEST-MRI pH imaging. J Magn Reson 287:1–9. https://doi.org/10.1016/j.jmr.2017.12.007
54. Song X, Walczak P, He X, Yang X, Pearl M, Bulte JW, Pomper MG, McMahon MT, Janowski M (2016) Salicylic acid analogues as chemical exchange saturation transfer MRI contrast agents for the assessment of brain perfusion territory and blood-brain barrier opening after intra-arterial infusion. J Cereb Blood Flow Metab 36(7):1186–1194. https://doi.org/10.1177/0271678X16637882
55. Song X, Yang X, Ray Banerjee S, Pomper MG, McMahon MT (2015) Anthranilic acid analogs as diamagnetic CEST MRI contrast agents that feature an intramolecular-bond shifted hydrogen. Contrast Media Mol Imaging 10 (1):74–80. https://doi.org/10.1002/cmmi.1597
56. Yang X, Song X, Li Y, Liu G, Ray Banerjee S, Pomper MG, McMahon MT (2013) Salicylic acid and analogues as diaCEST MRI contrast agents with highly shifted exchangeable proton frequencies. Angew Chem Int Ed Engl 52 (31):8116–8119. https://doi.org/10.1002/anie.201302764
57. Yang X, Song X, Ray Banerjee S, Li Y, Byun Y, Liu G, Bhujwalla ZM, Pomper MG, McMahon MT (2016) Developing imidazoles as CEST MRI pH sensors. Contrast Media Mol Imaging 11(4):304–312. https://doi.org/10.1002/cmmi.1693
58. Zhang S, Merritt M, Woessner DE, Lenkinski RE, Sherry AD (2003) PARACEST agents: modulating MRI contrast via water proton exchange. Acc Chem Res 36(10):783–790. https://doi.org/10.1021/ar020228m
59. Hancu I, Dixon WT, Woods M, Vinogradov E, Sherry AD, Lenkinski RE (2010) CEST and PARACEST MR contrast agents. Acta Radiol 51(8):910–923. https://doi.org/10.3109/02841851.2010.502126
60. Liu G, Ali MM, Yoo B, Griswold MA, Tkach JA, Pagel MD (2009) PARACEST MRI with improved temporal resolution. Magn Reson Med 61(2):399–408. https://doi.org/10.1002/mrm.21863
61. Aime S, Delli Castelli D, Terreno E (2005) Highly sensitive MRI chemical exchange saturation transfer agents using liposomes. Angew Chem Int Ed Engl 44(34):5513–5515. https://doi.org/10.1002/anie.200501473
62. Srivastava K, Ferrauto G, Harris SM, Longo DL, Botta M, Aime S, Pierre VC (2018) Complete on/off responsive ParaCEST MRI contrast agents for copper and zinc. Dalton Trans 47(33):11346–11357. https://doi.org/10.1039/c8dt01172a
63. Woods M, Woessner DE, Sherry AD (2006) Paramagnetic lanthanide complexes as PARACEST agents for medical imaging. Chem Soc Rev 35(6):500–511. https://doi.org/10.1039/b509907m
64. Vinogradov E, He H, Lubag A, Balschi JA, Sherry AD, Lenkinski RE (2007) MRI detection of paramagnetic chemical exchange effects in mice kidneys in vivo. Magn Reson Med 58 (4):650–655. https://doi.org/10.1002/mrm.21393
65. Wu Y, Soesbe TC, Kiefer GE, Zhao P, Sherry AD (2010) A responsive europium(III) chelate that provides a direct readout of pH by MRI. J Am Chem Soc 132(40):14002–14003. https://doi.org/10.1021/ja106018n

66. Wu Y, Zhang S, Soesbe TC, Yu J, Vinogradov E, Lenkinski RE, Sherry AD (2016) pH imaging of mouse kidneys in vivo using a frequency-dependent paraCEST agent. Magn Reson Med 75(6):2432–2441. https://doi.org/10.1002/mrm.25844
67. Sun PZ, Cheung JS, Wang E, Benner T, Sorensen AG (2011) Fast multislice pH-weighted chemical exchange saturation transfer (CEST) MRI with unevenly segmented RF irradiation. Magn Reson Med 65(2):588–594. https://doi.org/10.1002/mrm.22628
68. Sheth VR, Li Y, Chen LQ, Howison CM, Flask CA, Pagel MD (2012) Measuring in vivo tumor pHe with CEST-FISP MRI. Magn Reson Med 67(3):760–768. https://doi.org/10.1002/mrm.23038
69. Zaiss M, Ehses P, Scheffler K (2018) Snapshot-CEST: optimizing spiral-centric-reordered gradient echo acquisition for fast and robust 3D CEST MRI at 9.4 T. NMR Biomed 31 (4):e3879. https://doi.org/10.1002/nbm.3879
70. Zhu H, Jones CK, van Zijl PC, Barker PB, Zhou J (2010) Fast 3D chemical exchange saturation transfer (CEST) imaging of the human brain. Magn Reson Med 64 (3):638–644. https://doi.org/10.1002/mrm.22546
71. Sun PZ, Murata Y, Lu J, Wang X, Lo EH, Sorensen AG (2008) Relaxation-compensated fast multislice amide proton transfer (APT) imaging of acute ischemic stroke. Magn Reson Med 59(5):1175–1182. https://doi.org/10.1002/mrm.21591
72. Randtke EA, Granados JC, Howison CM, Pagel MD, Cardenas-Rodriguez J (2017) Multislice CEST MRI improves the spatial assessment of tumor pH. Magn Reson Med 78 (1):97–106. https://doi.org/10.1002/mrm.26348
73. Wang F, Kopylov D, Zu Z, Takahashi K, Wang S, Quarles CC, Gore JC, Harris RC, Takahashi T (2016) Mapping murine diabetic kidney disease using chemical exchange saturation transfer MRI. Magn Reson Med 76 (5):1531–1541. https://doi.org/10.1002/mrm.26045
74. Longo DL, Busato A, Lanzardo S, Antico F, Aime S (2013) Imaging the pH evolution of an acute kidney injury model by means of iopamidol, a MRI-CEST pH-responsive contrast agent. Magn Reson Med 70(3):859–864. https://doi.org/10.1002/mrm.24513
75. Longo DL, Cutrin JC, Michelotti F, Irrera P, Aime S (2017) Noninvasive evaluation of renal pH homeostasis after ischemia reperfusion injury by CEST-MRI. NMR Biomed 30(7). https://doi.org/10.1002/nbm.3720
76. Walker-Samuel S, Ramasawmy R, Torrealdea F, Rega M, Rajkumar V, Johnson SP, Richardson S, Goncalves M, Parkes HG, Arstad E, Thomas DL, Pedley RB, Lythgoe MF, Golay X (2013) In vivo imaging of glucose uptake and metabolism in tumors. Nat Med 19 (8):1067–1072. https://doi.org/10.1038/nm.3252
77. Xu X, Chan KW, Knutsson L, Artemov D, Xu J, Liu G, Kato Y, Lal B, Laterra J, McMahon MT, van Zijl PC (2015) Dynamic glucose enhanced (DGE) MRI for combined imaging of blood-brain barrier break down and increased blood volume in brain cancer. Magn Reson Med 74 (6):1556–1563. https://doi.org/10.1002/mrm.25995
78. Chan KW, McMahon MT, Kato Y, Liu G, Bulte JW, Bhujwalla ZM, Artemov D, van Zijl PC (2012) Natural D-glucose as a biodegradable MRI contrast agent for detecting cancer. Magn Reson Med 68(6):1764–1773. https://doi.org/10.1002/mrm.24520
79. Kentrup D, Bovenkamp P, Busch A, Schuette-Nuetgen K, Pawelski H, Pavenstadt H, Schlatter E, Herrmann KH, Reichenbach JR, Loffler B, Heitplatz B, Van Marck V, Yadav NN, Liu G, van Zijl PCM, Reuter S, Hoerr V (2017) GlucoCEST magnetic resonance imaging in vivo may be diagnostic of acute renal allograft rejection. Kidney Int 92(3):757–764. https://doi.org/10.1016/j.kint.2017.04.015

2

Preparation and Monitoring of Small Animals in Renal MRI

Tamas Kaucsar, Adam Hosszu, Erdmann Seeliger, Henning M. Reimann, and Andrea Fekete

Abstract

Renal diseases remain devastating illnesses with unacceptably high rates of mortality and morbidity worldwide. Animal models are essential tools to better understand the pathomechanism of kidney-related illnesses and to develop new, successful therapeutic strategies. Magnetic resonance imaging (MRI) has been actively explored in the last decades for assessing renal function, perfusion, tissue oxygenation as well as the degree of fibrosis and inflammation. This chapter aims to provide an overview of the preparation and monitoring of small animals before, during, and after surgical interventions or MR imaging. Standardization of experimental settings such as body temperature or hydration of animals and minimizing pain and distress are essential for diminishing nonexperimental variables as well as for conducting ethical research.

This publication is based upon work from the COST Action PARENCHIMA, a community-driven network funded by the European Cooperation in Science and Technology (COST) program of the European Union, which aims to improve the reproducibility and standardization of renal MRI biomarkers.

Key words Magnetic resonance imaging (MRI), Kidney, Rodent surgery, Anesthesia

1 Introduction

Renal diseases are devastating illnesses with unacceptably high rates of mortality and morbidity worldwide. End-stage renal disease is the final stage of chronic kidney disease (CKD) characterized by complete loss of kidney function. Global prevalence is estimated to be 8–16% and the overall years of life lost due to premature death is third behind AIDS and diabetes mellitus [1]. Kidney diseases create a huge burden on healthcare systems; thus, the social and economic impact of prevention and early treatment would be enormous. Several publications have highlighted the need for new, effective therapies as well as superior diagnostic tools.

At present, diagnosis of kidney disease is difficult and often involves invasive procedures. Conventional markers of renal function such as serum creatinine and blood urea nitrogen are poorly sensitive and poorly selective, as they represent a delayed indication

Andreas Pohlmann and Thoralf Niendorf (eds.), *Preclinical MRI of the Kidney: Methods and Protocols*, Methods in Molecular Biology, vol. 2216, https://doi.org/10.1007/978-1-0716-0978-1_3, © The Author(s) 2021

of functional change that lags behind structural deterioration during the early stage of acute kidney injury (AKI). Currently kidney biopsy is the single method to assess renal microstructure in humans, but it is an invasive procedure and sampling bias can alter results. Thus, noninvasive, in vivo imaging methods are crucial for the adequate assessment of kidney function, oxygenation, and structure in both preclinical and clinical setups. Importantly, state-of-the-art functional MRI techniques are available to determine tissue oxygenation, perfusion, fibrosis, inflammation, or tissue edema that can be used as biomarkers of renal disease [2]. MRI affords full kidney coverage, soft tissue contrast that helps to differentiate the renal layers, second-to-minute temporal resolution, support of longitudinal studies and high anatomical detail without the use of ionizing radiation [3, 4].

However, imaging rodents can be challenging because in contrast to human studies, imaging of animals requires anesthesia to physically restrain the animals and minimize their gross motion. Anesthetic agents can profoundly alter physiology of the experimental animal and may thus influence the image data acquired. It is therefore necessary to use the most appropriate anesthetic compound and to monitor the physiology of anesthetized animals during image acquisition [5–7].

It is essential that researchers use animals in scientifically, technically, and humanely appropriate ways. Effective and appropriate animal care before, during, and after experimentation not only is important for the enhancement of animal well-being but can also have a major effect on the quality of research. Hydration status, the type of anesthesia used, or body temperature of the animals during surgery or MRI measurements, as well as postoperative care are all factors that can affect results, and thus should be carefully planned prior to the intervention. Standard protocols can be modified, but should not compromise the well-being of the animals.

This chapter summarizes preoperative procedures, advantages and disadvantages of different anesthetic agents, monitoring of physiological functions during surgical or imaging procedures, and how these challenges can be successfully addressed.

This chapter is part of the book Pohlmann A, Niendorf T (eds) (2020) Preclinical MRI of the Kidney—Methods and Protocols. Springer, New York.

2 Hydration

Animals can experience considerable fluid loss during surgery mainly due to evaporation from open body cavities or blood loss. Rodents are particularly vulnerable to intraoperative fluid loss because of their small size and relatively small total body fluid content. Warm, sterile isotonic fluids should be administered at 3–5% of the body weight subcutaneously or intraperitoneally prior to and at the end of surgery. Alternatively, isotonic fluid can be continuously administered via intravenous infusion or even via intra-arterial infusion in case a catheter has already been placed into an artery for monitoring of blood pressure and heart rate. The operative field should be irrigated with warm saline and drying out of tissues should be avoided [8, 9]. In any case, quantity of hydration has to be logged and/or standardized to eliminate non-experimental variable factors. For example, with proper hydration tubular reabsorption, an energy-dependent process can be spared. Hence, some procedures such as ischemia will have less effect on renal injury in well hydrated animals. Intraoperative fluid replacement is also important because during the recovery phase water intake is usually reduced, even though ad libitum water access is usually ensured after surgery.

An ophthalmic lubricating ointment should be applied to the eyes to protect the cornea from drying out.

3 Anesthesia

The use of anesthetics for surgical or in vivo imaging procedures comes with an inevitable autonomic nervous system depression, causing cardiovascular and respiratory depression, hypothermia, and altered metabolism [10]. Different anesthetics influence these physiological processes differently; thus, various anesthetic agents should be selected for different experimental models. For example, anesthesia used during renal ischemia–reperfusion injury (IRI) surgery has an important impact on the extent of injury. Numerous studies showed that anesthetics are renoprotective due to their anti-inflammatory, antiapoptotic, or antinecrotic effect, independently of the way of administration. Also different anesthetics impose different effects on vasomotion (dilation and constriction). Vasomotion, in turn, has a direct impact on local renal blood volume fraction, which affects the measure T_2*. Furthermore, it influences perfusion, which affects the blood oxygenation and ultimately T_2* as well. R_2*—the transverse relaxation rate—can vary by more than 100% depending on the anesthetic regimen [11]. In animal experiments inhalable and injectable anesthetics are both popular. Advantage of inhalable anesthetics (e.g., halothane or fluranes) are that they are rapidly eliminated through the lungs; therefore, incidence of fatal events is lower and fast recovery can be achieved. On the other hand, they are frequently irritant, and it is hard to set a precise dosage; hence, it is easier to cause hypoxia, and if apnea occurs loss of consciousness will last longer. Injectable anesthetics (barbiturates, ketamine, propofol, etc.) promote a quick loss of consciousness with better control of cardiopulmonary function and induce anesthesia at a lower dose. They frequently influence blood pressure, and hypothermia can also develop. Although barbiturates can be precisely dosed through intravenous administration, the intraperitoneal, subcutaneous, or intramuscular injection of other injectable anesthetics may lead to variable levels of anesthesia. Because of the short time of action (with the exception of urethane) repeated dosing or constant infusion of injectable anesthetics is sometimes needed, prolonging recovery time [12]. During procedures respiratory rate and alertness of the animal should be followed. Anesthesia should be intensified at the first signs of alertness such as movement of whiskers or reflex triggered by pinching the toes outside the MR environment. It should be noted that deeper anesthesia is needed for surgical interventions than for MRI alone.

3.1 Injectable Anesthetics

Ketamine is one of the safest and most widely used injectable anesthetics in animal surgeries because it does not require intravenous access and cardiorespiratory depression occurs only at a much higher dose than what is needed for anesthesia [13]. Ketamine is frequently used in combination with other anesthetics like α2 agonists (xylazine) or benzodiazepines to prevent muscle rigidity and produce more stable anesthesia [7]. In these cases, the dose of ketamine can be reduced. However, ketamine may reduce IRI in rats in low doses, when its antioxidant capacity is the greatest [14]. On the other hand, ketamine may be harmful at higher doses due to its sympathomimetic effect [15]. Despite the low cardiovascular and respiratory influence of ketamine alone [16], cardiac influences, like hypotension with minimal respiratory depression must also be considered when using ketamine together with xylazine [17]. Substantial cardiovascular effects (bradycardia, hypotension) were observed when acepromazine, buprenorphine, or carprofen was also added to the ketamine–xylazine combination. Nevertheless, the addition of acepromazine led to stable hemodynamic parameters while sustaining adequate anesthesia for performing surgical procedures [18]. Cerebral hemodynamics are also affected by ketamine–xylazine combinations, which may cause reduction of cerebral blood flow thus affecting brain oxygenation and leading to interferences with several imaging procedures [19]. Metabolic changes could also occur during ketamine–xylazine anesthesia. Decreased insulin secretion by pancreatic β cells together with the blockade of ATP-dependent potassium channels may cause elevated levels of blood glucose and potassium [20].

Short and ultrashort acting barbiturates (pentobarbital and thiopental, respectively) are also frequently used in animal experiments. They are relatively inexpensive and have a rapid and smooth onset of action as well as recovery [21]. On the other hand, they have small therapeutic margin and even though they can be precisely dosed via intravenous administration, the risk of fatal events is much higher than for ketamine [22]. However, their use is limited in renal ischemia–reperfusion surgery, since they reduce blood pressure and thus blood flow to the kidney. Although by lowering pentobarbital dose there are less cardiovascular side effects, poor anesthetic depth, and serious respiratory depression with low oxygen saturation can be expected during pentobarbital monoanesthesia [17]. Thiopental decreased malondialdehyde levels and reduced histopathologic damage to the kidneys after IRI in subanesthetic doses [15]. Moreover, clinically high doses of thiopental effectively protected against renal IRI [23]. What may lie behind this renoprotective effect is that thiopental is also an antioxidant [24] and inhibits neutrophil function [25]. Thiopental might also depress brain metabolism and thus elevate brain glucose content in the cortex [26]; however, pentobarbital has no effect on blood glucose levels [20].

Propofol is a rapid acting anesthetic, with short recovery duration, thus convenient for short procedures [10]. Propofol has a serious respiratory depressant effect and decrease in cerebral blood flow and intracranial pressure have also been reported [27]. The renoprotective effect of propofol via reduced production of proinflammatory cytokines, less neutrophil infiltration, and hence lower reactive oxygen species accumulation is well documented [15, 28, 29]. Due to its renoprotective effect, propofol is currently not used in experimental models of renal injury.

Urethane is extensively used alone or in combination with ketamine and xylazine in nonrecovery procedures. Advantages are its long-lasting (several hours) surgical plane of anesthesia [30, 31] and least effects on cardiovascular and respiratory control compared to other anesthetics [32, 33]. At least 8 h of fasting of the animals is recommended before urethane anesthesia.

3.2 Inhalable Anesthetics

Halogenated ethers are the preferred volatile anesthetics during animal experiments. Due to their rapid onset and short recovery time and low metabolism the side effects of inhalation anesthesia can be well controlled [10]. For example, isoflurane is preferred in cardiovascular studies, since it causes less hemodynamic depression than injectable anesthetics [17, 34]. It also reduces peripheral resistance thus hypotension might occur [35]. On the other hand, the rate of respiratory depression is higher than by injectable anesthetics; therefore, respiratory rate monitoring is indispensable when adjusting gas concentration. By maintaining high tidal volumes a stable oxygen saturation may be achieved during isoflurane anesthesia [17]. Yet isoflurane-induced respiratory depression results in hypercapnia, leading to substantial vasodilation in the brain and increased baseline cerebral blood flow [36]. To maintain physiological cerebral blood flow mechanical ventilation of the animal is recommended. In contrast, hypercapnia has only negligible effects on vasomotion in the kidney [37]. However, vasodilatory effects of isoflurane may be reflected in renal T_2^* that has been found substantially higher compared to other anesthetics [11]. Metabolic changes have also been reported: isoflurane decreases insulin production, thus leads to higher blood glucose levels [20].

There is increasing evidence that halogenated ethers provide significant protection against renal IRI, which effect is differential: desflurane being less protective than isoflurane or sevoflurane [38]. Moreover, anesthesia with isoflurane has a preconditioning effect on renal IRI, with the involvement of JNK and ERK protein kinases [39]. When compared to propofol, isoflurane provided the same level of protection against ischemia reperfusion injury and therefore should be used with caution [40].

4 Physiological Monitoring

4.1 Body Temperature

Due to their large surface to body weight ratio rodents lose heat rapidly especially if the abdominal cavity is exposed. Hypothermia might further be exacerbated by the use of cold, dry gases, hair clipping, or the administration of cold fluids. Hairless strains and neonates which are considered exothermic in the early stages of life are especially susceptible to hypothermia because of their diminished insulation. Hypothermia poses multiple risks during anesthesia and recovery, including infection, bleeding complications and cardiac dysfunction. These factors may be the difference between life and death and if the animal survives, the difference between good and unreliable data; therefore, it is highly recommended that an external heat source be used during surgery. Adjustable heating pads or circulating warm water blankets usually allow a good maintenance of body temperature. Homogeneous warming of large surface areas of the animal's body—instead of using planar heating pads that provide comparably smaller contact areas—permits to reduce the heating temperature and allows for better maintenance of overall physiological body temperature [41]. For accurate control, a thermometer should be used to measure the temperature rectally and—if abdominal surgery is part of the procedure—also a second temperature probe placed close to the kidney should be used. Here it is important to consider the possible interactions of the temperature probe with the MRI. Conventional resistive probes with metallic cables may suffer from electrical currents induced by the time-varying magnetic field gradients used during imaging. This might disturb the temperature measurement and even heat up the cables. Use of fiber optical probes helps to avoid these issues but some optical probes experience a sizable offset in the measured temperature with a very strong magnetic field. For instance, a negative offset of 4.7 °C at a magnetic field strength of 9.4T was observed with GaAs-based probes. Some heating pads can automatically regulate the temperature with the help of a thermostat [42]. Too high temperatures can cause protein denaturation and tissue injury, which might result in death.

Kidney temperature during ischemia significantly influences IRI. Body temperature drops after anesthesia, which mitigates IRI

[9]. Therefore, close control and maintenance of body temperature is needed in order to perform reproducible AKI. Ischemia should only be initiated if the desired stable temperature is set and maintained.

4.2 Respiration

Respiratory monitoring can be achieved by observation of chest motion, depth and character of respiration during surgical interventions. Direct visualization of the animal is not feasible during imaging; therefore, respiratory motion detection systems that are compatible with and safe to use for most imaging modalities should be employed. These systems typically detect breathing motion by compressions of a respiratory sensor placed in contact with the chest.

During MRI, breathing often causes motion artefacts, which can severely compromise imaging acquisitions and hence measures to reduce or eliminate such artefacts should be taken. Gating techniques allow for the synchronization of data acquisition with the respiratory cycle. The largest movement of the abdomen occurs between inspiration and expiration; therefore, this period should be excluded from data acquisition.

4.3 Cardiovascular System

Heart rate can be monitored using an electrocardiograph system. Heart rate usually correlates with anesthetic depth. A pulse oximeter can be used to measure arterial O_2 saturation, pulse strength, breath rate and blood flow in real time, and can thus detect hypoventilation, airway obstruction, or other problems during anesthesia. Pulse oximeters are not remarkably accurate in rodents, but can detect trends and are nevertheless valuable tools. Whenever possible, cardiovascular monitoring should include continuous blood pressure measurement. For nonrecovery experiments, direct blood pressure (and heart rate) monitoring via a catheter in the femoral or carotid artery connected to a pressure transducer is preferred. Alternatively, an inflatable tail pressure cuff can be used noninvasively [10].

5 Recovery

Proper postoperative care is needed to minimize the loss of animals, to reduce intraexperimental variation and to offer humane conditions for recovery [8]. Body temperature should be maintained within physiological limits until the end of anesthesia, when the animal starts to be active.

5.1 Analgesia

If activity is resumed, analgesics may be given without the risk of further respiratory depression. Opioids are most commonly used for this purpose [9]; however, some of them can protect against IRI. For example, morphine and naloxone inhibited superoxide anion production after renal IRI in rabbits [43] and naloxone alone can also improve warm renal IRI in dogs [44]. However, buprenorphine, a mixed partial μ-opioid receptor agonist and κ-and δ-opioid receptor antagonist improved animal health by reducing postsurgical stress response, without interfering with renal IRI [45].

Other analgesics, like α2-agonists are proven to have benefic effect on renal IRI [46, 47]. Nonsteroidal anti-inflammatory drugs also interfere with the renal IRI model [48, 49].

5.2 Antibiotics

Although there is a risk for postoperative infections after surgery, there is no indication for empiric use of antibiotic prevention [50]. Focus has to be placed on aseptic surgical infrastructure, cautious animal handling, and well-managed animal facilities (SPF, etc.). If systemic antibiotic use is inevitable, then fluoroquinolones and the trimethoprim–sulfonamide combination are generally recommended, since they are not harmful to the symbiotic intestinal bacterial population of mice [51]. Gentamicin is reported to ameliorate IRI mostly during the reperfusion phase and should not be used in such experiments [52]. Antibiotic administration should be delayed until complete anesthetic recovery takes place because of hypotension and prolonged anesthesia due to their calcium blocking action [51].

Acknowledgments

This chapter is based upon work from COST Action PARENCHIMA, supported by European Cooperation in Science and Technology (COST). COST (www.cost.eu) is a funding agency for research and innovation networks. COST Actions help connect research initiatives across Europe and enable scientists to enrich their ideas by sharing them with their peers. This boosts their research, career, and innovation.

PARENCHIMA (renalmri.org) is a community-driven Action in the COST program of the European Union, which unites more than 200 experts in renal MRI from 30 countries with the aim to improve the reproducibility and standardization of renal MRI biomarkers.

References

1. US Renal Data System Annual Report 2016. (2016). https://www.usrds.org/adr.aspx
2. Selby NM, Blankestijn PJ, Boor P, Combe C, Eckardt KU, Eikefjord E, Garcia-Fernandez N, Golay X, Gordon I, Grenier N, Hockings PD, Jensen JD, Joles JA, Kalra PA, Kramer BK, Mark PB, Mendichovszky IA, Nikolic O, Odudu A, Ong ACM, Ortiz A, Pruijm M, Remuzzi G, Rorvik J, de Seigneux S, Simms RJ, Slatinska J, Summers P, Taal MW, Thoeny HC, Vallee JP, Wolf M, Caroli A, Sourbron S (2018) Magnetic resonance imaging biomarkers for chronic kidney disease: a position paper from the European Cooperation in

Science and Technology Action PARENCHIMA. Nephrol Dial Transplant 33(suppl_2): ii4–ii14. https://doi.org/10.1093/ndt/gfy152

3. Prasad PV (2006) Functional MRI of the kidney: tools for translational studies of pathophysiology of renal disease. Am J Physiol Renal Physiol 290(5):F958–F974. https://doi.org/10.1152/ajprenal.00114.2005
4. Haque M, Franklin T, Prasad P (2011) Renal oxygenation changes during water loading as evaluated by BOLD MRI: effect of NOS inhibition. J Magn Reson Imaging 33 (4):898–901. https://doi.org/10.1002/jmri.22509
5. Tremoleda JL, Macholl S, Sosabowski JK (2018) Anesthesia and monitoring of animals during MRI studies. Methods Mol Biol 1718:423–439. https://doi.org/10.1007/978-1-4939-7531-0_25
6. Herrmann K, Flecknell P (2019) Retrospective review of anesthetic and analgesic regimens used in animal research proposals. ALTEX 36 (1):65–80. https://doi.org/10.14573/altex.1804011
7. Reimann HM, Niendorf T (2020) The (un)-conscious mouse as a model for human brain functions: key principles of anesthesia and their impact on translational neuroimaging. Front Syst Neurosci 14:8. https://doi.org/10.3389/fnsys.2020.00008
8. Wei Q, Dong Z (2012) Mouse model of ischemic acute kidney injury: technical notes and tricks. Am J Physiol Renal Physiol 303(11): F1487–F1494. https://doi.org/10.1152/ajprenal.00352.2012
9. Le Clef N, Verhulst A, D'Haese PC, Vervaet BA (2016) Unilateral renal ischemia-reperfusion as a robust model for acute to chronic kidney injury in mice. PLoS One 11 (3):e0152153. https://doi.org/10.1371/journal.pone.0152153
10. Tremoleda JL, Kerton A, Gsell W (2012) Anaesthesia and physiological monitoring during in vivo imaging of laboratory rodents: considerations on experimental outcomes and animal welfare. EJNMMI Res 2(1):44. https://doi.org/10.1186/2191-219x-2-44
11. Niles DJ, Gordon JW, Fain SB (2015) Effect of anesthesia on renal R2 * measured by blood oxygen level-dependent MRI. NMR Biomed 28(7):811–817. https://doi.org/10.1002/nbm.3314
12. Furtado KS, Andrade FO (2013) Comparison of the beneficial and adverse effects of inhaled and injectable anaesthetics: a mini-review. OA Anaesthetics 1(2):20. https://doi.org/10.13172/2052-7853-1-2-1006
13. Hedenqvist P, Hellebrekers L (2003) Laboratory animal analgesia, anesthesia, and euthanasia
14. Demirkiran H, Senoglu N, Oksuz H, Dogan Z, Yüzbaşıoğu F, Bulbuloglu E, Inanc Tolun F, Aral M, Ciralik H, Goksu M, Yardimci C (2019) The effects of different doses ketamine on the renal ischemia/reperfusion injury in rats. Eastern J Med 24(2):194–199. https://doi.org/10.5505/ejm.2019.48658
15. Yuzer H, Yuzbasioglu MF, Ciralik H, Kurutas EB, Ozkan OV, Bulbuloglu E, Atlı Y, Erdogan O, Kale IT (2009) Effects of intravenous anesthetics on renal ischemia/reperfusion injury. Ren Fail 31(4):290–296. https://doi.org/10.1080/08860220902779962
16. Hau J, Schapiro SJ (2010) Handbook of laboratory animal science, volume I: essential principles and practices. CRC Press, Boca Raton
17. Tsukamoto A, Serizawa K, Sato R, Yamazaki J, Inomata T (2015) Vital signs monitoring during injectable and inhalant anesthesia in mice. Exp Anim 64(1):57–64. https://doi.org/10.1538/expanim.14-0050
18. Buitrago S, Martin TE, Tetens-Woodring J, Belicha-Villanueva A, Wilding GE (2008) Safety and efficacy of various combinations of injectable anesthetics in BALB/c mice. J Am Assoc Lab Anim Sci 47(1):11–17
19. Lei H, Grinberg O, Nwaigwe CI, Hou HG, Williams H, Swartz HM, Dunn JF (2001) The effects of ketamine-xylazine anesthesia on cerebral blood flow and oxygenation observed using nuclear magnetic resonance perfusion imaging and electron paramagnetic resonance oximetry. Brain Res 913(2):174–179. https://doi.org/10.1016/s0006-8993(01)02786-x
20. Ochiai Y, Iwano H, Sakamoto T, Hirabayashi M, Kaneko E, Watanabe T, Yamashita K, Yokota H (2016) Blood biochemical changes in mice after administration of a mixture of three anesthetic agents. J Vet Med Sci 78(6):951–956. https://doi.org/10.1292/jvms.15-0474
21. Ilkiw JE (1992) Advantages and guidelines for using ultrashort barbiturates for induction of anesthesia. Vet Clin North Am Small Anim Pract 22(2):261–264
22. Lopez-Munoz F, Ucha-Udabe R, Alamo C (2005) The history of barbiturates a century after their clinical introduction. Neuropsychiatr Dis Treat 1(4):329–343
23. Dogan Z, Yuzbasioglu MF, Kurutas EB, Yildiz H, Coskuner I, Senoglu N, Oksuz H, Bulbuloglu E (2010) Thiopental improves renal ischemia-reperfusion injury. Ren Fail 32 (3):391–395. https://doi.org/10.3109/08860221003611752

24. Almaas R, Saugstad OD, Pleasure D, Rootwelt T (2000) Effect of barbiturates on hydroxyl radicals, lipid peroxidation, and hypoxic cell death in human NT2-N neurons. Anesthesiology 92(3):764–774. https://doi.org/10.1097/00000542-200003000-00020
25. Nishina K, Akamatsu H, Mikawa K, Shiga M, Maekawa N, Obara H, Niwa Y (1998) The inhibitory effects of thiopental, midazolam, and ketamine on human neutrophil functions. Anesth Analg 86(1):159–165. https://doi.org/10.1097/00000539-199801000-00032
26. Lei H, Duarte JM, Mlynarik V, Python A, Gruetter R (2010) Deep thiopental anesthesia alters steady-state glucose homeostasis but not the neurochemical profile of rat cortex. J Neurosci Res 88(2):413–419. https://doi.org/10.1002/jnr.22212
27. Bruns A, Kunnecke B, Risterucci C, Moreau JL, von Kienlin M (2009) Validation of cerebral blood perfusion imaging as a modality for quantitative pharmacological MRI in rats. Magn Reson Med 61(6):1451–1458. https://doi.org/10.1002/mrm.21779
28. Yuzbasioglu MF, Aykas A, Kurutas EB, Sahinkanat T (2010) Protective effects of propofol against ischemia/reperfusion injury in rat kidneys. Ren Fail 32(5):578–583. https://doi.org/10.3109/08860220903548940
29. Sanchez-Conde P, Rodriguez-Lopez JM, Nicolas JL, Lozano FS, Garcia-Criado FJ, Cascajo C, Gonzalez-Sarmiento R, Muriel C (2008) The comparative abilities of propofol and sevoflurane to modulate inflammation and oxidative stress in the kidney after aortic cross-clamping. Anesth Analg 106(2):371–378, table of contents. https://doi.org/10.1213/ane.0b013e318160580b
30. Liu X, Li R, Yang Z, Hudetz AG, Li SJ (2012) Differential effect of isoflurane, medetomidine, and urethane on BOLD responses to acute levo-tetrahydropalmatine in the rat. Magn Reson Med 68(2):552–559. https://doi.org/10.1002/mrm.23243
31. Aizawa N, Ogawa S, Sugiyama R, Homma Y, Igawa Y (2015) Influence of urethane-anesthesia on the effect of resiniferatoxin treatment on bladder function in rats with spinal cord injury. Neurourol Urodyn 34(3):274–279. https://doi.org/10.1002/nau.22549
32. Maggi CA, Meli A (1986) Suitability of urethane anesthesia for physiopharmacological investigations in various systems. Part 1: general considerations. Experientia 42(2):109–114. https://doi.org/10.1007/bf01952426
33. Ganjoo P, Farber NE, Schwabe D, Kampine JP, Schmeling WT (1996) Desflurane attenuates the somatosympathetic reflex in rats. Anesth Analg 83(1):55–61. https://doi.org/10.1097/00000539-199607000-00010
34. Kober F, Iltis I, Cozzone PJ, Bernard M (2004) Cine-MRI assessment of cardiac function in mice anesthetized with ketamine/xylazine and isoflurane. MAGMA 17(3–6):157–161. https://doi.org/10.1007/s10334-004-0086-0
35. Kersten JR, Lowe D, Hettrick DA, Pagel PS, Gross GJ, Warltier DC (1996) Glyburide, a KATP channel antagonist, attenuates the cardioprotective effects of isoflurane in stunned myocardium. Anesth Analg 83(1):27–33. https://doi.org/10.1097/00000539-199607000-00006
36. van Alst TM, Wachsmuth L, Datunashvili M, Albers F, Just N, Budde T, Faber C (2019) Anesthesia differentially modulates neuronal and vascular contributions to the BOLD signal. NeuroImage 195:89–103. https://doi.org/10.1016/j.neuroimage.2019.03.057
37. Grosenick D, Cantow K, Arakelyan K, Wabnitz H, Flemming B, Skalweit A, Ladwig M, Macdonald R, Niendorf T, Seeliger E (2015) Detailing renal hemodynamics and oxygenation in rats by a combined near-infrared spectroscopy and invasive probe approach. Biomed Opt Express 6(2):309–323. https://doi.org/10.1364/BOE.6.000309
38. Lee HT, Ota-Setlik A, Fu Y, Nasr SH, Emala CW (2004) Differential protective effects of volatile anesthetics against renal ischemia-reperfusion injury in vivo. Anesthesiology 101(6):1313–1324. https://doi.org/10.1097/00000542-200412000-00011
39. Hashiguchi H, Morooka H, Miyoshi H, Matsumoto M, Koji T, Sumikawa K (2005) Isoflurane protects renal function against ischemia and reperfusion through inhibition of protein kinases, JNK and ERK. Anesth Analg 101(6):1584–1589. https://doi.org/10.1213/01.Ane.0000184044.51749.B8
40. Carraretto AR, Vianna Filho PT, Castiglia YM, Golim Mde A, Souza AV, Carvalho LR, Deffune E, Vianna PT (2013) Do propofol and isoflurane protect the kidney against ischemia/reperfusion injury during transient hyperglycemia? Acta Cir Bras 28(3):161–166
41. Reimann HM, Hentschel J, Marek J, Huelnhagen T, Todiras M, Kox S, Waiczies S, Hodge R, Bader M, Pohlmann A, Niendorf T (2016) Normothermic mouse functional MRI of acute focal Thermostimulation for probing

nociception. Sci Rep 6:17230. https://doi.org/10.1038/srep17230

42. Delbridge MS, Shrestha BM, Raftery AT, El Nahas AM, Haylor JL (2007) The effect of body temperature in a rat model of renal ischemia-reperfusion injury. Transplant Proc 39(10):2983–2985. https://doi.org/10.1016/j.transproceed.2007.04.028
43. Blaszczyk J, Kedziora J, Luciak M, Sibinska E, Trznadel K, Pawlicki L (1994) Effect of morphine and naloxone on oxidative metabolism during experimental renal ischemia and reperfusion. Exp Nephrol 2(6):364–370
44. Elkadi HK, Nghiem DD, Southard JH, Kelly KM, Olson CL (1987) Naloxone in renal ischemia: a functional and microanatomical study. J Surg Res 42(6):675–692
45. Deng J, St Clair M, Everett C, Reitman M, Star RA (2000) Buprenorphine given after surgery does not alter renal ischemia/reperfusion injury. Comp Med 50(6):628–632
46. Gonullu E, Ozkardesler S, Kume T, Duru LS, Akan M, Guneli ME, Ergur BU, Meseri R, Dora O (2014) Comparison of the effects of dexmedetomidine administered at two different times on renal ischemia/reperfusion injury in rats. Braz J Anesthesiol 64(3):152–158. https://doi.org/10.1016/j.bjane.2013.06.002
47. Ma J, Chen Q, Li J, Zhao H, Mi E, Chen Y, Yi B, Ning J, Ma D, Lu K, Gu J (2018) Dexmedetomidine-mediated prevention of renal ischemia-reperfusion injury depends in part on cholinergic anti-inflammatory mechanisms. Anesth Analg 130(4):1054–1062. https://doi.org/10.1213/ANE.0000000000003820
48. Zhu SH, Zhou LJ, Jiang H, Chen RJ, Lin C, Feng S, Jin J, Chen JH, Wu JY (2014) Protective effect of indomethacin in renal ischemia-reperfusion injury in mice. J Zhejiang Univ Sci B 15(8):735–742. https://doi.org/10.1631/jzus.B1300196
49. Calistro Neto JP, Torres Rda C, Goncalves GM, Silva LM, Domingues MA, Modolo NS, Barros GA (2015) Parecoxib reduces renal injury in an ischemia/reperfusion model in rats. Acta Cir Bras 30(4):270–276. https://doi.org/10.1590/SC102-865020150040000006
50. Narver HL (2017) Antimicrobial stewardship in laboratory animal facilities. J Am Assoc Lab Anim Sci 56(1):6–10
51. Gargiulo S, Greco A, Gramanzini M, Esposito S, Affuso A, Brunetti A, Vesce G (2012) Mice anesthesia, analgesia, and care, part II: anesthetic considerations in preclinical imaging studies. ILAR J 53(1):E70–E81. https://doi.org/10.1093/ilar.53.1.70
52. Zager RA (1992) Gentamicin effects on renal ischemia/reperfusion injury. Circ Res 70(1):20–28. https://doi.org/10.1161/01.res.70.1.20

3

Dynamic Contrast Enhancement (DCE) MRI–Derived Renal Perfusion and Filtration: Basic Concepts

Michael Pedersen, Pietro Irrera, Walter Dastrù, Frank G. Zöllner, Kevin M. Bennett, Scott C. Beeman, G. Larry Bretthorst, Joel R. Garbow, and Dario Livio Longo

Abstract

Dynamic contrast-enhanced (DCE) MRI monitors the transit of contrast agents, typically gadolinium chelates, through the intrarenal regions, the renal cortex, the medulla, and the collecting system. In this way, DCE-MRI reveals the renal uptake and excretion of the contrast agent. An optimal DCE-MRI acquisition protocol involves finding a good compromise between whole-kidney coverage (i.e., 3D imaging), spatial and temporal resolution, and contrast resolution. By analyzing the enhancement of the renal tissues as a function of time, one can determine indirect measures of clinically important single-kidney parameters as the renal blood flow, glomerular filtration rate, and intrarenal blood volumes. Gadolinium-containing contrast agents may be nephrotoxic in patients suffering from severe renal dysfunction, but otherwise DCE-MRI is clearly useful for diagnosis of renal functions and for assessing treatment response and posttransplant rejection.

Here we introduce the concept of renal DCE-MRI, describe the existing methods, and provide an overview of preclinical DCE-MRI applications to illustrate the utility of this technique to measure renal perfusion and glomerular filtration rate in animal models.

This publication is based upon work from the COST Action PARENCHIMA, a community-driven network funded by the European Cooperation in Science and Technology (COST) program of the European Union, which aims to improve the reproducibility and standardization of renal MRI biomarkers. This introduction is complemented by two separate publications describing the experimental procedure and data analysis.

Key words Magnetic resonance imaging (MRI), Dynamic contrast-enhanced (DCE), Kidney, Mice, Rats, T_1 mapping, Contrast agent, Perfusion, Glomerular filtration rate (GFR)

1 Introduction

Glomerular filtration rate (GFR) is a standard measure of kidney function. In past decades, simplified plasma clearance employing radiopharmaceuticals (51Cr-EDTA, 125I-iothalamate, 99mTc-DTPA) was introduced and validated to provide very accurate estimates of total GFR [1–4]. Later, alternative techniques have

Andreas Pohlmann and Thoralf Niendorf (eds.), *Preclinical MRI of the Kidney: Methods and Protocols*, Methods in Molecular Biology, vol. 2216, https://doi.org/10.1007/978-1-0716-0978-1_12,

been evaluated, using minute doses of nonradioactive contrast agents, including iothalamate and iohexol [5]. Plasma clearance of such compounds has also been applied to measure renal function. Renal blood flow (RBF) is another important measure of the functional status of a kidney. The standard tracer-based technique for quantifying RBF is to measure clearance of substances such as hippurate or of radiopharmaceuticals [6].

Dynamic contrast enhanced (DCE-MRI) is an alternative to these techniques that uses gadolinium chelates as contrast agents (CAs), providing functional information analogous to that obtained from radionuclide studies [7, 8]. These chelates are generally considered glomerular filtration markers, since they are removed from the circulation exclusively by glomerular filtration.

DCE-MRI measures T_1-weighted signal intensity changes in tissues over time after bolus administration of a contrast agent. Dynamic data acquisition allows for monitoring of the contrast agent in the renal cortex, the medulla, and the collecting system, providing a renographic representation with underlying information about the renal perfusion, filtration, and vascularization [9–12]. Postprocessing analyses of these signal-vs-time curves reveal kidney functionality in terms of filtration and perfusion, including both heuristic nonmodel approaches and model-based quantitative methods [13, 14]. However, while DCE-MRI is a promising tool in animal models, its clinical utility is hampered by the risk of developing nephrogenic systemic fibrosis in renal patients with severely reduced glomerular filtration capacity [15]. In this chapter, we will address the basic concept of DCE-MRI with the emphasis on kidney disease models in rodents.

This introduction chapter is complemented by two separate chapters describing the experimental procedure and data analysis, which are part of this book.

This chapter is part of the book Pohlmann A, Niendorf T (eds) (2020) Preclinical MRI of the Kidney—Methods and Protocols. Springer, New York.

2 Measurement Concept

2.1 Basic Concept of DCE

The standard acquisition scheme of a DCE-MRI experiment is based on repeated T_1-weighted images before and after the injection of a Gadolinium-based CA. In this way, a dynamic curve of the signal enhancement in the kidney is recorded in a time window wide enough (5–10 min) to see the contrast range from the vascular peak enhancement to the wash-out phase. An injection dose of 0.1 mmol Gd/kg is considered standard [16], and lower doses are occasionally exploited to reduce concomitant T_2* effects in vessels.

2.2 Gadolinium-Based Contrast Agents

In DCE-MRI, the gadolinium agents have two main advantages, one attributed to the properties of the gadolinium-ion in response to a magnetic field, and one attributed to the chelate that has a biodistribution in the body which favors measurements of renal clearance. In physical terms, the gadolinium ion is chosen having seven unpaired electrons in its orbitals resulting in strong paramagnetism [17–19]. Furthermore, the symmetry of the electron configuration of the trivalent gadolinium ion is a hospitable environment for electron spins, contributing to the rise of the crucial nuclear magnetic resonance parameter called relaxation. For these reasons, gadolinium (Gd^{3+}) is the most common metal ion used in paramagnetic contrast agent and its relationship is given by $1/T_{1\ (\text{Measured})} = 1/T_{1\ (\text{Water})} + r_1\,[\text{Gd}]$. The relaxivity is dependent on the magnetic field and temperature [20–22]. Due to its toxicity as free ion, Gd is trapped in a molecular structure defined by the closed/open ring that chelates the metal. These macrocyclic and linear CAs may possess different r_1, osmolarity, and molecular size [23–25]. In addition to clinical contrast agents, several other Gd complexes have been investigated for providing higher relaxivity or contrast efficiency [26–31]. All the contrast agents used for mapping kidney perfusion are small molecular weight extracellular agents and are administered intravenously [32].

2.3 Conversion of Signal into Contrast Agent Concentration

Contrary to nuclear medicine modalities, MRI unfortunately does not measure changes in signal intensity in a straightforward way. This means that measurements of injected contrast agent concentration is difficult, which again severely hinders the possibility to calculate important parameters in absolute units such as ml/min or ml/min/g. Previous studies have taken this constraint into account in three different ways: (1) by assuming that the signal intensity is linearly related to the concentration of contrast agent, (2) by making calibration of water doped with contrast agent and then assume the same signal-vs-concentration can be applied in the living tissue, and (3) by introducing the mathematical complex relationship between signal and concentration. These three approaches are here ordered with increasing difficulties in which they can be performed, meaning that the third method is by far the most ambitious. To be able to convert signal intensities into concentration, we present a step-by-procedure. First, the mathematical equation that relates the signal into concentration relies on both well-known constants, the employed MR imaging technique and the pulse sequence parameters (echo-time, recovery time, flip angle, etc.). Due to the paramagnetic properties of the contrast agent, the magnetic relaxation time (T_1) decreases in the presence of the contrast agent. Conversion of acquired signal (enhancement) to changes in T_1 needs some mathematical understanding. In a simple setup, DCE-MRI is performed with a T_1-weighted-2D-spoiled gradient-echo train (Fig. 1).

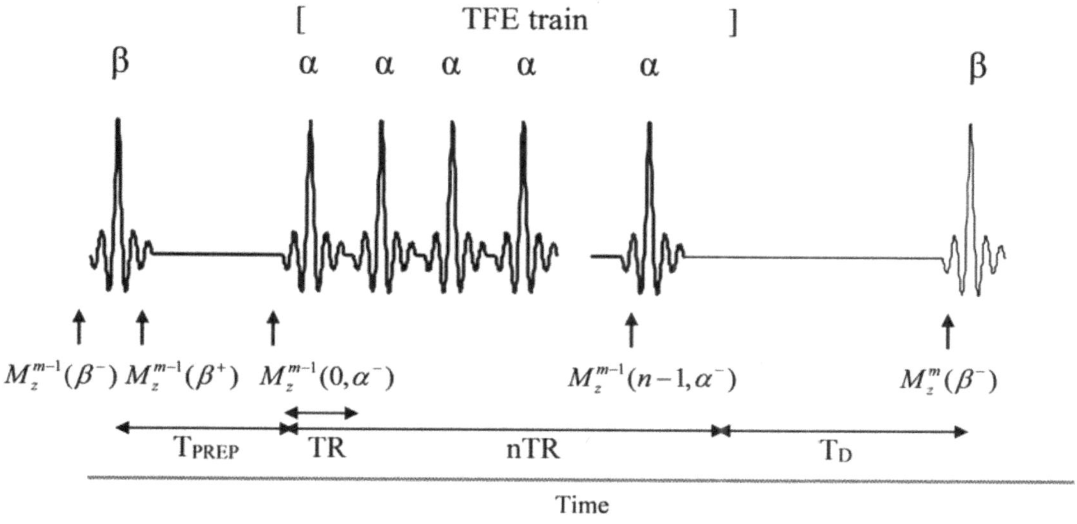

Fig. 1 Pulse train for dynamic MRI using a spoiled gradient-echo sequence

First, we consider the spoiled gradient echo sequence (TFE) without prepulses. The longitudinal component of the magnetization is denoted M_z, which relaxes back to its equilibrium M_0 due to a characteristic relaxation time (T_1). The magnetization M_z is derived by the Bloch equation, given as follows:

$$\frac{dM_z}{dt} = \frac{M_0 - M_z}{T_1} \tag{1}$$

where M_0 denotes the bulk longitudinal magnetization, and T_1 is the longitudinal relaxation time. Integration of Eq. 1 returns the time-dependent $M_z(t)$:

$$\int_0^{M_z} \frac{dM_z}{M_0 - M_z} = \int_0^t \frac{dt}{T_1} \Rightarrow M_z(t) - M_0 = Ae^{-t/T_1} \tag{2}$$

Giving the notation that $M_z(t = 0)$ is $M_z(0)$, we define the constraint:

$$M_z(0) = M_0 + A \Rightarrow A = M_z(0) - M_0 \tag{3}$$

Resolving Eq. 2 gives the following:

$$\begin{aligned} M_z(t) &= M_0 + [M_z(0) - M_0]e^{-t/T_1} \\ &= M_0\left[1 - e^{-t/T_1}\right] + M_z(0^+)e^{-t/T_1} \end{aligned} \tag{4}$$

The magnetization just before the n'th pulse (denoted as $n\text{TR}^-$) can now be determined:

$$\begin{aligned} M_z(n\mathrm{TR}^-) &= M_0\left[1 - e^{-\mathrm{TR}/T_1}\right] + M_z((n-1)\mathrm{TR}^+)e^{-\mathrm{TR}/T_1} \\ &= M_0[1 - E_1] + M_z((n-1)\mathrm{TR}^-)\cos\alpha E_1 \end{aligned} \tag{5}$$

where $E = e^{-\mathrm{TR}/T_1}$, and $M_z((n-1)\mathrm{TR}^-)$ represents the magnetization just after a time $(n - 1)$TR. Eq. 5 can be developed recursively:

$$\begin{aligned} M_z(n\mathrm{TR}^-) &= M_0[1 - E_1] + [M_0[1 - E_1] + M_z((n-2)\mathrm{TR}^-)\cos\alpha E_1]\cos\alpha E_1 \\ &= M_0[1 - E_1] + M_0[1 - E_1]\cos\alpha E_1 + M_z((n-2)\mathrm{TR}^-)[\cos\alpha E_1]^2 \\ &= \sum\nolimits_{i=0}^{n-1} M_0[1 - E_1][\cos\alpha E_1]^i + M_z(0^-)[\cos\alpha E_1]^n \\ &= M_0[1 - E_1]\frac{1 - [\cos\alpha E_1]^n}{1 - \cos\alpha E_1} + M_0^{\mathrm{eq}}[\cos\alpha E_1]^n \end{aligned} \tag{6}$$

Herein, the geometric series is assumed:

$$M_z^{\mathrm{eq}} = \lim_{n\to\infty} M_z(n\mathrm{TR}) \to M_0\frac{1 - E_1}{1 - \cos\alpha E_1} \tag{7}$$

The steady-state condition can then be described as follows:

$$M_z^{\mathrm{eq}} = M_0^{\mathrm{eq}}\frac{1 - E_1}{1 - E_1\cos\alpha} \tag{8}$$

Taking into account that steady-state condition must be fulfilled in presence of a delay T_{D}, employed between the TFE train and the subsequent RF pulse, the following must apply:

$$M_z^{\mathrm{eq}} = M_z^{\mathrm{eq},0}\left[1 - e^{-T_{\mathrm{D}}/T1}\right] + M_z^{\mathrm{eq}}e^{-T_{\mathrm{D}}/T1} \tag{9}$$

Now, let us introduce the preparation pulse (with flip-angle β) applied a time T_{PREP} before the excitation pulse. M_0^{eq} is taken into account by solving:

$$M_z^0 = M_0^{\mathrm{eq}}\left[1 - e^{-T_{\mathrm{PREP}}/T1}\right] + M_z(\beta^+)e^{-T_{\mathrm{PREP}}/T1} \tag{10}$$

where $M_z(\beta^+)$ represents the magnetization just after the β pulse. The magnetization before the n'th α-pulse, denoted as $M_z(n,\alpha^-)$, is given as the combination of Eqs. 6 and 10:

$$\begin{aligned} M_z^-(n,\alpha) = &\left[M_0^{\mathrm{eq}}\left(1 - e^{-T_{\mathrm{PREP}}/T1}\right) + M_z^{\mathrm{eq},0}e^{-T_{\mathrm{PREP}}/T1}\cos\beta\right][E_1\cos\alpha]^n \\ &+ M_0^{\mathrm{eq}}[1 - E_1]\frac{1 - [E_1\cos\alpha]^n}{1 - E_1\cos\alpha} \end{aligned} \tag{11}$$

Therefore, using a heavily T_1-weighted pulse sequence, changes in signal intensity are then almost entirely dependent on changes of T_1. In these circumstances, it can be shown that M_z^{eq} is almost linearly dependent on T_1 relaxation rate. Note again that the specific magnetic relaxivity of the gadolinium-agent (r) defines the characteristic enhancement property by the equation: $[Gd] = (1/T_1 - 1/T_{1(0)})/r$, where $T_{1(0)}$ is the bulk relaxation time in the tissue without the presence of contrast agent, and [Gd] is the concentration of contrast (gadolinium) agent. In principle, this means that a precontrast measurement of T_1 (T_1-mapping) should be performed before injection of the contrast agent. One important factor contributing to erroneous measurements of $T_{1(0)}$ of blood is the inflow effect, because the coherent movement of flowing fluid can alter T_1 of the signal arising from spins therein. Placing the central-encoding lines within the low blood flow window within the cardiac cycle can, to some extent, minimize the problems of the inflow effect.

2.4 Imaging Readout

For dynamic acquisitions, two factors must be taken into consideration: the time resolution and the contrast resolution required. For quantitative studies of renal perfusion and GFR, based on the first-pass of the contrast agent, a high temporal resolution is particularly important to accurately sample the vascular phase of the kidney (especially for renal perfusion studies) in order to measure the arterial input function (AIF). The AIF is the signal-time-curve usually observed in the suprarenal abdominal aorta or in a renal artery and is used in different kinetic models in order to compensate for the non-instantaneous bolus injected into the blood. The request for a high temporal resolution explains why some studies have been performed using a single slice acquisition scheme and not as multislice or 3D techniques. However, the required extrapolation of functional data from one slice to the whole kidney is not always valid if the renal disease is irregularly or focally distributed.

Most of the exploited sampling techniques are gradient echo imaging, echo-planar imaging and spiral imaging. Differences in the sequence are represented by the ability to cover the image space, from conventional approaches that acquire a portion of the space every TR to entire space acquisition in every TR step. Among them, other subtechniques exist with little changes in the sampling approach like spoiled gradient echo, segmental echo planar imaging, keyhole imaging or parallel imaging [33].

2.4.1 Gradient-Echo

Gradient echo (also "gradient recalled echo," GRE)-based sequences are the most commonly used sequences for DCE-MRI studies, where fast GRE sequences can be implemented in different ways, including unbalanced, balanced steady-state, and RF-spoiled sequences [34]. Notably, standard (unbalanced) and balanced gradient echo sequences are sensitive to T_2 effects that result in signal decreases upon the accumulation of the contrast agent in the region of interest. Therefore, spoiled GRE sequences are mostly used since they are more sensitive to T_1 effects leading to higher contrast enhancements. A drawback of these sequences is the low SNR (signal to noise ratio) that can be compensated by the use of 3D acquisitions.

2.4.2 Echo-Planar Imaging

Echo planar imaging (EPI) allows fast image acquisition in combination with high temporal and spatial resolution, with acquisition of several images per second [35]. On the other hand, EPI sequences are difficult to exploit in abdomen and thorax regions since they are sensitive to susceptibility and motion effects. These artifacts can however be reduced by using segmented EPI sequences with a concomitant loss in temporal resolution.

2.4.3 Keyhole Imaging

Since central lines of the K-space are more sensitive to image contrast in comparison to peripheral lines, keyhole imaging is exploited for accelerating imaging acquisition by acquiring multiple central K-space lines. This high-contrast but low-spatial resolution image can then be combined with a high-resolution image to restore the spatial information. Consequently, temporal resolution can be increased up to three- to fourfold, despite some problems that can be encountered in areas with large physiological movements. Several partial K-space sampling techniques have been developed and exploited in a variety of applications [36].

2.5 T_1 Mapping

T_1 measurements can be performed along the dynamic acquisition (precontrast and postcontrast) at every repetition time or before and after the bolus administration using T_1 mapping techniques. Applying a radiofrequency (RF) pulse, spins will change their magnetization status according to the design of the pulse. The magnetization can be inverted or saturated (nulled), and T_1-weighted images are acquired after the inversion or time after saturation pulse. Since the T_1 calculation is the time that magnetization takes to restore to its equilibrium (which is considered fully restored after 5 times the T_1), the two models of RF pulses are called inversion recovery and saturation recovery. Another way to perturb the magnetization is achieved by manipulating the flip angle of the RF pulse at every sequence acquisition, sampling the T_1 relaxation for different angle values.

2.5.1 Saturation Recovery

A 90° saturation pulse effectively nulls the magnetization independently of its state before the saturation pulse. In this way, keeping the repetition time lower than the T_1, the system is unable to fully recover to equilibrium and is said to be saturated. Thus, the T_1 measurements are performed by varying the TR constantly ranging from 0 to, at least, 2–3 times the longest T_1 value expected in the sample. The result is that saturation recovery is a very fast method but with the drawback of a limited dynamic range and limited T_1 range.

2.5.2 Inversion Recovery

Inversion recovery consists of a 180° inversion pulse which rotates the longitudinal magnetization to give the classical decay with a 90° pulse. The inversion recovery pulse sequence is repeated continuously, each time applying the same inversion pulse, followed by different waiting times (time of inversion). The principle of this method implies that the repetition time of the sequence must be greater than the longest T_1 since the magnetization needs to be fully recovered before applying another inversion pulse. Inversion recovery is a method for T_1 map acquisition which produces maps with good accuracy and intensity dynamic range but with the drawback of being time-consuming.

2.5.3 Variable Flip Angle (VFA)

Variable flip angle is used to acquire 3D T_1 maps, and the technique uses two or more repeated sequences with different flip angles (ranging from a few degrees to even more than 90°), sampling the T_1 relaxation for different angle values. The method is relatively sensitive to B_1 inhomogeneities; hence a field map should be acquired. Recently, magnetization transfer effects were identified as an additional source of variability in the obtained VFA data, which can be reduced dramatically by use of tailored composite RF pulses that apply the same power to the bound proton pool for all flip angles [37].

2.6 Renal Handling of Contrast Agents

Before analysis of the acquired DCE-MRI data, it is important to understand how the renal segments handle the gadolinium agent during DCE-MRI. Following an i.v. (intravenous) bolus of contrast agent, the arterial concentration is promptly increased following a steady decline over time, reflecting the input and output of the agent over time. Figure 2 shows an example of dynamic

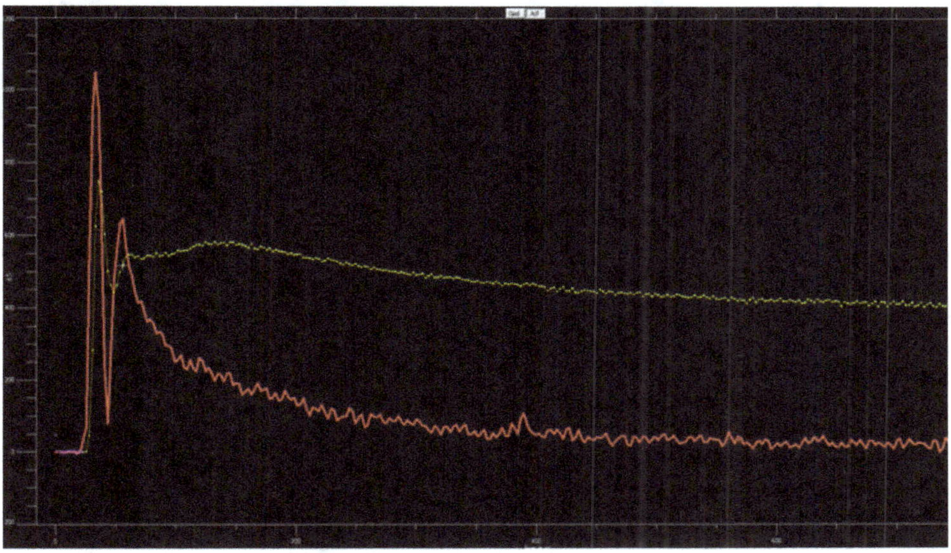

Fig. 2 Dynamic uptake curve (enhancement) in the aorta (red) and renal whole-parenchyma (yellow) following iv bolus of a gadolinium agent. Purple dots indicate baseline values prior to bolus administration. *See* Fig. 3 text for MRI sequence parameters. The aorta curve shows a rapid increase followed by a decline over time (0–800 s). The renal curve shows a first-pass vascular uptake, followed by a pattern with decreasing vascular gadolinium-content combined with a glomerular handling of the contrast agent

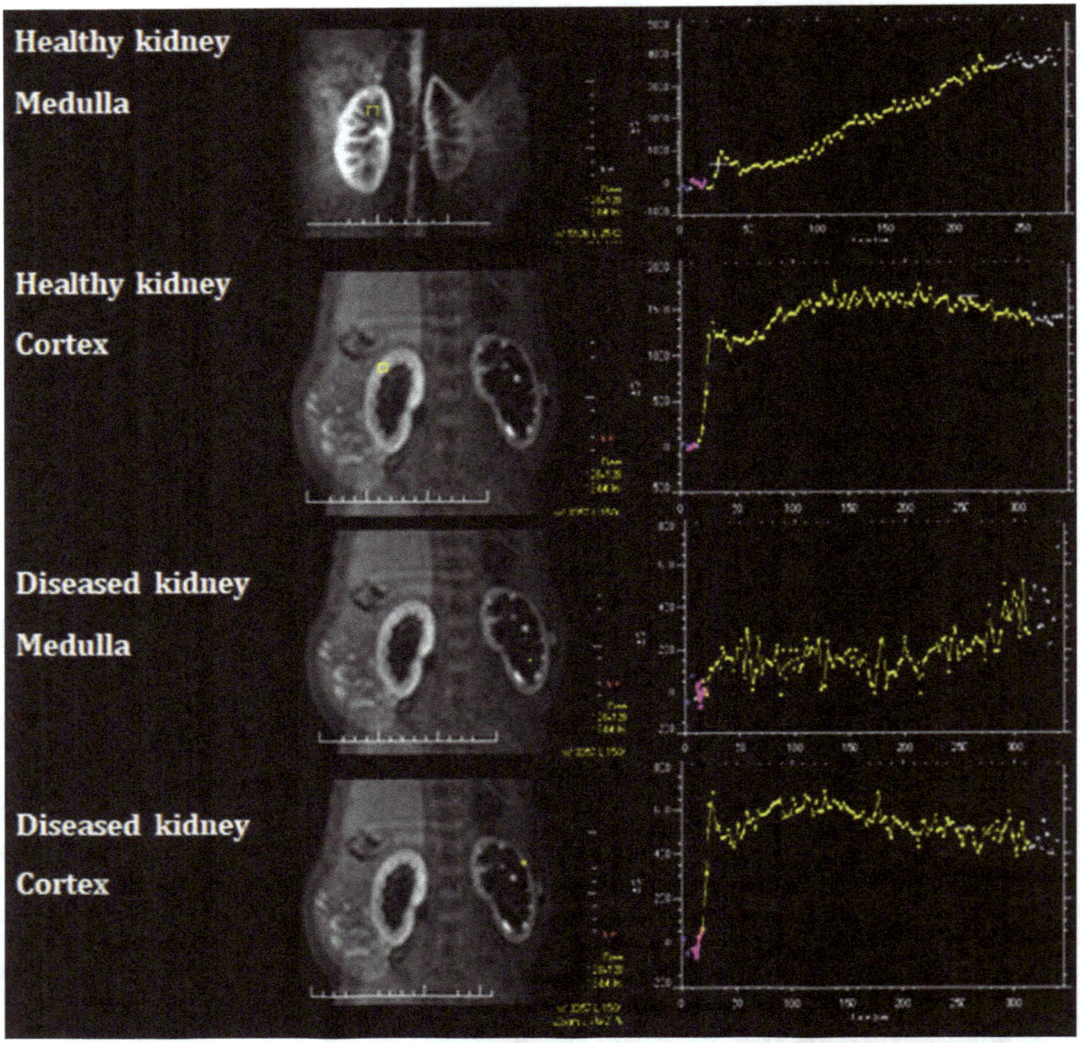

Fig. 3 Example of MR renogram, the result of DCE-MRI of pig kidneys with healthy (left) and diseased (right) kidneys. The yellow ROIs are shown to illustrate where the dynamic curves were drawn. The data were obtained as follows: the anaesthetized pig was placed supine in the magnet, and a surface radiofrequency coil was used for data reception. Fast multislice anatomical images were initially acquired to localize both kidneys. Next, an MRI renography pulse sequence was employed. The whole kidney was covered using a mutlislice (3.0 mm thickness with zero gap) fast 3D gradient echo sequence. Other parameters included: matrix = 128 × 128, field of view = 220 × 220 mm^2, TR = 4.3 ms, TE = 1.5 ms. This scan was accompanied by an intravenous injection of 0.05 ml/kg of Gd-DTPA-BMA (Omniscan®; GE Healthcare, Oslo, Norway) was performed as a single bolus administered by hand 10 s after start of a dynamic gradient-echo sequence, with a single phase acquisition time of 2.2 s. A total of 700 dynamic phases were acquired during 7 min

enhancement following a bolus of a gadolinium agent, and Fig. 3 shows the handling of a gadolinium agent in the healthy and diseased (ureteric obstructed) kidneys. Graphical presentation of the renal enhancement is denoted as an MR renogram.

The MR renogram typically consists of vascular, parenchymal, and excretory phases [38]. The vascular phase occurs almost immediately after contrast injection and provides the first segment of the renographic curve, which is reflected by a steep linear rise. In the cortex, this is followed by the parenchymal phase, characterized by continuous uptake, which is represented in the intensity–time curve as a slower linear increase up to a second peak. In the excretory phase, contrast material is released into the collecting system calices and constitutes the third segment of the renographic curve.

2.7 Analysis Methods

While the experimental design of DCE-MRI is simple, extracting true morphological or physiological parameters from a DCE time course is extraordinarily difficult, due to a number of factors, including intravoxel heterogeneity in tissue microstructure and the need for pharmacokinetic (model-based) or empirical (non-model based) modeling of the DCE-MRI signal [16, 38]. Tissue heterogeneity depends upon the organ of interest and image resolution, which are typically not varied in a single experiment. Pharmacokinetic and empirical modeling, however, are active areas of investigation.

2.7.1 Semiquantitative Analysis

As a descriptive approach, the dynamic time-vs-time curve of DCE-MRI data provides information with parameters like time-to-peak enhancement, uptake slope, area-under-the-curve and wash-out rate. These heuristic enhancement parameters may have some relation to physiologic parameters although they also depend on the particular MRI system and acquisition settings, including pulse sequence, sequence parameters, system manufacturer, and contrast agent employed [39]. Figure 4 shows an example of such parameters.

2.7.2 Quantitative—Pharmacokinetic Models

Alternatively, various physiological pharmacokinetic models have been proposed, usually based on long-term experiences in nuclear medicine. These models are often attributed to situations where the capillary bed (e.g., the blood–brain barrier) is compromised, resulting in extravasation of the contrast agent through the leaky capillaries. For example, modeling the dynamic extravasation of MRI contrast agent can provide a measure of the extravascular uptake. Overall, applying pharmacokinetic models allow calculation of several measures: (1) physiologic properties (transendothelial permeability, capillary surface area, lesion leakage space), (2) pharmacokinetic parameters (compartmental transfer and rate constants, leakage space), and (3) pathological measures (microvessel density and vascular endothelial growth factor) [13, 16]. Measurements of these parameters using modeling are now considered diagnostically important in tumor evaluation (grade classification) and to recognize the onset of stroke by indirect measurements of rCBF, rCBV, and MTT, although they usually provide limited

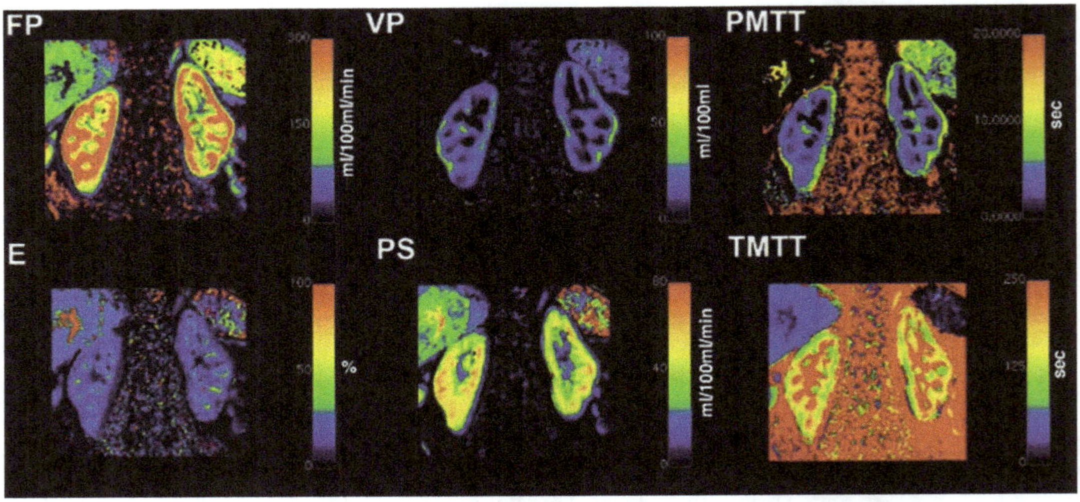

Fig. 4 Example of parameters estimated from DCE-MRI in kidneys. Top row from left to right: plasma flow (FP), plasma volume (VP), plasma mean transit time (PMTT). Lower row from left to right: extraction fraction (E), permeable surface area product (PS), and tubular mean transit time (TMMT). The maps are reproduced with permission from Zöllner et al. [39]

insight into the underlying pathophysiology of the brain tumor or stroke [40]. It is therefore likely that similar parameters can be measured in the kidney. The quantitative models require additional postprocessing steps, including contrast agent concentration calculation (e.g., based on linearity assumption between concentration and signal changes or in previously acquired T_1 maps), selection of a major artery to derive the AIF curve, selection of the pharmacokinetic model (as well as of the number of the compartments and how they are connected) to be used. In addition, the focus of the application as well as the quality of the data will guide the selection of the more appropriate model. Besides, the temporal resolution, protocol injection, and acquisition time can influence the quality of the outcomes, making it necessary to have appropriate and optimized measurement protocols.

2.7.3 Model Selection

All data analysis, including analysis of DCE-MRI data, involves either explicit or implicit comparison to a model. The data are typically considered to be the sum of the signal and noise, and the estimated signal model parameters are of primary interest. In the ideal case, the underlying principles of the measurement and the signal response form the basis of the signal model. Often, however, there are several potential signal models. The analyst must decide which of these competing models best represents the data without "over fitting" (i.e., fitting the noise). Even when the correct signal model is known, the signal-to-noise ratio of the data may not support the complexity of the correct model, requiring that simpler models be considered.

Here, we consider the problem of model selection in DCE-MRI experiments in the kidney. The importance of selecting an appropriate DCE tracer kinetic model to measure tissue perfusion and capillary permeability has already been examined in tumors in previous reports [41, 42]. Model selection algorithms, including Chi-square [43], Akaike information criterion (AIC) [44–46], F-test [47–49], and the Durbin–Watson statistic [45, 50], have been applied to evaluate tracer kinetic models commonly used in DCE-MRI.

2.7.4 Bayesian Probability Theory

An elegant solution to the model selection problem using Bayesian probability theory-based methods has recently been described [51–53]. Bayesian probability theory [54] provides a rigorous formalism for model selection. To determine the optimal model amongst a cohort of competing models, it is necessary to balance the accuracy with which the model recapitulates the data (the goodness of fit, characterized by the residuals) against the number of free parameters in each model (the complexity). Cox's theorem [55] and its further elaboration by Jaynes [56], state that Bayesian probability theory is the only method of ranking hypotheses concerning model selection that is consistent and can incorporate all of the available prior information. Advances in computational power and the development of Markov-chain Monte Carlo (MCMC) methods have greatly increased the applicability of Bayesian inference to a range of problems.

Bayesian probability theory seeks to assign a probability to the truth of a specific hypothesis. Using a Bayesian approach, the model selection problem treats the model itself as a parameter, for which the posterior probability of a model, given the data and prior information, is computed [51–53]. The posterior probability of each model is calculated by:

$$P(M|DI) = \frac{P(M|I)P(D|MI)}{P(D|I)} \tag{12}$$

where $P(M|DI)$ is the posterior probability for any one of M models. The vertical bar "|" means "given the data, D and the prior information, I." On the right-hand side, $P(M|I)$ is the prior probability for each of the M different models, assigned in this calculation as a uniform prior probability. $P(D|MI)$ is the probability for the data, given model M and prior information I. Finally, the denominator, $P(D|I)$ is a normalization constant that ensures the total probability over all of the models sums to one.

An example of a joint Bayesian approach to model selection in DCE-MRI was described recently by Beeman et al. [57], applied to models of blood flow in cortex in a mouse model of three different renal perfusion rates. The three cohorts of mice studied were: (1) Control; (2) Losartan-treated (high renal blood flow); (3) L-NAME-treated (low renal blood flow). DCE-MRI data were analyzed on a voxel-by-voxel basis. Four models and model parameters were compared in each voxel. Two of the models, the Patlak–Rutland model [58] and the two-compartment model were pharmacokinetic and two, the cumulative log-logistic model with either monoexponential decay with a constant offset or biexponential decay, were empirical. A Markov-chain Monte Carlo simulation was run to compute the posterior probability for the parameters and the model. The estimated probabilities of the parameters of the biexponential model, obtained using this approach, are shown in Fig. 5.

The importance of signal-to-noise in model selection in DCE-MRI was described recently by Duan et al. [51] In their paper, the authors considered four established kinetic models for analyzing DCE-MRI data collected from patients enrolled in the EMBRACE study, an international study of MRI-guided brachytherapy in locally advanced cervical cancer. The models were (1) Toft's (TM), (2) Extended Toft's (ETM), (3) Two-Site Exchange (2CXM), and (4) Compartment Tissue Uptake (CTUM). To demonstrate the importance of signal-to-noise in DCE data analysis, noise-free in silico DCE data sets were generated for each of the four models. The temporal resolution and total data acquisition times were identical to those of the clinical DCE-MRI protocol, using patient-derived tissue parameters.

As expected, Bayesian model selection chose the "correct" signal model for each of these noise-free data sets. Increasing amounts of normally distributed (Gaussian) noise were then added to each data set. At each noise power, 100 independent MCMC simulations (i.e., different noise sets) were performed and the number of "correct" selections, in which model selection chose the model used to simulate the data, was recorded. The number of correct model selections varied as a function of both model complexity and noise power. With increasing levels of noise, simpler data representations were preferred relative to more complex models (Fig. 6a). Figure 6b shows model selection results for in silico data created based on the 2XCM. The number of correct model selections dropped rapidly with increasing noise, with a concomitant increase in the selection of the CTUM, a simplified version of the 2XCM. Figure 6c, d shows how the accuracy and uncertainty of estimations of extravascular, extracellular volume (ve), the only common parameter between the simplest model (TM) and the most complex model (2XCM), vary with added noise. At every noise level, the uncertainties of the estimated ve are much smaller for the TM, relative to the 2CXM.

2.8 Practical Considerations

The main advantage of T_1-weighted DCE-MRI is that both tissue blood flow and filtration (permeability surface) can be measured simultaneously. One important element in the T_1-weighted DCE-MRI is the underlying model from which the calculated parameters are derived. Many assumptions about the tissue system

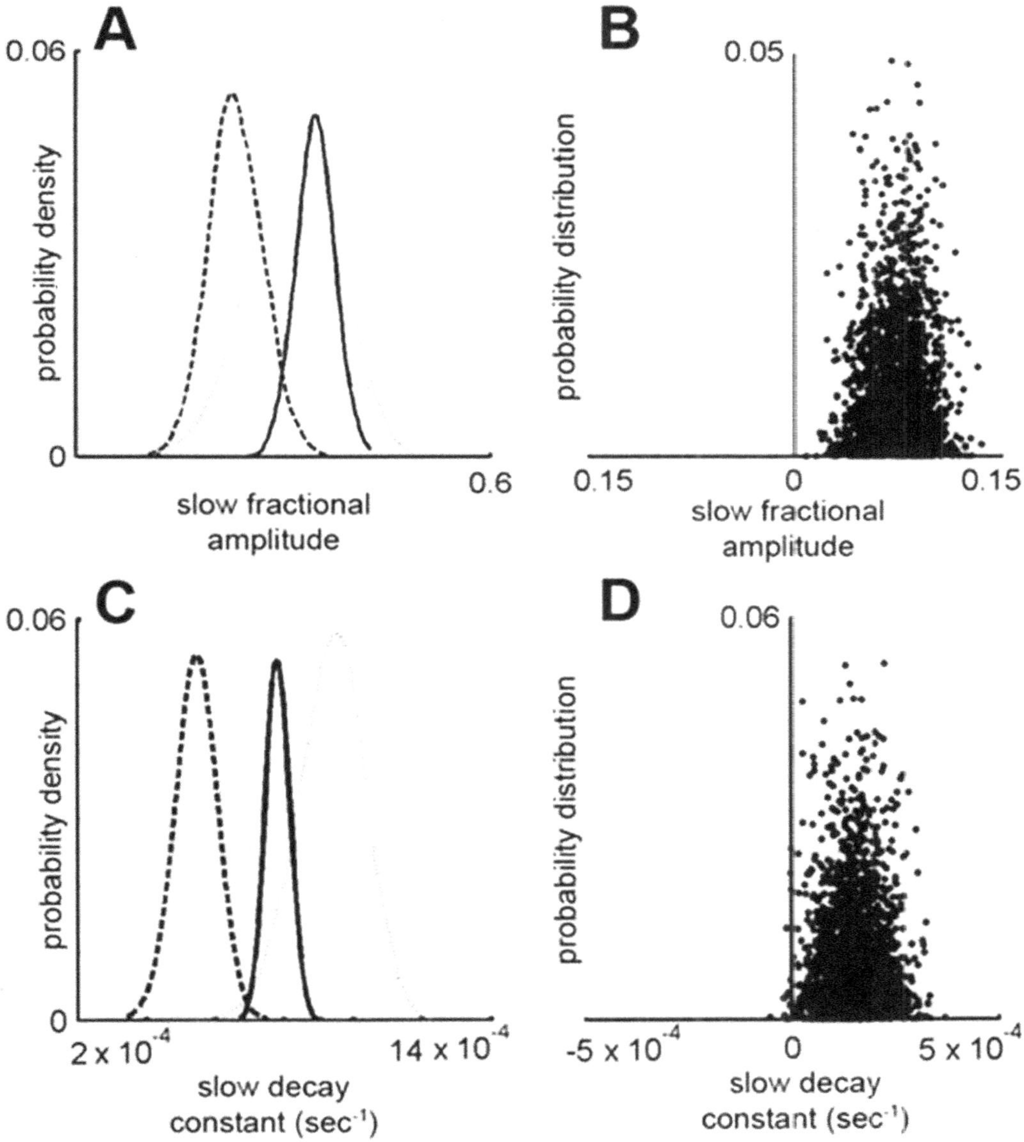

Fig. 5 (**a**, **c**) Bayesian-estimated posterior probability densities of the empirical biexponential model's joint fractional amplitudes of the washout and joint slow decay-rate constants, respectively, for each cohort. The Losartan-treated (high renal blood flow) group is represented by the solid black line, the L-NAME (low renal blood flow group) by the dashed black line, and the control group by the dotted gray line. (**b**, **d**) The difference in the posterior probability distributions for the joint fractional amplitudes of the washout and joint slow decay-rate constants, respectively, calculated on the high and low flow cohorts. From among the empirical/biexponential model joint parameter estimates, the fractional amplitudes of the washout terms (**a**) and the slow decay-rate constants (**c**) differed between mouse cohorts of high and low flow; that is, the 95% confidence interval of the difference in the probability distributions did not overlap with 0 (**b** and **d**). (Adapted, with permission, from Beeman, et al. [57])

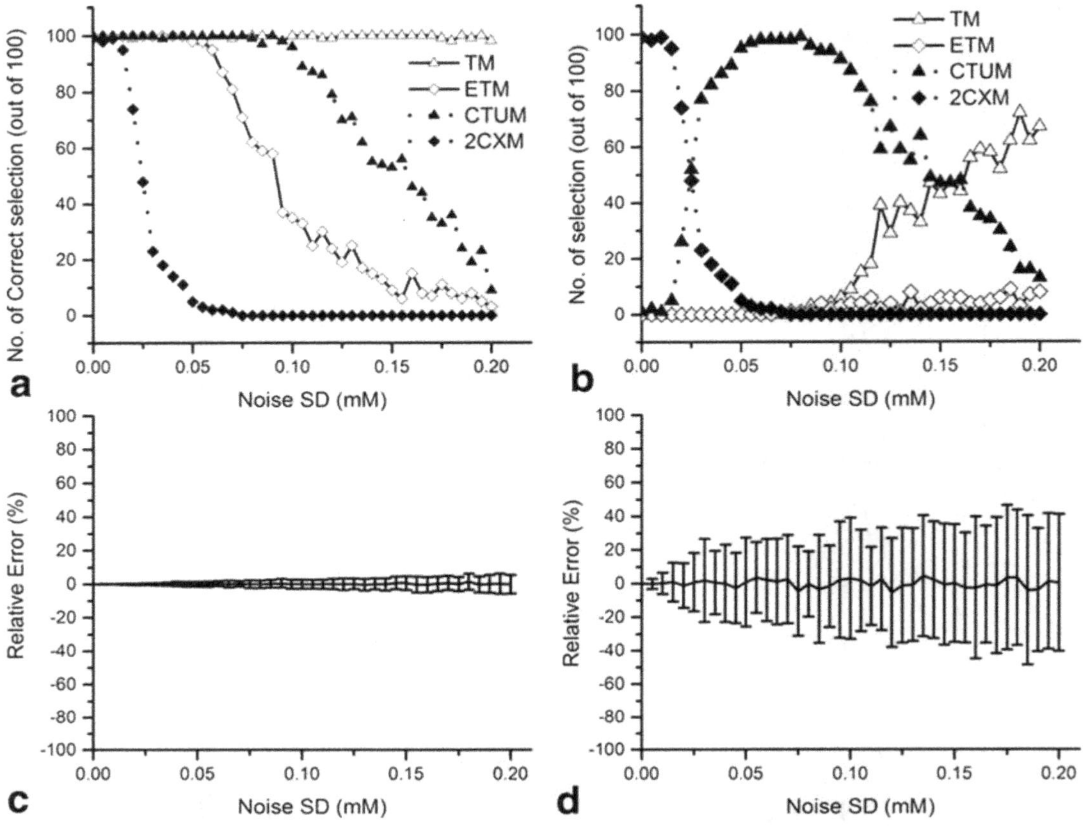

Fig. 6 Bayesian DCE-MRI model-selection and parameter-estimation results for in silico datasets created based on the whole-tumor averaged ROI DCE time course from a single patient in the EMBRACE study. (**a**) For each of the four in silico DCE-MRI data models, the number of "correct" model selections (out of 100 different noise representations), as a function of the noise standard deviation (SD). (**b**) For the two-compartment exchange in silico DCE-MRI data model (the most complex model of the four models examined), the number of times a given model was selected (out of 100 different noise representations) as a function of the noise SD. (**c**, **d**) Relative percent error of v_e (extracellular-extravascular volume fraction) estimated from initially noiseless simulated TM (**c**) and 2CXM (**d**) data as a function of added noise. (Adapted with permission from Duan et al. [51])

are made with respect to the nature of contrast agent kinetic modeling, and these assumptions may affect the accuracy of the parameter calculations. In practice, a compromise must be struck between reality and the precision of the measured data (signal-to noise ratio, temporal resolution, etc.). The different models proposed by leading experts in this field have unfortunately been presented with a variety of quantities, meaning that comparisons between different groups are almost impossible. Consequently, a standardization of quantities associated with analysis of T_1-weighted DCE-MRI has been proposed in the review by Tofts et al. [59], and later by Sourbron [42] as part of building up a common language for the estimation and description of physiologic parameters in the kidney.

For all methods proposed, the calculation of renal parameters requires knowledge of the arterial input function, which in practice is derived from the abdominal aorta or a renal artery with the assumption that this represents the exact input to the renal tissue. Delay and dispersion of the bolus that are introduced during its passage from the site of arterial input function estimation to the renal tissue will therefore introduce an error in the quantification of RBF or GFR, and this error could very well vary from one region to another because of the differences in the amount of delay and dispersion for different kidney regions. Thus, some general approximations seem useful: (1) DCE-MRI is performed under a steady-state condition. (2) The renal relaxivity of the gadolinium-agent is known. (3) Some conversion to gadolinium concentration can be made. (4) An input curve is defined. (5) A mathematical analytical model can be approximated.

Today, little is known about the potential of gadolinium-enhanced MRI for the assessment of the regional renal blood flow and the regional glomerular filtration rate. Nor do we know the limitations and accuracy of this technique under different pathological and pathophysiological conditions. Thirdly, we do not know the clinical applicability of DCE-MRI and the role it may have in clinical diagnosis. A step-by-step procedure should therefore be initiated to exploit the abovementioned fundamental questions: (1) The methodologies should be further validated against standard methods to obtain reproducible results in agreements to those obtained by clinical non-MRI techniques. (2) Further animal studies should be performed to examine the accuracy and availability under different pathological and pathophysiological conditions. (3) Experimental studies in humans, where the DCE-MRI methods are validated against a standard reference method.

3 Overview of Applications

3.1 DCE-MRI Validation Studies in Animal Models

Several studies investigated DCE-MRI approaches for assessing renal filtration in animal models. Annet et al. estimated the GFR in rabbit kidneys by applying a compartment model and compared the MRI-derived estimate with the measured plasma clearance of 51Cr-EDTA [60]. Although MRI-based GFR values were lower than those measured experimentally, a marked correlation was observed between the two techniques. Winter et al. compared renal perfusion values obtained by arterial spin labeling (ASL) or DCE-MRI in healthy rats, with absolute renal cortex perfusion estimates in close agreement with those obtained by ASL [61].

Zimmer et al. performed an inter- and intramethodical comparison by measuring differences in renal blood flow (RBF) in five rats with unilateral ischemic acute kidney injury with both ASL and DCE-MRI. Both, the FAIR-ASL approach and DCE-MRI

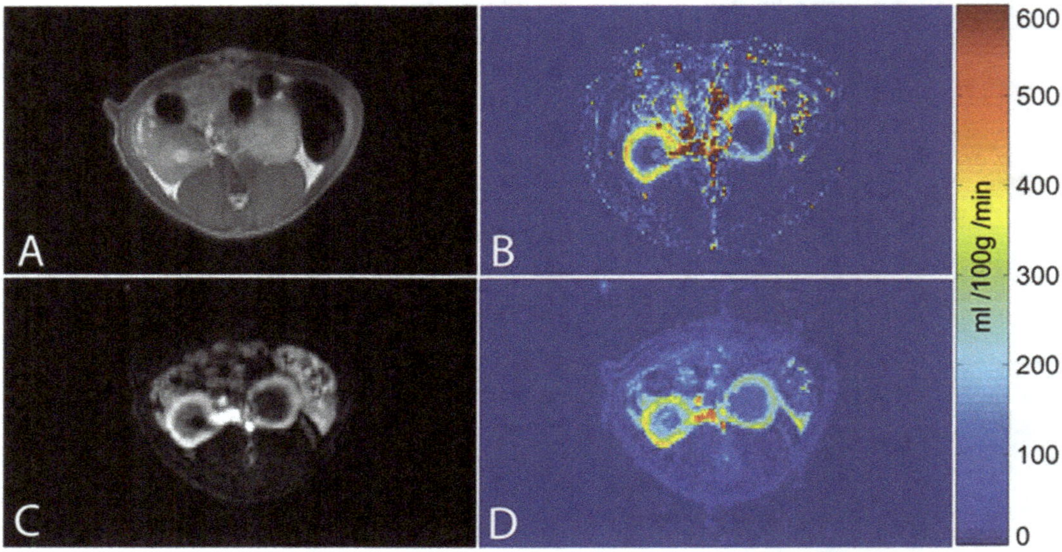

Fig. 7 Exemplary illustration of perfusion MRI of a rat with left-side AKI and perfusion maps. (**a**) True-FISP M_0 image of an ASL measurement and the corresponding perfusion map (**b**). (**c**) TWIST post–contrast agent injection image and the corresponding RBF map (**d**). All drawings show the same rat and the same axial slice. Differences between the kidney with AKI and the contralateral kidney are clearly visible on the MRI images as well as on the perfusion maps. (Reproduced with permission from Zimmer et al. [62])

deconvolution technique showed significant differences in RBF between healthy and diseased kidneys as shown in Fig. 7 [62]. The validation of MRI-based GFR estimation by optical imaging was proposed by Sadick et al. [63]. GFR estimation was performed by DCE-MRI on a 3 T whole body scanner using a dedicated animal rat volume coil and by clearance using a fluorescent tracer (FITC-sinistrin) and an optical imaging device. However, the correlation between optical GFR and MRI-based GFR was poor, probably due to the fact that measurements were performed on different days involving two anesthesia thus affecting the physiology of the animals. Zöllner et al. recently showed a simultaneous measurement of optical and MR-based GFR in healthy rats and rats with unilateral nephrectomy (UNX) [64]. A two-compartment filtration model was employed to calculate a map of the tubular flow. Subsequent, taking the cortex volume into account single kidney GFR values were calculated with a good correlation observed between the two methods. The reduction of GFR in the UNX rats was about 50% and observed for both techniques.

The role played by the binding to serum proteins in the calculation of DCE-MRI derived estimates was investigated by Notohamiprodjo et al. by administering Gadolinium-based contrast agents with different chemical structure [65]. The two investigated contrast agents, Gd-BOPTA and Gd-DTPA differ in their binding affinity toward serum albumin, hence affecting both the relaxivity and the pharmacokinetic properties [66–68]. In fact, binding to the serum protein results in longer circulation times (hence reduced filtration) and higher contrast capability that are easily observed at low magnetic fields (0.5–1.5 T) [69–73]. Therefore, whereas similar renal perfusion values were obtained by both the two contrast agents, GFR estimates were not accurate when obtained with the albumin-binding one (Gd-BOPTA), thus indicating that even low albumin binding may affect GFR estimates.

3.2 DCE-MRI for Assessing Kidney Damages in Animal Models

In the preclinical panorama, DCE-MRI has been widely used to assess kidney function in renovascular and parenchymal diseases that may lead to chronic kidney failure but also in acute events like ischemia–reperfusion, toxicity, infections, or surgery. Thus, different animal models have been explored ranging from classical acute kidney injury (AKI) and chronic kidney disease (CKD) to posttransplant rejection, nephrectomy, and assessment of drug treatment [74–80]. In a murine model of unilateral renal artery stenosis (RAS), measurements of single kidney GFR and perfusion by a modified two-compartment model were compared to those obtained from fluorescein isothiocyanate (FITC)-inulin clearance and ASL, respectively. Both renal GFR and perfusion measurements were in close agreement with the FITC-inulin clearance and ASL methods, with a marked reduction in GFR and perfusion estimates for the stenotic as compared to the control kidneys [81]. Ischemia–reperfusion injury has been exploited to model acute kidney damages and DCE-MRI approaches have been investigated for assessing single-kidney function in both mice and rats [82, 83]. Significant reduction in single kidney GFR (calculated by applying a two compartment renal filtration model) was observed for ischemic kidneys in comparison to contralateral ones in rats [84]. Conversely, for all the other DCE-MRI derived functional parameters (mean transit times and renal blood volume) differences were present, but were not significant between diseased and contralateral kidneys of ischemic rats.

DCE-MRI studies have also been exploited in murine renal transplantations studies for assessing acute rejection and evaluation of immunosuppressive therapy [85]. In this study, a deconvolution approach was applied to the DCE-MRI data and the plasma flow estimate provided restored organ perfusion under Ciclosporin A therapy in syngeneic transplants compared to controls.

Acknowledgments

The Italian Ministry for Education and Research (MIUR) is gratefully acknowledged for yearly FOE funding to the Euro-BioImaging Multi-Modal Molecular Imaging Italian Node (MMMI).

This publication is based upon work from COST Action PARENCHIMA, supported by European Cooperation in Science and Technology (COST). COST (www.cost.eu) is a funding agency for research and innovation networks. COST Actions help connect research initiatives across Europe and enable scientists to enrich their ideas by sharing them with their peers. This boosts their research, career, and innovation.
PARENCHIMA (renalmri.org) is a community-driven Action in the COST program of the European Union, which unites more than 200 experts in renal MRI from 30 countries with the aim to improve the reproducibility and standardization of renal MRI biomarkers.

References

1. Hauser W, Atkins HL, Nelson KG, Richards P (1970) Technetium-99m DTPA: a new radiopharmaceutical for brain and kidney scanning. Radiology 94(3):679–684. https://doi.org/10.1148/94.3.679
2. Taylor A (1999) Radionuclide renography: a personal approach. Semin Nucl Med 29 (2):102–127
3. Gaspari F, Perico N, Remuzzi G (1997) Measurement of glomerular filtration rate. Kidney Int Suppl 63:S151–S154
4. Barbour GL, Crumb CK, Boyd CM, Reeves RD, Rastogi SP, Patterson RM (1976) Comparison of inulin, iothalamate, and 99mTc-DTPA for measurement of glomerular filtration rate. J Nucl Med 17(4):317–320
5. Soveri I, Berg UB, Bjork J, Elinder CG, Grubb A, Mejare I, Sterner G, Back SE, SBU GFR Review Group (2014) Measuring GFR: a systematic review. Am J Kidney Dis 64 (3):411–424. https://doi.org/10.1053/j.ajkd.2014.04.010
6. Peters AM (1991) Quantification of renal haemodynamics with radionuclides. Eur J Nucl Med 18(4):274–286
7. Suto Y, Caner BE, Tamagawa Y, Matsuda T, Nakashima T, Matsushita T, Odori T, Ishii Y, Torizuka K (1989) Assessment of magnetic resonance contrast enhancement with Gd-DTPA: comparison with the uptake of Tc-99m-DTPA. Radiat Med 7(5):209–213
8. Prato FS, Wisenberg G, Marshall TP, Uksik P, Zabel P (1988) Comparison of the biodistribution of gadolinium-153 DTPA and technetium-99m DTPA in rats. J Nucl Med 29(10):1683–1687
9. Choyke PL, Frank JA, Girton ME, Inscoe SW, Carvlin MJ, Black JL, Austin HA, Dwyer AJ (1989) Dynamic Gd-DTPA-enhanced MR imaging of the kidney: experimental results. Radiology 170(3 Pt 1):713–720. https://doi.org/10.1148/radiology.170.3.2916025
10. Fransen R, Muller HJ, Boer WH, Nicolay K, Koomans HA (1996) Contrast-enhanced dynamic magnetic resonance imaging of the rat kidney. J Am Soc Nephrol 7(3):424–430
11. Wen JG, Chen Y, Ringgaard S, Frokiaer J, Jorgensen TM, Stodkilde-Jorgensen H, Djurhuus JC (2000) Evaluation of renal function in normal and hydronephrotic kidneys in rats using gadolinium diethylenetetramine-pentaacetic acid enhanced dynamic magnetic resonance imaging. J Urol 163(4):1264–1270
12. Kikinis R, von Schulthess GK, Jager P, Durr R, Bino M, Kuoni W, Kubler O (1987) Normal and hydronephrotic kidney: evaluation of renal function with contrast-enhanced MR imaging. Radiology 165(3):837–842. https://doi.org/10.1148/radiology.165.3.3685363
13. Sourbron SP, Michaely HJ, Reiser MF, Schoenberg SO (2008) MRI-measurement of perfusion and glomerular filtration in the human kidney with a separable compartment model. Investig Radiol 43(1):40–48. https://doi.org/10.1097/RLI.0b013e31815597c5
14. Pedersen M, Shi Y, Anderson P, Stodkilde-Jorgensen H, Djurhuus JC, Gordon I, Frokiaer J (2004) Quantitation of differential renal blood flow and renal function using dynamic contrast-enhanced MRI in rats. Magn Reson Med 51(3):510–517. https://doi.org/10.1002/mrm.10711
15. Elmholdt TR, Pedersen M, Jorgensen B, Sondergaard K, Jensen JD, Ramsing M, Olesen AB (2011) Nephrogenic systemic fibrosis is found only among gadolinium-exposed patients with renal insufficiency: a case-control study from Denmark. Br J Dermatol 165

(4):828–836. https://doi.org/10.1111/j.1365-2133.2011.10465.x

16. Grenier N, Mendichovszky I, de Senneville BD, Roujol S, Desbarats P, Pedersen M, Wells K, Frokiaer J, Gordon I (2008) Measurement of glomerular filtration rate with magnetic resonance imaging: principles, limitations, and expectations. Semin Nucl Med 38(1):47–55. https://doi.org/10.1053/j.semnuclmed.2007.09.004
17. Aime S, Botta M, Terreno E (2005) Gd(III)-based contrast agents for MRI. Adv Inorg Chem 57(57):173–237. https://doi.org/10.1016/S0898-8838(05)57004-1
18. Caravan P, Ellison JJ, McMurry TJ, Lauffer RB (1999) Gadolinium(III) chelates as MRI contrast agents: structure, dynamics, and applications. Chem Rev 99(9):2293–2352
19. Aime S, Botta M, Fasano M, Crich SG, Terreno E (1996) Gd(III) complexes as contrast agents for magnetic resonance imaging: a proton relaxation enhancement study of the interaction with human serum albumin. J Biol Inorg Chem 1(4):312–319. https://doi.org/10.1007/s007750050059
20. Lauffer RB (1987) Paramagnetic metal complexes as water proton relaxation agents for NMR imaging: theory and design. Chem Rev 87(5):901–927
21. Werner EJ, Datta A, Jocher CJ, Raymond KN (2008) High-relaxivity MRI contrast agents: where coordination chemistry meets medical imaging. Angew Chem Int Ed Engl 47(45):8568–8580. https://doi.org/10.1002/anie.200800212
22. Burtea C, Laurent S, Vander Elst L, Muller RN (2008) Contrast agents: magnetic resonance. Handb Exp Pharmacol (185 Pt 1):135-165. https://doi.org/10.1007/978-3-540-72718-7_7
23. Aime S, Caravan P (2009) Biodistribution of gadolinium-based contrast agents, including gadolinium deposition. J Magn Reson Imaging 30(6):1259–1267. https://doi.org/10.1002/jmri.21969
24. Baranyai Z, Palinkas Z, Uggeri F, Maiocchi A, Aime S, Brucher E (2012) Dissociation kinetics of open-chain and macrocyclic gadolinium (III)-aminopolycarboxylate complexes related to magnetic resonance imaging: catalytic effect of endogenous ligands. Chemistry 18(51):16426–16435. https://doi.org/10.1002/chem.201202930
25. Baranyai Z, Uggeri F, Giovenzana GB, Benyei A, Brucher E, Aime S (2009) Equilibrium and kinetic properties of the lanthanoids (III) and various divalent metal complexes of the heptadentate ligand AAZTA. Chemistry 15(7):1696–1705. https://doi.org/10.1002/chem.200801803
26. Sherry AD, Caravan P, Lenkinski RE (2009) Primer on gadolinium chemistry. J Magn Reson Imaging 30(6):1240–1248. https://doi.org/10.1002/jmri.21966
27. Wahsner J, Gale EM, Rodriguez-Rodriguez A, Caravan P (2019) Chemistry of MRI contrast agents: current challenges and new frontiers. Chem Rev 119(2):957–1057. https://doi.org/10.1021/acs.chemrev.8b00363
28. Dastru W, Longo D, Aime S (2011) Contrast agents and mechanisms. Drug Discov Today 8(2–4):e109–e115. https://doi.org/10.1016/j.ddtec.2011.11.013
29. Terreno E, Dastru W, Delli Castelli D, Gianolio E, Geninatti Crich S, Longo D, Aime S (2010) Advances in metal-based probes for MR molecular imaging applications. Curr Med Chem 17(31):3684–3700
30. Avedano S, Botta M, Haigh JS, Longo DL, Woods M (2013) Coupling fast water exchange to slow molecular tumbling in Gd3+ chelates: why faster is not always better. Inorg Chem 52(15):8436–8450. https://doi.org/10.1021/ic400308a
31. Longo DL, Arena F, Consolino L, Minazzi P, Geninatti-Crich S, Giovenzana GB, Aime S (2016) Gd-AAZTA-MADEC, an improved blood pool agent for DCE-MRI studies on mice on 1 T scanners. Biomaterials 75:47–57. https://doi.org/10.1016/j.biomaterials.2015.10.012
32. Pierre VC, Allen MJ, Caravan P (2014) Contrast agents for MRI: 30+ years and where are we going? J Biol Inorg Chem 19(2):127–131. https://doi.org/10.1007/s00775-013-1074-5
33. Paschal CB, Morris HD (2004) K-space in the clinic. J Magn Reson Imaging 19(2):145–159. https://doi.org/10.1002/jmri.10451
34. Markl M, Leupold J (2012) Gradient echo imaging. J Magn Reson Imaging 35(6):1274–1289. https://doi.org/10.1002/jmri.23638
35. Tsao J (2010) Ultrafast imaging: principles, pitfalls, solutions, and applications. J Magn Reson Imaging 32(2):252–266. https://doi.org/10.1002/jmri.22239
36. Oesterle C, Strohschein R, Kohler M, Schnell M, Hennig J (2000) Benefits and pitfalls of keyhole imaging, especially in first-pass perfusion studies. J Magn Reson Imaging 11(3):312–323
37. Teixeira RPAG, Malik SJ, Hajnal JV (2019) Fast quantitative MRI using controlled

saturation magnetization transfer. Magn Reson Med 81(2):907–920. https://doi.org/10.1002/mrm.27442

38. Grenier N, Pedersen M, Hauger O (2006) Contrast agents for functional and cellular MRI of the kidney. Eur J Radiol 60 (3):341–352. https://doi.org/10.1016/j.ejrad.2006.06.024
39. Zollner FG, Daab M, Sourbron SP, Schad LR, Schoenberg SO, Weisser G (2016) An open source software for analysis of dynamic contrast enhanced magnetic resonance images: UMM-Perfusion revisited. BMC Med Imaging 16:7. https://doi.org/10.1186/s12880-016-0109-0
40. Roldan-Valadez E, Gonzalez-Gutierrez O, Martinez-Lopez M (2012) Diagnostic performance of PWI/DWI MRI parameters in discriminating hyperacute versus acute ischaemic stroke: finding the best thresholds. Clin Radiol 67(3):250–257. https://doi.org/10.1016/j.crad.2011.08.020
41. Ewing JR, Bagher-Ebadian H (2013) Model selection in measures of vascular parameters using dynamic contrast-enhanced MRI: experimental and clinical applications. NMR Biomed 26(8):1028–1041. https://doi.org/10.1002/nbm.2996
42. Sourbron SP, Buckley DL (2013) Classic models for dynamic contrast-enhanced MRI. NMR Biomed 26(8):1004–1027. https://doi.org/10.1002/nbm.2940
43. Abrikossova N, Skoglund C, Ahren M, Bengtsson T, Uvdal K (2012) Effects of gadolinium oxide nanoparticles on the oxidative burst from human neutrophil granulocytes. Nanotechnology 23(27):275101. https://doi.org/10.1088/0957-4484/23/27/275101
44. Kallehauge JF, Tanderup K, Duan C, Haack S, Pedersen EM, Lindegaard JC, Fokdal LU, Mohamed SM, Nielsen T (2014) Tracer kinetic model selection for dynamic contrast-enhanced magnetic resonance imaging of locally advanced cervical cancer. Acta Oncol 53 (8):1064–1072. https://doi.org/10.3109/0284186X.2014.937879
45. Li X, Welch EB, Chakravarthy AB, Xu L, Arlinghaus LR, Farley J, Mayer IA, Kelley MC, Meszoely IM, Means-Powell J, Abramson VG, Grau AM, Gore JC, Yankeelov TE (2012) Statistical comparison of dynamic contrast-enhanced MRI pharmacokinetic models in human breast cancer. Magn Reson Med 68(1):261–271. https://doi.org/10.1002/mrm.23205
46. Naish JH, Kershaw LE, Buckley DL, Jackson A, Waterton JC, Parker GJ (2009) Modeling of contrast agent kinetics in the lung using T1-weighted dynamic contrast-enhanced MRI. Magn Reson Med 61 (6):1507–1514. https://doi.org/10.1002/mrm.21814
47. Bagher-Ebadian H, Jain R, Nejad-Davarani SP, Mikkelsen T, Lu M, Jiang Q, Scarpace L, Arbab AS, Narang J, Soltanian-Zadeh H, Paudyal R, Ewing JR (2012) Model selection for DCE-T1 studies in glioblastoma. Magn Reson Med 68 (1):241–251. https://doi.org/10.1002/mrm.23211
48. Chwang WB, Jain R, Bagher-Ebadian H, Nejad-Davarani SP, Iskander AS, VanSlooten A, Schultz L, Arbab AS, Ewing JR (2014) Measurement of rat brain tumor kinetics using an intravascular MR contrast agent and DCE-MRI nested model selection. J Magn Reson Imaging 40(5):1223–1229. https://doi.org/10.1002/jmri.24469
49. Donaldson SB, West CM, Davidson SE, Carrington BM, Hutchison G, Jones AP, Sourbron SP, Buckley DL (2010) A comparison of tracer kinetic models for T1-weighted dynamic contrast-enhanced MRI: application in carcinoma of the cervix. Magn Reson Med 63 (3):691–700. https://doi.org/10.1002/mrm.22217
50. Draper NR, Smith H (1998) Applied regression analysis, 3rd edn. Wiley, New York
51. Duan C, Kallehauge JF, Bretthorst GL, Tanderup K, Ackerman JJ, Garbow JR (2017) Are complex DCE-MRI models supported by clinical data? Magn Reson Med 77 (3):1329–1339. https://doi.org/10.1002/mrm.26189
52. Meinerz K, Beeman SC, Duan C, Bretthorst GL, Garbow JR, Ackerman JJH (2018) Bayesian modeling of NMR data: quantifying longitudinal relaxation in vivo, and in vitro with a tissue-water-relaxation mimic (crosslinked bovine serum albumin). Appl Magn Reson 49 (1):3–24
53. Quirk JD, Bretthorst GL, Garbow JR, Ackerman JJ (2019) Magnetic resonance data modeling: the Bayesian analysis toolbox. Concepts Magn Reson Part A 47A:e21467
54. Bayes T, Price R (1763) An essay toward solving a problem in the doctrine of chance. Philos Trans R Soc Lond 53:370–418
55. Cox RT (1961) The algebra of probable inference. Johns Hopkins University Press, Baltimore, MD
56. Jaynes ET (1988) Optimal information-processing and Bayes theorem - comment. Am Stat 42(4):280–281. https://doi.org/10.2307/2685144

57. Beeman SC, Osei-Owusu P, Duan C, Engelbach J, Bretthorst GL, Ackerman JJH, Blumer KJ, Garbow JR (2015) Renal DCE-MRI model selection using Bayesian probability theory. Tomography 1(1):61–68. https://doi.org/10.18383/j.tom.2015.00133
58. Patlak CS, Blasberg RG, Fenstermacher JD (1983) Graphical evaluation of blood-to-brain transfer constants from multiple-time uptake data. J Cereb Blood Flow Metab 3(1):1–7. https://doi.org/10.1038/jcbfm.1983.1
59. Tofts PS, Brix G, Buckley DL, Evelhoch JL, Henderson E, Knopp MV, Larsson HB, Lee TY, Mayr NA, Parker GJ, Port RE, Taylor J, Weisskoff RM (1999) Estimating kinetic parameters from dynamic contrast-enhanced T(1)-weighted MRI of a diffusable tracer: standardized quantities and symbols. J Magn Reson Imaging 10(3):223–232. https://doi.org/10.1002/(SICI)1522-2586(199909)10:3<223::AID-JMRI2>3.0.CO;2-S
60. Annet L, Hermoye L, Peeters F, Jamar F, Dehoux JP, Van Beers BE (2004) Glomerular filtration rate: assessment with dynamic contrast-enhanced MRI and a cortical-compartment model in the rabbit kidney. J Magn Reson Imaging 20(5):843–849. https://doi.org/10.1002/jmri.20173
61. Winter JD, St Lawrence KS, Cheng HL (2011) Quantification of renal perfusion: comparison of arterial spin labeling and dynamic contrast-enhanced MRI. J Magn Reson Imaging 34(3):608–615. https://doi.org/10.1002/jmri.22660
62. Zimmer F, Zollner FG, Hoeger S, Klotz S, Tsagogiorgas C, Kramer BK, Schad LR (2013) Quantitative renal perfusion measurements in a rat model of acute kidney injury at 3T: testing inter- and intramethodical significance of ASL and DCE-MRI. PLoS One 8(1):e53849. https://doi.org/10.1371/journal.pone.0053849
63. Sadick M, Attenberger U, Kraenzlin B, Kayed H, Schoenberg SO, Gretz N, Schock-Kusch D (2011) Two non-invasive GFR-estimation methods in rat models of polycystic kidney disease: 3.0 tesla dynamic contrast-enhanced MRI and optical imaging. Nephrol Dial Transplant 26(10):3101–3108. https://doi.org/10.1093/ndt/gfr148
64. Zollner FG, Schock-Kusch D, Backer S, Neudecker S, Gretz N, Schad LR (2013) Simultaneous measurement of kidney function by dynamic contrast enhanced MRI and FITC-sinistrin clearance in rats at 3 tesla: initial results. PLoS One 8(11):e79992. https://doi.org/10.1371/journal.pone.0079992
65. Notohamiprodjo M, Pedersen M, Glaser C, Helck AD, Lodemann K-P, Jespersen B, Fischereder M, Reiser MF, Sourbron SP (2011) Comparison of Gd-DTPA and Gd-BOPTA for studying renal perfusion and filtration. J Magn Reson Imaging 34(3):595–607. https://doi.org/10.1002/jmri.22640
66. Laurent S, Elst LV, Muller RN (2006) Comparative study of the physicochemical properties of six clinical low molecular weight gadolinium contrast agents. Contrast Media Mol Imaging 1(3):128–137. https://doi.org/10.1002/cmmi.100
67. Caravan P, Cloutier NJ, Greenfield MT, McDermid SA, Dunham SU, Bulte JW, Amedio JC Jr, Looby RJ, Supkowski RM, Horrocks WD Jr, McMurry TJ, Lauffer RB (2002) The interaction of MS-325 with human serum albumin and its effect on proton relaxation rates. J Am Chem Soc 124(12):3152–3162
68. Aime S, Barge A, Botta M, Terreno E (2003) Interactions of lanthanides and their complexes with proteins. Conclusions regarding magnetic resonance imaging. Met Ions Biol Syst 40:643–682
69. Caravan P, Parigi G, Chasse JM, Cloutier NJ, Ellison JJ, Lauffer RB, Luchinat C, McDermid SA, Spiller M, McMurry TJ (2007) Albumin binding, relaxivity, and water exchange kinetics of the diastereoisomers of MS-325, a gadolinium(III)-based magnetic resonance angiography contrast agent. Inorg Chem 46(16):6632–6639. https://doi.org/10.1021/ic700686k
70. Botta M, Avedano S, Giovenzana GB, Lombardi A, Longo D, Cassino C, Tei L, Aime S (2011) Relaxometric study of a series of monoaqua Gd-III complexes of rigidified EGTA-like chelators and their noncovalent interaction with human serum albumin. Eur J Inorg Chem (6):802–810. https://doi.org/10.1002/ejic.201001103
71. Gianolio E, Giovenzana GB, Longo D, Longo I, Menegotto I, Aime S (2007) Relaxometric and modelling studies of the binding of a lipophilic Gd-AAZTA complex to fatted and defatted human serum albumin. Chemistry 13(20):5785–5797. https://doi.org/10.1002/chem.200601277
72. Avedano S, Tei L, Lombardi A, Giovenzana GB, Aime S, Longo D, Botta M (2007) Maximizing the relaxivity of HSA-bound gadolinium complexes by simultaneous optimization of rotation and water exchange. Chem Commun (Camb) (45):4726–4728. https://doi.org/10.1039/b714438e

73. Aime S, Gianolio E, Longo D, Pagliarin R, Lovazzano C, Sisti M (2005) New insights for pursuing high relaxivity MRI agents from modelling the binding interaction of Gd(III) chelates to HSA. Chembiochem 6 (5):818–820. https://doi.org/10.1002/cbic.200400364
74. Egger C, Cannet C, Gérard C, Debon C, Stohler N, Dunbar A, Tigani B, Li J, Beckmann N (2015) Adriamycin-induced nephropathy in rats: functional and cellular effects characterized by MRI. J Magn Reson Imaging 41 (3):829–840. https://doi.org/10.1002/jmri.24603
75. Laurent D, Poirier K, Wasvary J, Rudin M (2002) Effect of essential hypertension on kidney function as measured in rat by dynamic MRI. Magn Reson Med 47(1):127–134
76. Hermoye L, Annet L, Lemmerling P, Peeters F, Jamar F, Gianello P, Van Huffel S, Van Beers BE (2004) Calculation of the renal perfusion and glomerular filtration rate from the renal impulse response obtained with MRI. Magn Reson Med 51(5):1017–1025. https://doi.org/10.1002/mrm.20026
77. Zhang YD, Wang J, Zhang J, Wang X, Jiang X (2014) Effect of iodinated contrast media on renal function evaluated with dynamic three-dimensional MR renography. Radiology 270 (2):409–415. https://doi.org/10.1148/radiol.13122495
78. Liu X, Murphy MP, Xing W, Wu H, Zhang R, Sun H (2018) Mitochondria-targeted antioxidant MitoQ reduced renal damage caused by ischemia-reperfusion injury in rodent kidneys: longitudinal observations of T. Magn Reson Med 79(3):1559–1567. https://doi.org/10.1002/mrm.26772
79. Sari-Sarraf F, Pomposiello S, Laurent D (2008) Acute impairment of rat renal function by L-NAME as measured using dynamic MRI. MAGMA 21(4):291–297. https://doi.org/10.1007/s10334-008-0130-6
80. Privratsky JR, Wang N, Qi Y, Ren J, Morris BT, Hunting JC, Johnson GA, Crowley SD (2019) Dynamic contrast-enhanced MRI promotes early detection of toxin-induced acute kidney injury. Am J Physiol Renal Physiol 316(2): F351–F359. https://doi.org/10.1152/ajprenal.00416.2018
81. Jiang K, Tang H, Mishra PK, Macura SI, Lerman LO (2017) Measurement of murine single-kidney glomerular filtration rate using dynamic contrast-enhanced MRI. Magn Reson Med 79(6):2935–2943. https://doi.org/10.1002/mrm.26955
82. Zollner FG, Zimmer F, Klotz S, Hoeger S, Schad LR (2014) Renal perfusion in acute kidney injury with DCE-MRI: deconvolution analysis versus two-compartment filtration model. Magn Reson Imaging 32(6):781–785. https://doi.org/10.1016/j.mri.2014.02.014
83. Oostendorp M, de Vries EE, Slenter JM, Peutz-Kootstra CJ, Snoeijs MG, Post MJ, van Heurn LW, Backes WH (2011) MRI of renal oxygenation and function after normothermic ischemia-reperfusion injury. NMR Biomed 24 (2):194–200. https://doi.org/10.1002/nbm.1572
84. Zöllner FG, Zimmer F, Klotz S, Hoeger S, Schad LR (2015) Functional imaging of acute kidney injury at 3 tesla: investigating multiple parameters using DCE-MRI and a two-compartment filtration model. Z Med Phys 25(1):58–65. https://doi.org/10.1016/j.zemedi.2014.01.002
85. Notohamiprodjo M, Kalnins A, Andrassy M, Kolb M, Ehle B, Mueller S, Thomas MN, Werner J, Guba M, Nikolaou K, Andrassy J (2016) Multiparametric functional MRI: a tool to uncover subtle changes following allogeneic renal transplantation. PLoS One 11 (11):e0165532. https://doi.org/10.1371/journal.pone.0165532

4

Preparation of Ex Vivo Rodent Phantoms for Developing, Testing, and Training MR Imaging of the Kidney and Other Organs

Jason M. Millward, João S. Periquito, Paula Ramos Delgado, Christian Prinz, Thoralf Niendorf, and Sonia Waiczies

Abstract

Here we describe a simple and inexpensive protocol for preparing ex vivo rodent phantoms for use in MR imaging studies. The experimental animals are perfused and fixed with formaldehyde, and then wrapped with gauze and sealed with liquid latex. This yields a phantom that preserves all organs in situ, and which avoids the need to keep fixed animals and organs in containers that have dimensions very different from living animals. This is especially important for loading in MR detectors, and specifically the RF coils, they are usually used with. The phantom can be safely stored and conveniently reused, and can provide MR scientists with a realistic phantom with which to establish protocols in preparation for preclinical in vivo studies—for renal, brain, and body imaging. The phantom also serves as an ideal teaching tool, for trainees learning how to perform preclinical MRI investigations of the kidney and other target organs, while avoiding the need for handling living animals, and reducing the total number of animals required.

This protocol chapter is part of the PARENCHIMA initiative "MRI Biomarkers for CKD" (CA16103), a community-driven Action of the European Cooperation in Science and Technology (COST) program of the European Union, which aims to improve the reproducibility and standardization of renal MRI biomarkers.

Key words Ex vivo methods, Rat, Mouse, Phantom, Magnetic resonance imaging (MRI), Kidney

1 Introduction

Prior to starting any preclinical in vivo MRI study, it is essential to invest time to test novel imaging techniques, optimize MR pulse sequence parameters and develop a workflow tailored to address the specific scientific questions at hand [1]. Much of this work can be done without using living animals, by constructing synthetic phantoms using materials that have similar MR properties as the tissue of interest (e.g., agarose). Ultimately, a point is reached when the limitations of synthetic phantoms impede progress, and phantoms that are more biologically realistic are needed. In some cases this

Andreas Pohlmann and Thoralf Niendorf (eds.), *Preclinical MRI of the Kidney: Methods and Protocols*, Methods in Molecular Biology, vol. 2216, https://doi.org/10.1007/978-1-0716-0978-1_5,

can be accomplished using ex vivo tissue samples removed from experimental animals postmortem. The tissues are chemically fixed (usually with formaldehyde), and samples embedded in tubes or containers for imaging. However, this removes the organs from their surrounding environment. In the case of renal MR, it is advantageous to image the kidney in situ, within its biological context, including the surrounding organs and perirenal fat. The typical solution for this problem is to use ex vivo phantoms, which consist of the intact experimental animal (usually rats or mice) placed inside a sealed container along with the fixation solution. This solution is suboptimal. The containers used generally have a cylindrical or rectangular shape, which is substantially different from the shape of an animal. This can be problematic given the space constraints of the MR hardware (e.g., RF coil diameter, size of the animal holding bed). In some cases the container size may mean that a larger field of view needs to be acquired than would otherwise be necessary for a living animal. It may also be difficult, or impossible, to use surface RF coils to scan samples embedded in a container. For example, when scanning the brain or the kidney, positioning the sample such that the target organ is as close as possible to the RF coil could be problematic if the container is in the way. Furthermore, the additional mass of the fixation liquid in a container with a rat or mouse body can substantially change the loading in the coil, which could cause problems with matching and tuning. The shape of the container can also cause other problems; the curved and conical shapes of typical laboratory plastic tubes can interfere with shimming the main magnetic field B_0.

Here we describe a simple and inexpensive method to prepare ex vivo phantoms using mice or rats that are perfused and chemically fixed, covered in gauze and sealed with latex. This solution results in a phantom that preserves the biological context of the organs of interest, and which is much more similar to the original animal in terms of dimensions and loading. It avoids the use of containers of toxic formaldehyde solution. The phantoms can be readily used by imaging scientists and scientists from related fields who are not trained in the handling of living experimental animals. This makes the phantom an ideal teaching tool for educating trainees learning how to perform preclinical studies, while also avoiding the confounding effects of motion artifacts. Finally, the phantoms can be easily stored and reused for extended periods of time. This will substantially reduce the total number of animals required for developing new MRI methods, and will facilitate more efficient and effective in vivo studies, thus consistent with the 3R principles of animal research [2, 3].

This chapter is part of the book Pohlmann A, Niendorf T (eds) (2020) Preclinical MRI of the Kidney—Methods and Protocols. Springer, New York.

2 Materials

2.1 Animals

The method described here can be used for any animal strain. The choice of strain depends on the specific needs of the researcher. Ideally, the specific rat or mouse strain should be consistent with the strain that will be used for the corresponding in vivo experiments. Most importantly the size and geometry of the animal should be comparable to that of the animal used for in vivo experiments, to ensure that the loading will be similar between phantom and in vivo experiments.

2.2 Perfusion and Dissection

All steps of the protocol should be conducted in accordance with procedures approved by the local Animal Welfare Department and authorities and conform to guidelines to minimize discomfort to animals (86/609/EEC).

The perfusion should be done in a lab environment equipped for dealing with hazardous fumes, using a chemical fume hood (alternatively fume extraction dome hoods) due to the respiratory hazards of formaldehyde. The lab should also have appropriate mechanisms in place for disposing of formaldehyde liquid waste, solid materials contaminated with formaldehyde (e.g., paper tissues), as well as animal carcasses (e.g., freezer for temporary storage; capacity for incineration).

1. Anesthesia (e.g., ketamine–xylazine various suppliers). Or alternative for terminal anesthesia, as per individual institutional experimental animal use guidelines.
2. Surgical instruments (scissors, rongeurs, forceps, hemostat).
3. Syringes (1 ml, 20 ml, 60 ml); needles (26 Gauge, 23 Gauge Butterfly).
4. 70% ethanol in a spray bottle.
5. Solutions for perfusion: phosphate buffered saline (PBS); formaldehyde solution (e.g., 4% aq. paraformaldehyde [PFA]).
6. Airtight plastic container for storage of the animal during the post-fixation step (*see* **Note 1**).

2.3 Latex Covering

1. Liquid latex (e.g., 0.3% ammonia prevulcanized, low-viscosity—various suppliers).
2. Surgical gauze.
3. 3-O surgical suture (e.g., Ethicon.com, product code C003D).
4. Fine paintbrushes.
5. Hair dryer.

3 Methods

3.1 Perfusion and Fixation

1. Administer a terminal dose of anesthetic—here we used an intraperitoneal injection of a mixture of ketamine (100 mg/kg) and xylazine (5 mg/kg) diluted in 0.9% NaCl. We used the same dose for mouse and rat, adjusted for individual body weight.
2. Confirm that the animal has reached the required depth of anesthesia, for example by checking for absence of a reflex response to stimulation of the hind paws.
3. Place the animal in supine position on a work surface (e.g., Styrofoam covered with aluminum foil), and fix the extremities of the animal to the surface.
4. Apply 70% ethanol to the ventral surface, taking care not to spray the facial region.
5. With forceps, grasp the sternum, and make an incision into the thoracic cavity with large scissors.
6. Carefully expand the thoracic space with the scissors, taking care not to cut any major blood vessels. Cut down the ribs at the lateral sides to allow for blood drainage. Carefully separate the heart from the surrounding connective tissue. Cut through the diaphragm, and expose the inferior vena cava and the descending aorta. Attach a hemostat clamp to the sternum, and reflect backward to reveal the now opened thoracic cavity.
7. Visualize the separation between the left and right ventricles (slight color difference). Insert the needle into the **left ventricle** of the heart. Take care not to insert the needle too far, or you will enter the right ventricle. *MOUSE—inject a total volume of 20 ml PBS, using a 20 ml syringe with a 26G needle. *RAT—inject a total volume of 180 ml PBS, using 60 ml syringes attached to a tube connected to a 23G butterfly needle. After inserting the needle into the heart, use a hemostat to clamp the butterfly needle. Cut the inferior vena cava.
8. Start PBS perfusion by slowly depressing the plunger, alternatively use a perfusion pump if available. Observe the color change in the liver: as a sign that the perfusion is correct, the deep red color changes to dull brown as the blood is drained (*see* **Note 2**) *RAT—after finishing with the first 60 ml syringe, replace the empty syringe with a filled one. Repeat with a third syringe to complete the full 180 ml volume.
9. Start fixation by perfusing with 4% PFA (*see* **Note 3**) (this step should be done under a ventilation system, to avoid exposure to the hazardous PFA fumes). *MOUSE—switch from the 20 ml PBS syringe to a syringe filled with 20 ml PFA. Reinsert the needle in the left ventricle, into the same injection point,

used by the previous needle (look for a small dark spot). *RAT—attach the 60 ml syringe with PFA directly to the tube connected to the butterfly needle. At this point the exsanguination and perfusion is complete.

10. Postfixation. Place the animal body into a sealable plastic container and fill with PFA and stored at room temperature for approximately 1 week (*see* **Note 1**).

3.2 Disarticulation

Removal of the extremities (disarticulation) can be performed at the discretion of the researcher, depending on the objective, and depending on the space constraints of the specific hardware (RF coil diameter, dimensions of the animal holding bed) that the animal phantom is to be used with. In some cases it may be sufficient to secure the forelimb and hind limb into position by suturing them to the body, before wrapping the body with gauze. Regardless, the tail should be removed. In addition, it may be necessary to remove the skin, in order to tailor the size of the phantom to the hardware dimensions. Here we describe in detail how to perform the disarticulation on a rat. In the mouse, this is easily accomplished using standard surgical scissors.

1. Remove the skin around the joint of the forelimb and the shoulder (scapular joint) with surgical scissors. Using a scalpel, dissect the musculature around the scapula (Fig. 1a). Using the fingers, feel for the location of the joint (Fig. 1b). When the joint is exposed, use rongeurs to separate the scapula, and remove the entire forelimb (Fig. 1c). Repeat the process on the other side.
2. The procedure for the hind limbs is similar. Remove the skin around the joint of the femur and hip. Using a scalpel, dissect the musculature around the femur, and feel for the location of the ball and socket hip joint (where the femur fits in the acetabulum of the pelvis). When the joint is exposed, cut the tendons with a scalpel, or cut the bone directly using rongeurs (Fig. 1a). Repeat on the other side.
3. Use a scalpel to dissect the musculature of the tail at the proximal end. Expose the coccyx, and separate the tail using rongeurs. The disarticulation is now complete.
4. Proceed with removing the skin of the remaining body. Using scissors, cut through the skin at the level of the neck—the skin of the head can remain in place. Remove the skin and any extraneous tissue from the exposed thoracic cavity and the dorsal thoracic region. Use the fingers to separate the skin and expand the subcutaneous space in the dorsal lumbar region. Make a midline cut of the skin with scissors, and use a scalpel to separate the rest of the skin from the underlying

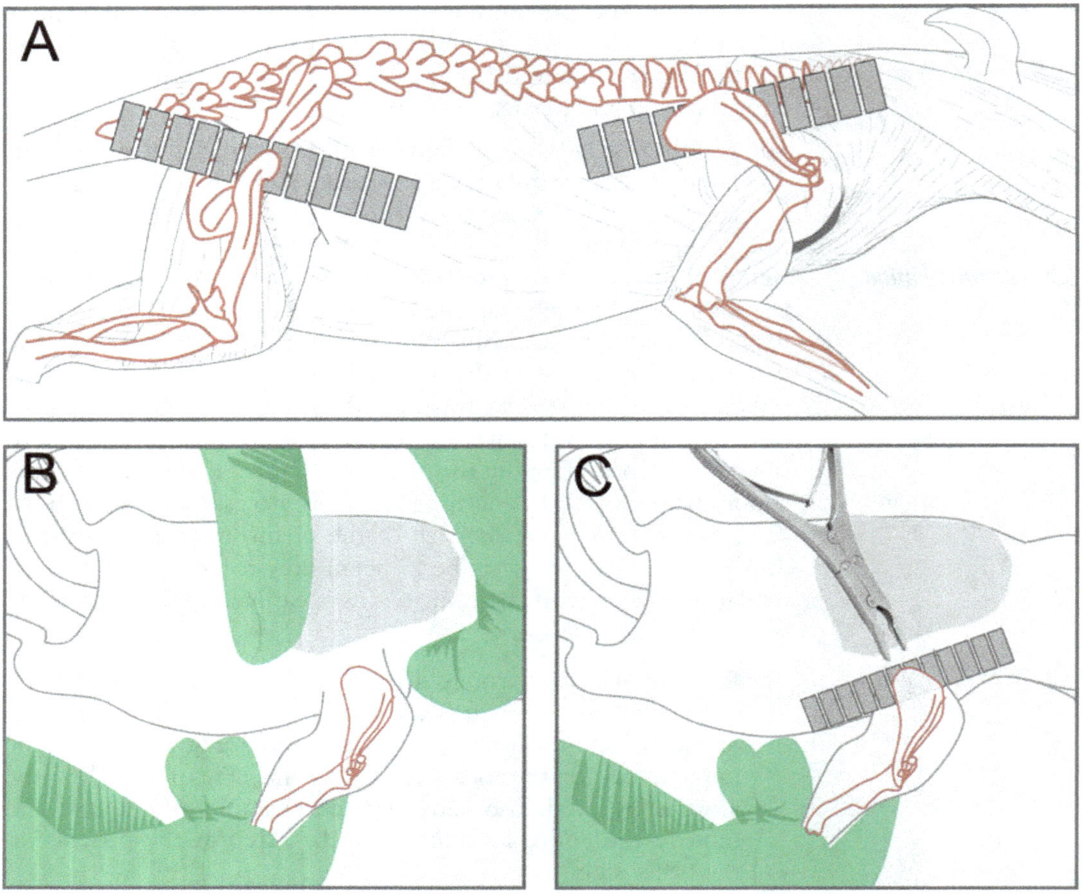

Fig. 1 Schematic for disarticulation. The location of the cut-points for removing the forelimb and hind limb is depicted by the gray lines (**a**). After cutting the overlying musculature, the joint of the scapula can be visualized (**b**). The forelimb is reflected back, and the joint cut using rongeurs (**c**)

tissue. Continue removing skin from the ventral lumbar region, taking care not to pierce the peritoneum.

5. The skin of the head can remain in place, since the head will not be covered with gauze. Remove the ears (exposing the auditory cavity), trim the whiskers and remove extraneous tissue from the lower mandible region.

3.3 Coating with Gauze and Latex

In the next steps the fixed and disarticulated body will be wrapped in gauze and covered in liquid latex.

1. Starting from the neck, tightly wrap the thoracic region with gauze. It may be necessary to fill part of the thoracic cavity that was opened during the perfusion step with gauze, in order to eliminate empty space and have a securely wrapped phantom. Continue wrapping the lumbar/sacral region with gauze; a

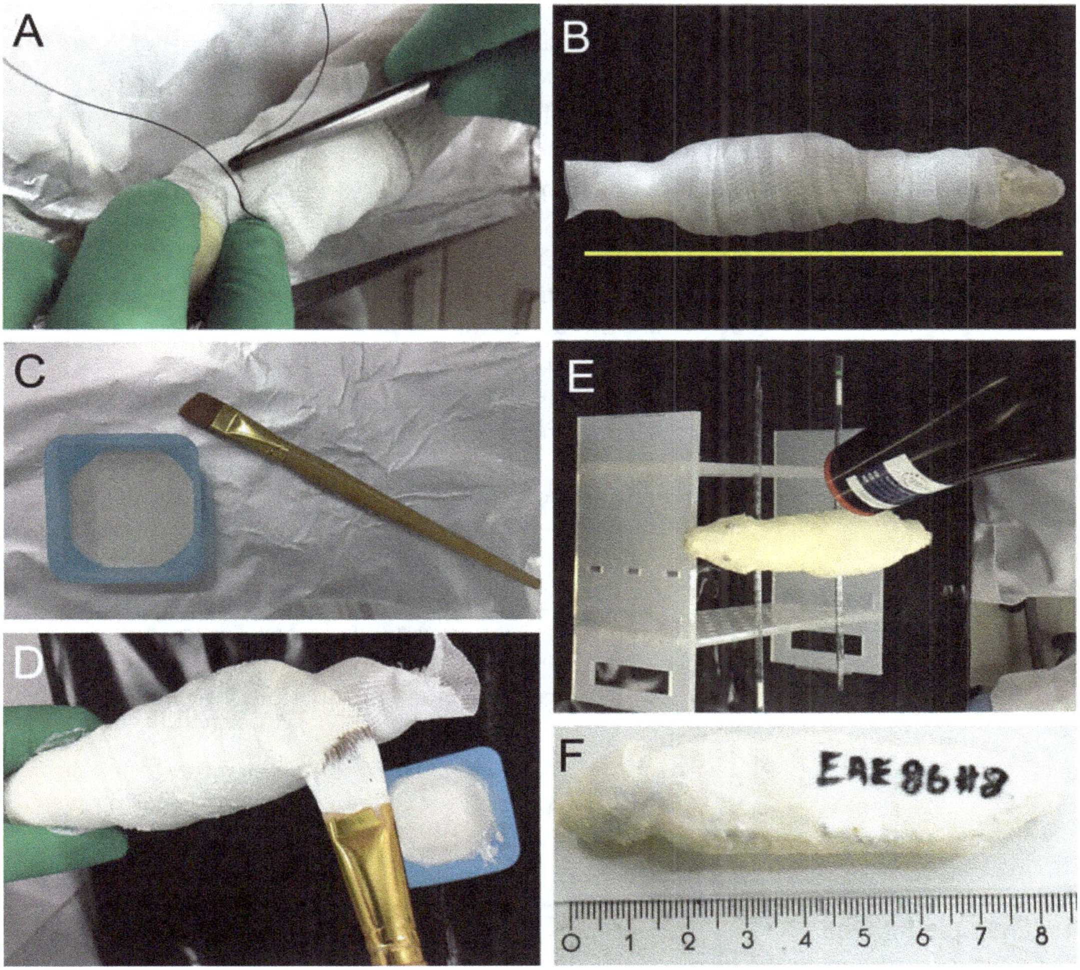

Fig. 2 Workflow for preparation of the phantom. The rat body is wrapped tightly with gauze, which is then fixed securely to the underlying musculature using surgical sutures (**a**). The entire body is covered with gauze, except for the head, which remains unwrapped (scale bar = 22 cm) (**b**). Liquid latex is applied directly to the surface of the phantom using a paintbrush (**c**, **d**). The phantom is place on an improvised holder, here a laboratory tube rack with pipettes. A hair dryer is used to accelerate the drying process (**e**). An example of a completed, labeled mouse phantom (**f**)

small extension of gauze can remain at the posterior end to serve as a grip when applying the latex.

2. Firmly attach the gauze to the underlying muscle tissue using standard surgical sutures (Fig. 2a). The phantom is now ready to be covered with latex (Fig. 2b).
3. Pour some liquid latex into a suitable container; for example, a plastic weigh boat used with a standard laboratory scale is ideal. Using a flat paintbrush, apply the first coat of latex directly to the gauze (Fig. 2b, c). All surfaces should be completely

covered, although avoid excessive latex. It is preferable to apply the latex with a brush, rather than simply submerging the phantom in latex.

4. Generously apply latex to the head, taking care to fill the auditory cavity and the oral cavity.
5. Place the phantom on a support to dry, allowing air to circulate. Here we improvised a support using a laboratory tube rack and pipettes (Fig. 2d).
6. Use a standard hair dryer to apply warm air (c. 5–10 min), to accelerate the drying of the latex (Fig. 2d). Allow additional time (c. 20 min) to dry at room temperature.
7. The phantom will be easier to handle once the first coat of latex is dry. Then, apply a second coat of liquid latex, ensuring that all gaps are completely covered. Make sure that the oral cavity is completely sealed. Apply the latex generously; the objective is to ensure that there is a complete watertight seal over the entire surface. Repeat the drying process with the hair dryer, and allow to air dry completely at room temperature.
8. The phantom is now finished. It is possible to write on the surface of the dry latex with a permanent felt-tipped marker, for example to record useful information about the animal (Fig. 2f).
9. The phantom can be used at room temperature, for example inside the MRI scanner, for extended periods. Long-term storage should be at 4 °C.

4 Example Images

In Fig. 3 we show representative images of MRI scans of the ex vivo phantoms. These scans were performed on a Bruker Biospec 9.4 Tesla USR94/20 animal MRI scanner (Bruker Biospin, Ettlingen, Germany).

4.1 Rat

MRI scans targeting the rat kidney were acquired in the coronal (Fig. 3a, b) and sagittal (Fig. 3d, e) planes. The identical MRI hardware setup (including the RF coils) and pulse sequence parameters were used to acquire the images of the ex vivo phantom (Fig. 3a, d) and an in vivo rat of the same strain and approximate mass as the animal used to prepare the phantom (Fig. 3b, e). The in vivo scans were done as described in the chapter by Pohlmann A et al. "Experimental Protocol for MRI Mapping of the Blood Oxygenation-Sensitive Parameters T_2^* and T_2 in the Kidney." The ex vivo and in vivo scans show a comparable level of detail, and the kidneys (denoted by "K") can be seen in relation to the surrounding tissues. MRI sequence parameters are listed in **Note 4**.

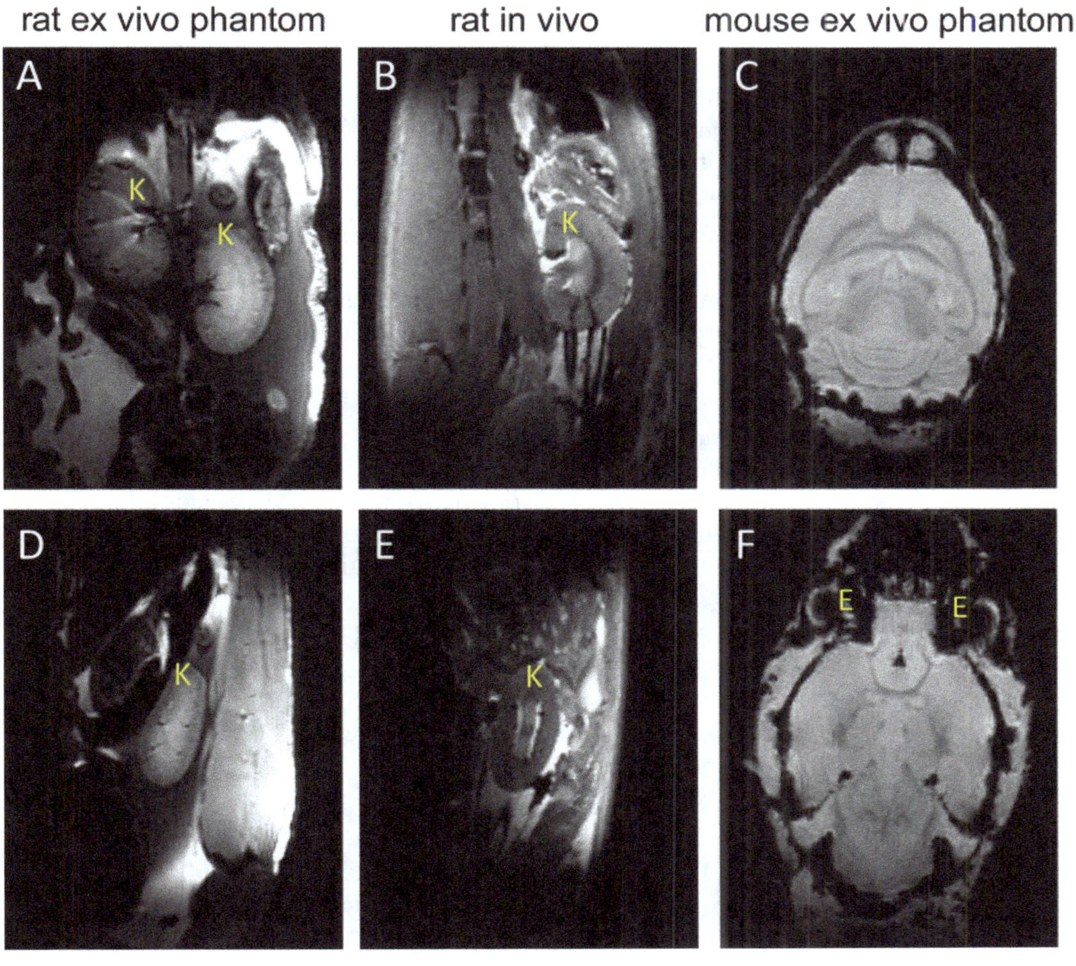

Fig. 3 Representative ex vivo and in vivo MR images. MRI scans targeting the rat kidney were acquired in the coronal (**a**, **b**) and sagittal (**d**, **e**) planes. Identical MRI hardware and pulse sequence parameters were used to acquire the images of the ex vivo phantom (**a**, **d**) and in vivo images of a rat of the same strain and approximate mass as the animal used to prepare the phantom (**b**, **e**). The kidneys are denoted by "K." MRI scans targeting the mouse brain were acquired in the coronal plane in the ex vivo phantom (**c**, **f**). Images show the brain in relation to surrounding structures such as the skull, and the eyes (denoted by "**e**")

4.2 Mouse

MRI scans targeting the mouse brain were acquired in the coronal plane in the ex vivo phantom (Fig. 3c, f). A mid-brain slice shows good contrast between gray matter and white matter structures, and the skull can be seen on the exterior of the brain (Fig. 3c). A lower brain slice (from a more inferior level) shows the brain in relation to surrounding tissue structures, for example the eyes (denoted by "E") (Fig. 3f). MRI sequence parameters are listed in **Note 5**.

5 Notes

1. The container should be large enough that the animal is completely submerged in the formaldehyde solution and also suited for preserving the shape of the animal (e.g., curvature of the body) during postfixation.
2. Ensure that no PBS leaks from the mouth and nose region: this is a sign that the needle has shifted position into the right ventricle (and that the PBS is being perfused into the respiratory circulation, not the systemic circulation). If this occurs, remove the needle and reposition into the left ventricle.
3. Formaldehyde fixation solutions such as 4% aq. PFA or 10% neutral buffered formalin are widely used, but other fixation solutions may be substituted, as suit the needs of the experimenter. One variation is to add 8 mM of gadolinium-based contrast agent, to change the relaxation properties of the tissue in the ex vivo preparation [4]. Another alternative is to use a zinc-based fixation solution [5].
4. MR images of the rat ex vivo and in vivo were acquired using a RARE sequence: TR = 540 ms, TE = 12 ms, FOV = 70 × 52 × 35 mm, matrix = 128 × 172 × 5, number of averages = 4, slice thickness = 0.7 mm. acquisition time = 1 min 9 s.
5. MR images of the mouse ex vivo phantom were acquired using a FLASH sequence: TR = 50 ms, TE = 8 ms, FOV = 20 × 20 × 12 mm, matrix = 160 × 160 × 96, number of averages = 4, slice thickness = 12 mm, acquisition time = 56 min 32 s.

Acknowledgments

This work was funded in part (Thoralf Niendorf, Sonia Waiczies, Joao Periquito) by the German Research Foundation (Gefoerdert durch die Deutsche Forschungsgemeinschaft (DFG), Projektnummer 394046635, SFB 1365, RENOPROTECTION. Funded by the Deutsche Forschungsgemeinschaft (DFG, German Research Foundation), Project number 394046635, SFB 1365, RENOPROTECTION).

This chapter is based upon work from COST Action PARENCHIMA, supported by European Cooperation in Science and Technology (COST). COST (www.cost.eu) is a funding agency for research and innovation networks. COST Actions help connect research initiatives across Europe and enable scientists to enrich their ideas by sharing them with their peers. This boosts their research, career, and innovation.

PARENCHIMA (renalmri.org) is a community-driven Action in the COST program of the European Union, which unites more than 200 experts in renal MRI from 30 countries with the aim to improve the reproducibility and standardization of renal MRI biomarkers.

References

1. Cunha L, Horvath I, Ferreira S, Lemos J, Costa P, Vieira D, Veres DS, Szigeti K, Summavielle T, Mathe D, Metello LF (2014) Preclinical imaging: an essential ally in modern biosciences. Mol Diagn Ther 18(2):153–173. https://doi.org/10.1007/s40291-013-0062-3
2. Graham ML, Prescott MJ (2015) The multifactorial role of the 3Rs in shifting the harm-benefit analysis in animal models of disease. European J Pharmacol 759:19–29. https://doi.org/10.1016/j.ejphar.2015.03.040
3. Russell WMS, Burch RL (1959) The principles of humane experimental technique. Methuen & Co. Ltd., London
4. Cleary JO, Wiseman FK, Norris FC, Price AN, Choy M, Tybulewicz VL, Ordidge RJ, Brandner S, Fisher EM, Lythgoe MF (2011) Structural correlates of active-staining following magnetic resonance microscopy in the mouse brain. NeuroImage 56(3):974–983. https://doi.org/10.1016/j.neuroimage.2011.01.082
5. Mori H, Soonsawad P, Schuetter L, Chen Q, Hubbard NE, Cardiff RD, Borowsky AD (2015) Introduction of zinc-salt fixation for effective detection of immune cell-related markers by immunohistochemistry. Toxicol Pathol 43(6):883–889. https://doi.org/10.1177/0192623315587593

5

MRI Mapping of Renal T_1: Basic Concept

Stefanie J. Hectors, Philippe Garteiser, Sabrina Doblas, Gwenaël Pagé, Bernard E. Van Beers, John C. Waterton, and Octavia Bane

Abstract

In renal MRI, measurement of the T_1 relaxation time of water molecules may provide a valuable biomarker for a variety of pathological conditions. Due to its sensitivity to the tissue microenvironment, T_1 has gained substantial interest for noninvasive imaging of renal pathology, including inflammation and fibrosis. In this chapter, we will discuss the basic concept of T_1 mapping and different T_1 measurement techniques and we will provide an overview of emerging preclinical applications of T_1 for imaging of kidney disease.

This chapter is based upon work from the COST Action PARENCHIMA, a community-driven network funded by the European Cooperation in Science and Technology (COST) program of the European Union, which aims to improve the reproducibility and standardization of renal MRI biomarkers. This introduction chapter is complemented by two separate chapters describing the experimental procedure and data analysis.

Key words Magnetic resonance imaging (MRI), Parametric imaging, T_1 mapping, Kidney, Preclinical

1 Introduction

Renal pathologies may result in structural and functional changes that could possibly be noninvasively detected by magnetic resonance imaging (MRI) [1]. While the MRI relaxometry parameter T_1, that is, the longitudinal relaxation time, is used quite extensively for assessment of other organs, for example in cardiac and brain MRI, its application for the assessment of renal pathology is relatively scarcely used. Several reports, both in the clinical [1] and preclinical setting [2–5], have shown promise of T_1 for detection and characterization of renal pathologies, including inflammation and fibrosis. These results warrant further investigation of this relaxation parameter for evaluation of renal pathology. In this chapter, we will discuss the basic concept of T_1 as well as emerging applications of this MRI parameter for noninvasive characterization of renal pathologies.

This introduction chapter is complemented by two separate chapters describing the experimental procedure and data analysis, which are part of this book.

Andreas Pohlmann and Thoralf Niendorf (eds.), *Preclinical MRI of the Kidney: Methods and Protocols*, Methods in Molecular Biology, vol. 2216, https://doi.org/10.1007/978-1-0716-0978-1_9,

This chapter is part of the book Pohlmann A, Niendorf T (eds) (2020) Preclinical MRI of the Kidney—Methods and Protocols. Springer, New York.

2 Measurement Concept

2.1 Basic Concept of T_1 Mapping

Magnetic resonance imaging (MRI) is based on the interaction of nuclear spins with three types of magnetic fields: main field B_0, radiofrequency field B_1, and linear gradient fields. MRI signal relies on the physical properties of atoms with an odd number of protons or neutrons, which possess a nuclear angular momentum (spin), that gives rise to a magnetic dipole moment. Using classical physics, the atom can be described as a charged sphere spinning about its axis and giving rise to a current loop that creates the magnetic dipole moment. Since MRI is concerned with the spin property of protons and neutrons, and their interactions with a large magnetic field, these particles will be referred to as "spins". Most MRI applications in biological specimens generate signal by manipulating the spin of single proton hydrogen (^1H), although it is feasible to generate MR images in biological samples from the signal of other nuclei such as sodium [6], or hyperpolarized gases.

$$\omega_0 = \gamma \mathbf{B}_0 \tag{1}$$

In the absence of a magnetic $\mathbf{B_0}$ field, nuclear spins are oriented randomly. The presence of an external magnetic field ($\mathbf{B_0}$) will have two effects on the spins: they will tend to align with the main magnetic field $\mathbf{B_0}$, to create a net macroscopic magnetic moment $\mathbf{M_0}$ in the direction of the field (the longitudinal direction, or conventionally, the z-direction), and they will precess around the main magnetic field at a well-defined frequency called the Larmor frequency (Eq. 1, Fig. 1) where γ, the gyromagnetic ratio, is a constant specific to each atom. Thus, a ^1H atom in a magnetic field of 1 tesla (T) $= 10^4$ gauss will precess about the field with a Larmor frequency of $\gamma/2\pi = 42.58$ MHz/tesla [7, 8].

The presence of the static magnetic field B_0 polarizes the sample of protons to a net magnetization $\mathbf{M_0}$ in the longitudinal direction. However, polarization is not sufficient to obtain a large, coherent MR signal for image reconstruction. To obtain the MR signal, a radiofrequency field $\mathbf{B_1}$ is applied as a pulse of a few milliseconds in the xy (transverse) plane. $\mathbf{B_1}$ is tuned to the resonant Larmor frequency of the spins, so it excites the spins out of equilibrium, tipping the $\mathbf{M_0}$ vector away from the z-axis by an angle known as flip angle, which is dependent on the amplitude and duration of the RF pulse (Fig. 2) [8]. The $\mathbf{B_1}$ induced rotation of the magnetization toward the transverse plane causes the longitudinal component of magnetization to decrease, and the transverse component to increase.

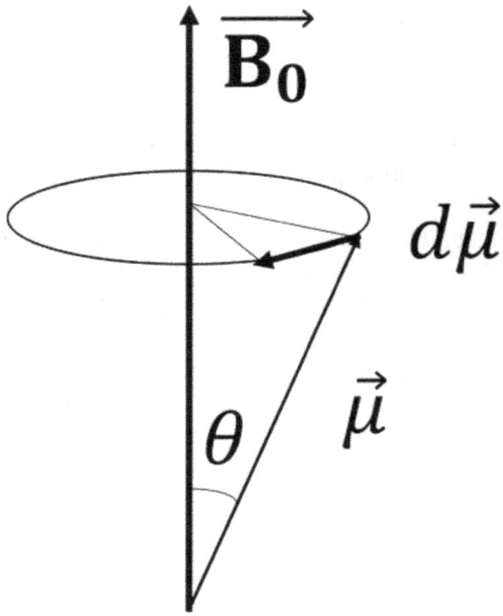

Fig. 1 B_0 interacts with the nuclear magnetic moment μ, producing a torque that causes the protons to precess around B_0. (From Dwight Nishimura, "Principles of Magnetic Resonance Imaging," Stanford University Press, Palo Alto, CA, 2010)

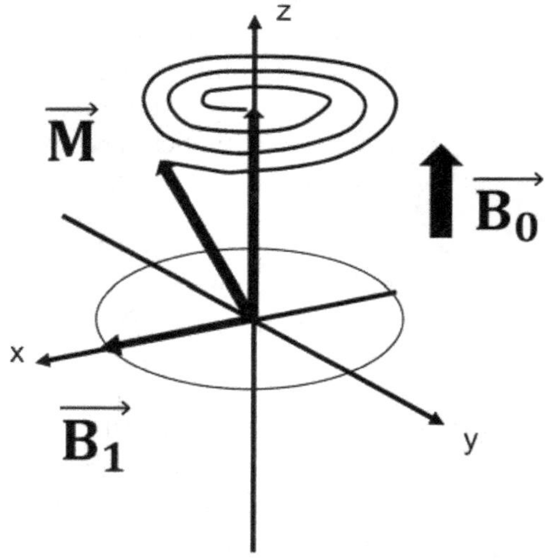

Fig. 2 Nutation at Larmor frequency of the magnetization vector around the RF pulse B_1 applied in the transverse plane. (From Dwight Nishimura, "Principles of Magnetic Resonance Imaging," Stanford University, Palo Alto, CA 2010)

When the RF $\mathbf{B_1}$ pulse is turned off, the magnetization precesses back to its equilibrium state, and the longitudinal component recovers, while the transverse component decays. The Bloch equation describes the behavior of the magnetization vector **M**, based on the T_1 and T_2 relaxation time constants and the magnetic fields applied:

$$\frac{d\mathbf{M}}{dt} = \mathbf{M} \times \gamma \mathbf{B} - \frac{M_x\mathbf{i} + M_y\mathbf{j}}{T_2} - \frac{(M_z - M_0)\mathbf{k}}{T_1} \tag{2}$$

Solving the z-axis component of the Bloch equation, we obtain an exponential expression for the recovery of M_z to the equilibrium M_0 magnetization (Eq. 3). The time constant T_1 is known as the spin-lattice or longitudinal relaxation time.

$$M_z(t) = M_0 + \left(M_{z\ (t=0)} - M_0\right) \exp\left(-\frac{t}{T_1}\right) \tag{3}$$

The reference standard method for measuring T_1 is the inversion-recovery spin echo method (IR-SE; see IR-SE signal curve in Fig. 3 top) that originated from early NMR experiments [9, 10]. It involves inversion of the magnetization M_0 by a 180° RF pulse in the z direction, followed by a time delay known as inversion time (TI) during which the equilibrium magnetization is allowed to decay. The TI ends after the application of a 90° RF pulse, which tips the magnetization in the x-y (transverse) plane for MR signal readout (receiving). A 180 pulse is then applied in the x direction, to rephase the precessing spins in a "spin echo" occurring at a fixed echo time TE.

After a long repetition time (TR) that allows for the magnetization to recover to equilibrium, the IR preparation is repeated with different subsequent inversion times. For accurate work, between 4 and 10 TI values should be used, although a T_1 can be calculated with as few as two TI values. TR is chosen to be much longer than the longest expected T_1 of interest in the tissue, in order to allow the magnetization to fully recover to equilibrium. For very accurate work this ratio TI/T_1 is as high as 5 or even 7, although for in vivo work 3 is more common. Signal decay and recovery can be observed on the images acquired with different TI's (Fig. 3 top), with signal nulling at $TI_{null} = T_1 \ln 2$, when the inversion preparation pulse is exactly 180° and the TR> > T_1 of tissue. If expected T_1 of the tissue is known, choosing a range of TI's before and after TI_{null} allows for acquisition of enough data points to fit the signal decay and recovery curve. Alternatively, performing a series of preliminary IR-SE experiments allows identification of the signal nulling time in the tissue of interest (TI_{null}), and choice of optimal range of TI values for measuring T_1.

IR-SE pulse sequences used currently in animal [2, 3] and human imaging differ from the reference standard IR-SE experiment described above by use of fast readout techniques. There are

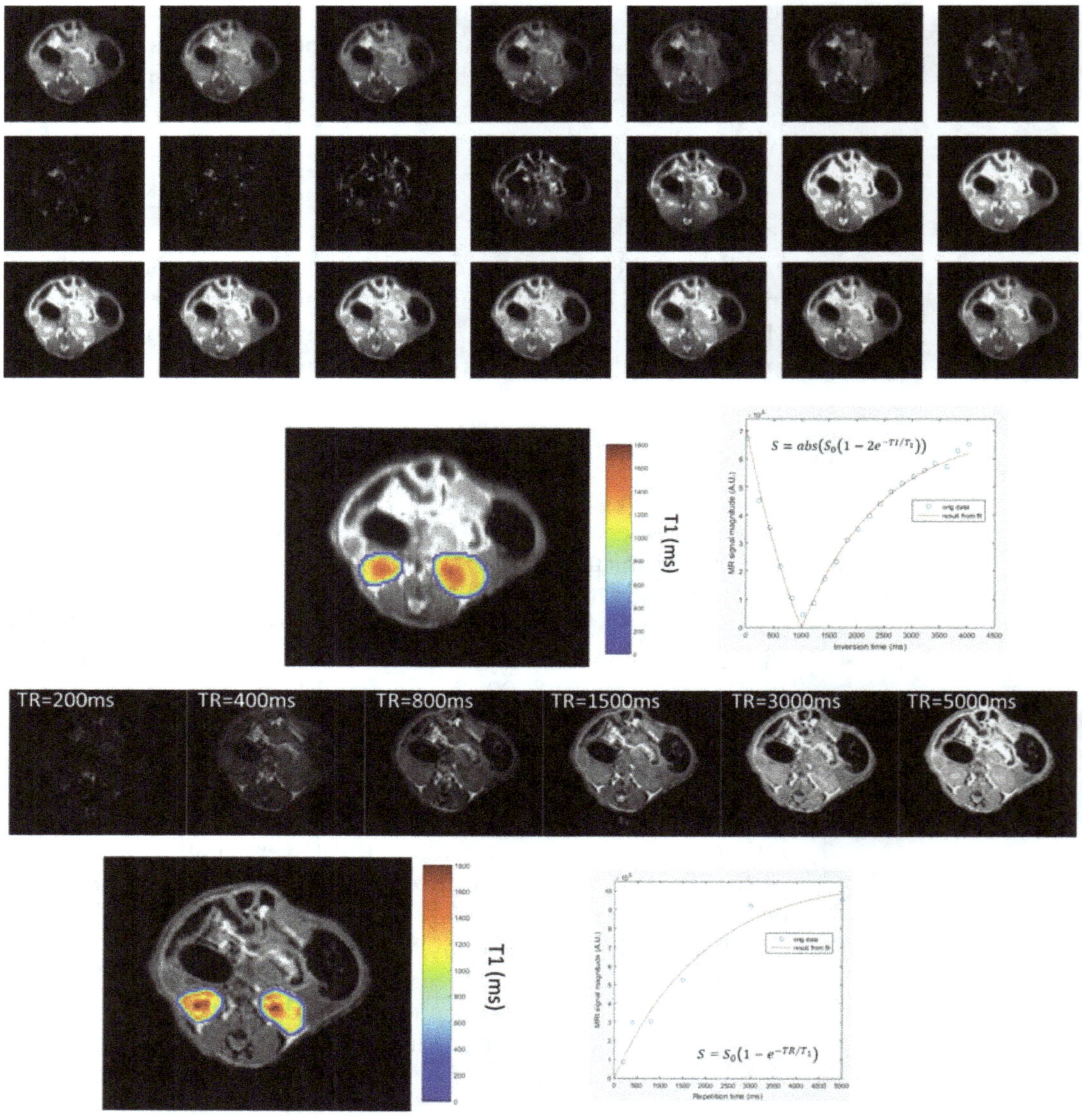

Fig. 3 T_1 mapping examples in the kidneys of a control mouse (c57bl6) imaged on a 7 T Bruker Pharmascan. Top: Inversion recovery experiment with a FAIR RARE pulse sequence, showing sequence of inversion times, T_1 color map and signal recovery curve: TE = 35.8 ms; recovery time = 10 s; NEX = 2; scan time 8 min 33 s; 21 inversion times (TI = 30 + $n \times$ 200 ms, n = 0 . . . 20); nonselective inversion slice; matrix 128 × 100; FOV 40 × 30 mm; single 1 mm-thick slice. Bottom: Variable TR experiment with a RARE VTR pulse sequence, showing 8 variable repetition times (200, 400, 800, 1500, 3000, 5000 ms), T_1 color map and signal recovery curve: TE 11 ms; NEX = 1; scan time 8 min 43 s; matrix 128 × 96; FOV = 40 × 30 mm; single 1 mm-thick slice; no fat suppression; shallow breathing; no motion compensation

various fast readout techniques that have been introduced for both inversion and saturation recovery pulse sequences:

1. The **Ra**pid Imaging with **R**efocused **E**choes (RARE) readout, also called fast or turbo spin-echo readout by clinical scanner manufacturers, uses several 180° refocusing pulses within the same TR to create an echo train. Within the echo train, each 180 pulse induces a refocused echo, comprising spin-echo and stimulated echo contributions, which is digitized, and each echo is acquired with a different phase encoding gradient, so that multiple lines of k-space (multiple phase encoding steps) can be acquired within the same TR. The number of 180° pulses is called the echo train length (ETL) or RARE factor: a typical value is 8.
2. **E**cho **p**lanar **i**maging (EPI) uses a single RF preparation (in the case of IR, 180°-TI-90°) and then acquire multiple gradient echoes by combining a high amplitude bipolar oscillating frequency encoding gradient with a low amplitude monopolar blip phase encoding gradient. This approach permits fast acquisition of k-space data in a single shot (all lines of k-space in the 2D plane are acquired for each RF preparation), or a few multiple shots (groups of k-space lines are acquired for each RF preparation).
3. A derivative of the IR methods, the Look–Locker inversion recovery (LL-IR) method, samples the magnetization recovery using rapid, small flip angle imaging readouts. More details and caveats on data acquisition and analysis with this method can be found in the chapters by Garteiser P et al. "Experimental Protocols for MRI Mapping of Renal T_1" and "Analysis Protocols for MRI Mapping of Renal T_1." In addition to EPI, LL-IR pulse sequences can employ other readout methods:
   - **F**ast **l**ow **a**ngle **sh**ots (FLASH) tips the magnetization to the transverse xy plane during the recovery period by a small angle, in order to sample it. Magnetization is spoiled before subsequent RF pulses. This readout method has the advantage of a short TR (~3 ms) that is compatible with low flip angles (<10°) [11]. As such, the longitudinal regrowth of the magnetization is perturbed only to a small extent. Use of a FLASH readout requires fitting the data with a modified version of the IR-SE equation, the Look–Locker equation (chapter by Garteiser P et al. "Analysis Protocols for MRI Mapping of Renal T_1"). FLASH can also be used in T_1 mapping methods that do not employ an inversion pulse, like variable flip angle (see next section).
   - Balanced readouts such as **s**teady-**s**tate **f**ree **p**recession (SSFP) can also be used, as they tend to yield higher signal to noise due to the reuse of magnetization from preceding shots [12]. Use of these types of readouts also requires

fitting the data with a Look–Locker equation or more complex equations that take into account the dependence of signal on both T_1 and T_2 decay. Details on acquisition and analysis with pulse sequences using an SSFP or FISP readout method can be found in the chapters by Garteiser P et al. "Experimental Protocols for MRI Mapping of Renal T_1" and "Analysis Protocols for MRI Mapping of Renal T_1."

2.2 Overview of T_1 Mapping Techniques

The longitudinal relaxation time T_1 can be measured by a variety of methods [13, 14]. The multiple delay inversion-recovery (IR) method can measure T_1 with high accuracy, however, it has long acquisition times (10–15 min with current EPI readouts [2, 3]), which makes it impractical for in vivo settings. There are several methods that have been developed for faster T_1 measurement: the saturation recovery or variable TR (VTR) method, the variable flip angle (VFA), the Look–Locker modified IR, and the proton density (PD) method. Comprehensive description of the most common pulse sequence implementations for each T_1 measurement method, acquisition protocols and corresponding analysis workflows for preclinical and clithe chapters by Garteiser P et al. "Experimental Protocols for MRI Mapping of Renal T_1" and "Analysis Protocols for MRI Mapping of Renal T_1."

2.2.1 The Saturation Recovery or VTR Method

The saturation recovery or variable TR (VTR) method, in which T_1-weighted signal is acquired with multiple TR values (Fig. 3b) shares the same limitations of limited spatial coverage and resolution as the IR method but allows shorter overall scan times [15]. The magnetization is tipped 90° (from the z to the xy plane) and the recovery is usually sampled by a RARE readout over several repetition times TR of different durations (Fig. 3b).

2.2.2 The VFA Method

In variable flip angle (VFA) methods [14–17], the RF flip angle is varied while keeping the TR constant in a 2D or 3D spoiled gradient echo (SPGR) acquisition. VFA is particularly useful in dynamic contrast-enhanced MRI (DCE-MRI) experiments, as VFA measurements allow for voxel-based baseline (precontrast enhancement) T_1 mapping with the same spatial resolution and coverage as the DCE-MRI scan in a short amount of time.

2.2.3 The Look–Locker Modified IR Method

The Look–Locker modified IR [18–21], decreases the acquisition time by sampling the signal recovery curve multiple times per TR after application of several low flip angle pulses during the acquisition. Despite shortened acquisition time, Look–Locker IR methods are still limited in spatial coverage.

2.2.4 The PD Method

In the proton density (PD) approach [22], T_1 is derived by comparing PD-weighted images with DCE baseline (precontrast) images acquired with an SPGR pulse sequence. More information on the use of T_1 for quantitative DCE-MRI measurements can be found in the chapters by Li L-P et al. "MRI Mapping of the Blood Oxygenation Sensitive Parameter T_2* in the Kidney: Basic Concept"; by Chuang K-H et al. "Renal Blood Flow Using Arterial Spin Labeling (ASL) MRI: Experimental Protocol and Principles"; and by Grist JT et al. "Analysis Protocol for Renal Sodium (23Na) MR Imaging," which cover the basic concept, experimental protocols, and analysis techniques of DCE-MRI, respectively.

2.2.5 MR Fingerprinting

Next to conventional T_1 mapping techniques, T_1 can also be extracted from magnetic resonance fingerprinting techniques, a novel MRI method that uses a pseudorandomized acquisition scheme to generate unique signal evolutions (or "fingerprints") for each tissue voxel dependent on the relaxation parameters [23].

3 Overview of Applications on Preclinical and Clinical MR Instruments

T_1 differs between different kidney components (cortex, medulla, urine, etc.); it decreases when paramagnetic contrast agents such as gadolinium chelates or oxygen (O_2) are present, and it may increase or decrease with pathology. In addition T_1 tends to increase with B_0, an important consideration since animal studies have been performed over more than an order of magnitude range in B_0.

The sensitivity of T_1 to the tissue microenvironment has been employed quite extensively to assess renal structure and function, both in clinical and preclinical studies. A comprehensive review of clinical T_1 (and T_2) applications in the kidney can be found here [24]. The use of T_1 for noninvasive assessment of renal pathology in preclinical models has already been explored in the 1980s, showing that various effects including ischemia, tubular obstruction and renal congestion may attribute to T_1 differences in rat models of acute and chronic renal failure [25, 26]. T_1 values can be affected by a wide variety of changes in the tissue environment, including inflammation and fibrosis. Inflammation can coexist with fibrosis in the kidney tissue [27], for example during rejection of transplanted kidneys. While clinical MRI studies are valuable for, for example, the grading of renal fibrosis in patients, preclinical studies with well-established animal models have the advantage of the possibility to assess dynamic changes in T_1 after the onset of pathology.

Hueper et al. performed longitudinal T_1 measurements on a 7 Tesla dedicated animal MR scanner in mice after transient unilateral clamping of the renal pedicle, causing moderate or severe acute kidney injury (AKI) dependent on the ischemia time [3]. T_1 values were significantly elevated after AKI, with a peak at 7 days after the ischemic event. In mice with severe AKI, the T_1 elevation persisted until at least a month after surgery. The initial peak in T_1 values is likely attributed to increased water content due to an acute

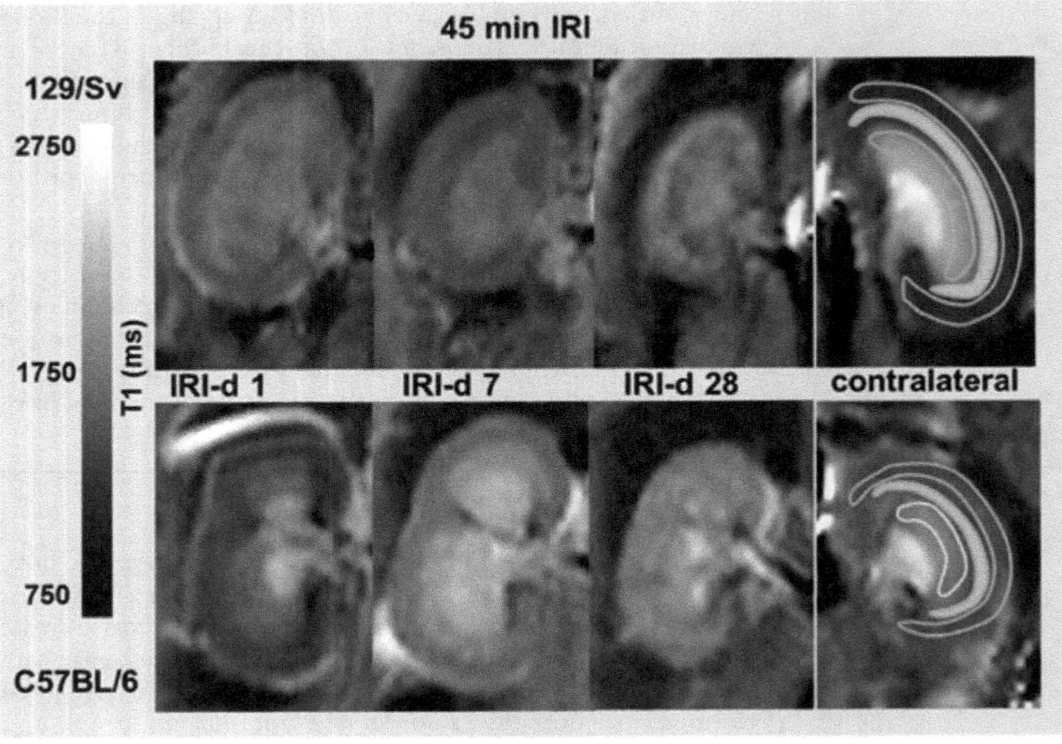

Fig. 4 T_1 maps after 45 min ischemia reperfusion injury (IRI) for 129/Sv (upper row) and C57BL/6 mice (lower row) at day 1, day 7 and day 28 are shown. In T_1 maps spatial differences can be measured by placing ROIs in the cortex and the outer stripe (OSOM) and inner stripe (ISOM) of the outer medulla, which is illustrated in the contralateral normal kidney. After severe acute kidney injury, differences of T_1-values between the two mouse strains were most pronounced on day 7: this example shows higher T_1-values in the ISOM and lower T_1-values in the renal cortex of C57BL/6 compared to 129/Sv mice. (Adapted from Tewes et al., "Functional MRI for characterization of renal perfusion impairment and edema formation due to acute kidney injury in different mouse strains" PloS One)

inflammation response. The persisting T_1 increase in severe AKI may at least partly be explained by development of fibrosis due to inadequate renal tissue regeneration and incomplete tubular repair. In a follow-up study, changes in T_1 (and arterial spin labeling perfusion parameters) after AKI was assessed in two mouse strains (C57BL/6 and 129/Sv) to investigate potential effects of different genetic backgrounds on the experimental study [5]. Overall, similar trends of increased T_1 were found in both animal models, except for a significantly higher T_1 increase in the cortex and outer stripe of the outer medulla (OSOM) of the 129/Sv vs. C57BL/6 mice at day 1 after moderate AKI and higher relative T_1 values in the cortex and lower relative T_1 values in the inner stripe of the outer medulla (ISOM) at day 7 after severe AKI in 129/Sv mice (Fig. 4) The same research team also assessed multiparametric MRI parameters, including T_1, in mouse models of allogenic and isogenic renal transplantation [2]. Acute allograft rejection was observed in allogenic kidney transplants. T_1 was significantly elevated in allogenic vs. isogenic allografts. Histopathological evaluation showed signification strong correlations of T_1 with presence of macrophages, T-cells and fibrosis (correlation coefficient r range 0.78–0.91, $P < 0.01$). These studies show that kidney T_1 is sensitive to several pathophysiological processes, including inflammation and fibrosis, which may occur simultaneously in events of kidney injury and rejection.

The findings of the group of Hueper et al. have also been observed by other research groups in independent studies. Jiang et al. employed longitudinal multiparametric MRI, including T_1 for evaluation of folic acid-induced AKI in mice [4]. The experiments were performed at a 16.4 T dedicated animal MR system (Bruker). T_1 was found to increase in both the renal cortex and medulla, most prominently at 2 weeks after treatment, while T_1 tended to regress at 4 weeks after treatment. Histopathological evaluation showed increased fluid content and association of tubular dilation at 2 weeks after treatment, explaining the T_1 elevation.

While dedicated preclinical MRI systems are highly suitable for high-resolution imaging of kidneys in small animals, clinical systems could also be used for preclinical renal T_1 studies. Ko et al. performed a longitudinal multiparametric MRI study after severe bilateral ischemic-reperfusion AKI in rat kidneys on a clinical 3 T MR scanner [28]. T_1 values were elevated in both the cortex and medulla after AKI, similar as reported in previous studies. No significant correlations of T_1 with histopathological evaluation of different markers including macrophages and collagen deposition were observed, possibly owing to complex pathological changes after AKI and multiple factors attributing to the T_1 changes. Hu et al. found significant positive correlations of T_1 with histological expression of Masson's trichrome (collagen) and alpha-smooth muscle actin in a multiparametric MRI study in a rat model of unilateral ureteral obstruction performed on a clinical 3 T MRI system [29]. Friedli et al. also found significant correlations of T_1 with histopathological inflammation and fibrosis in a rat model of unilateral ureteral obstruction. The latter study was performed on a 3 T MR system [20].

Gao et al. have reported feasibility of MR fingerprinting for imaging of healthy mouse kidneys on a preclinical 7 T MR system, showing inherent resistance of the MR fingerprinting technique to respiratory motion artifacts [30].

T_1 may also be used as baseline measurement for DCE-MRI acquisitions. More information on the use of T_1 for quantitative DCE-MRI measurements can be found in the chapters by Pedersen M et al. "Dynamic Contrast Enhancement (DCE) MRI–Derived Renal Perfusion and Filtration: Basic Concepts"; by Irrera P et al. "Dynamic Contrast Enhanced (DCE) MRI-Derived Renal

Perfusion and Filtration: Experimental Protocol"; and by Zöllner FG et al. "Analysis Protocol for Dynamic Contrast Enhanced (DCE) MRI of Renal Perfusion and Filtration," which cover the basic concept, experimental protocols, and analysis techniques of DCE-MRI, respectively.

In summary, several studies have demonstrated suitability of T_1 for assessment of renal pathology in preclinical models. These promising results warrant further investigation of this MRI relaxation technique both in the preclinical and clinical settings.

Acknowledgement

The experiments shown in Fig. 3 were performed on a platform member of France Life Imaging network (grant ANR-11-INBS-0006).

This chapter is based upon work from COST Action PARENCHIMA, supported by European Cooperation in Science and Technology (COST). COST (www.cost.eu) is a funding agency for research and innovation networks. COST Actions help connect research initiatives across Europe and enable scientists to enrich their ideas by sharing them with their peers. This boosts their research, career, and innovation.

PARENCHIMA (renalmri.org) is a community-driven Action in the COST program of the European Union, which unites more than 200 experts in renal MRI from 30 countries with the aim to improve the reproducibility and standardization of renal MRI biomarkers.

References

1. Selby NM, Blankestijn PJ, Boor P, Combe C, Eckardt KU, Eikefjord E, Garcia-Fernandez N, Golay X, Gordon I, Grenier N, Hockings PD, Jensen JD, Joles JA, Kalra PA, Kramer BK, Mark PB, Mendichovszky IA, Nikolic O, Odudu A, Ong ACM, Ortiz A, Pruijm M, Remuzzi G, Rorvik J, de Seigneux S, Simms RJ, Slatinska J, Summers P, Taal MW, Thoeny HC, Vallee JP, Wolf M, Caroli A, Sourbron S (2018) Magnetic resonance imaging biomarkers for chronic kidney disease: a position paper from the European Cooperation in Science and Technology action PARENCHIMA. Nephrol Dial Transplant 33(suppl_2):ii4–ii14. https://doi.org/10.1093/ndt/gfy152
2. Hueper K, Hensen B, Gutberlet M, Chen R, Hartung D, Barrmeyer A, Meier M, Li W, Jang MS, Mengel M, Wacker F, Rong S, Gueler F (2016) Kidney transplantation: multiparametric functional magnetic resonance imaging for assessment of renal allograft pathophysiology in mice. Investig Radiol 51(1):58–65. https://doi.org/10.1097/RLI.0000000000000205
3. Hueper K, Peperhove M, Rong S, Gerstenberg J, Mengel M, Meier M, Gutberlet M, Tewes S, Barrmeyer A, Chen R, Haller H, Wacker F, Hartung D, Gueler F (2014) T1-mapping for assessment of ischemia-induced acute kidney injury and prediction of chronic kidney disease in mice. Eur Radiol 24(9):2252–2260. https://doi.org/10.1007/s00330-014-3250-6
4. Jiang K, Ponzo TA, Tang H, Mishra PK, Macura SI, Lerman LO (2018) Multiparametric MRI detects longitudinal evolution of folic acid-induced nephropathy in mice. Am J Physiol Renal Physiol 315(5):F1252–F1260. https://doi.org/10.1152/ajprenal.00128.2018

5. Tewes S, Gueler F, Chen R, Gutberlet M, Jang MS, Meier M, Mengel M, Hartung D, Wacker F, Rong S, Hueper K (2017) Functional MRI for characterization of renal perfusion impairment and edema formation due to acute kidney injury in different mouse strains. PLoS One 12(3):e0173248. https://doi.org/10.1371/journal.pone.0173248
6. Maril N, Margalit R, Rosen S, Heyman SN, Degani H (2006) Detection of evolving acute tubular necrosis with renal 23Na MRI: studies in rats. Kidney Int 69(4):765–768. https://doi.org/10.1038/sj.ki.5000152
7. Haacke EM, Brown RW, Thompson MR, Venkatesan R (1999) Magnetic resonance imaging: physical principles and sequence design. Wiley, New York
8. Nishimura DG (1996) Principles of magnetic resonance imaging. Stanford University, Stanford, CA
9. Brown RW, Cheng Y-CN, Haacke EM, Thompson MR, Venkatesan R (2014) Magnetic resonance imaging: physical principles and sequence design, 2nd edn. Wiley-Blackwell, New York, NY
10. Berger S, Braun S (2004) 200 and more NMR experiments: a practical course, 1st edn. Wiley-VCH
11. Kierulf-Lassen C, Nielsen PM, Qi H, Damgaard M, Laustsen C, Pedersen M, Krag S, Birn H, Norregaard R, Jespersen B (2017) Unilateral nephrectomy diminishes ischemic acute kidney injury through enhanced perfusion and reduced pro-inflammatory and pro-fibrotic responses. PLoS One 12(12): e0190009. https://doi.org/10.1371/journal.pone.0190009
12. Little RA, Jamin Y, Boult JKR, Naish JH, Watson Y, Cheung S, Holliday KF, Lu H, McHugh DJ, Irlam J, West CML, Betts GN, Ashton G, Reynolds AR, Maddineni S, Clarke NW, Parker GJM, Waterton JC, Robinson SP, O'Connor JPB (2018) Mapping hypoxia in renal carcinoma with oxygen-enhanced MRI: comparison with intrinsic susceptibility MRI and pathology. Radiology 288(3):739–747. https://doi.org/10.1148/radiol.2018171531
13. Kingsley P (1999) Methods of measuring spin-lattice (t1) relaxation times: an annotated bibliography. Concepts Magn Reson 11:243–276. https://doi.org/10.1002/(SICI)1099-0534
14. Stikov N, Boudreau M, Levesque IR, Tardif CL, Barral JK, Pike GB (2015) On the accuracy of T1 mapping: searching for common ground. Magn Reson Med 73(2):514–522. https://doi.org/10.1002/mrm.25135
15. Fennessy FM, Fedorov A, Gupta SN, Schmidt EJ, Tempany CM, Mulkern RV (2012) Practical considerations in T1 mapping of prostate for dynamic contrast enhancement pharmacokinetic analyses. Magn Reson Imaging 30 (9):1224–1233. https://doi.org/10.1016/j.mri.2012.06.011
16. Aryal MP, Chenevert TL, Cao Y (2016) Impact of uncertainty in longitudinal T1 measurements on quantification of dynamic contrast-enhanced MRI. NMR Biomed 29(4):411–419
17. Schabel MC, Parker DL (2008) Uncertainty and bias in contrast concentration measurements using spoiled gradient echo pulse sequences. Phys Med Biol 53(9):2345–2373. https://doi.org/10.1088/0031-9155/53/9/010
18. Raman FS, Kawel-Boehm N, Gai N, Freed M, Han J, Liu CY, Lima JA, Bluemke DA, Liu S (2013) Modified Look-Locker inversion recovery T1 mapping indices: assessment of accuracy and reproducibility between magnetic resonance scanners. J Cardiovasc Magn Reson 15:64. https://doi.org/10.1186/1532-429x-15-64
19. Roujol S, Weingartner S, Foppa M, Chow K, Kawaji K, Ngo LH, Kellman P, Manning WJ, Thompson RB, Nezafat R (2014) Accuracy, precision, and reproducibility of four T1 mapping sequences: a head-to-head comparison of MOLLI, ShMOLLI, SASHA, and SAPPHIRE. Radiology 272(3):683–689. https://doi.org/10.1148/radiol.14140296
20. Friedli I, Crowe LA, Berchtold L, Moll S, Hadaya K, de Perrot T, Vesin C, Martin PY, de Seigneux S, Vallee JP (2016) New magnetic resonance imaging index for renal fibrosis assessment: a comparison between diffusion-weighted imaging and T1 mapping with histological validation. Sci Rep 6:30088. https://doi.org/10.1038/srep30088
21. Look DC, Locker D (1970) Time saving in measurement of NMR and EPR relaxation times. Rev Sci Instrum 41:250–251
22. Huang W, Wang Y, Panicek DM, Schwartz LH, Koutcher JA (2009) Feasibility of using limited-population-based average R10 for pharmacokinetic modeling of osteosarcoma dynamic contrast-enhanced magnetic resonance imaging data. Magn Reson Imaging 27 (6):852–858. https://doi.org/10.1016/j.mri.2009.01.020
23. Ma D, Gulani V, Seiberlich N, Liu K, Sunshine JL, Duerk JL, Griswold MA (2013) Magnetic resonance fingerprinting. Nature 495 (7440):187–192. https://doi.org/10.1038/nature11971

24. Wolf M, de Boer A, Sharma K, Boor P, Leiner T, Sunder-Plassmann G, Moser E, Caroli A, Jerome NP (2018) Magnetic resonance imaging T1- and T2-mapping to assess renal structure and function: a systematic review and statement paper. Nephrol Dial Transplant 33(suppl_2):ii41–ii50. https://doi.org/10.1093/ndt/gfy198

25. Abrashkin S, Weininger J, Griffel L, Schneider R, Iaina A (1987) Proton magnetic resonance in experimental acute and chronic renal failure in rats. Ren Fail 10(1):21–27

26. Iaina A, Abrashkin S, Weininger J (1986) Proton MR study of different types of experimental acute renal failure in rats. Magn Reson Imaging 4(3):241–244

27. Loupy A, Haas M, Solez K, Racusen L, Glotz D, Seron D, Nankivell BJ, Colvin RB, Afrouzian M, Akalin E, Alachkar N, Bagnasco S, Becker JU, Cornell L, Drachenberg C, Dragun D, de Kort H, Gibson IW, Kraus ES, Lefaucheur C, Legendre C, Liapis H, Muthukumar T, Nickeleit V, Orandi B, Park W, Rabant M, Randhawa P, Reed EF, Roufosse C, Seshan SV, Sis B, Singh HK, Schinstock C, Tambur A, Zeevi A, Mengel M (2017) The Banff 2015 kidney meeting report: current challenges in rejection classification and prospects for adopting molecular pathology. Am J Transplant 17(1):28–41. https://doi.org/10.1111/ajt.14107

28. Ko SF, Yip HK, Zhen YY, Lee CC, Lee CC, Huang SJ, Huang CC, Ng SH, Lin JW (2017) Severe bilateral ischemic-reperfusion renal injury: hyperacute and acute changes in apparent diffusion coefficient, T1, and T2 mapping with immunohistochemical correlations. Sci Rep 7(1):1725. https://doi.org/10.1038/s41598-017-01895-x

29. Hu G, Liang W, Wu M, Lai C, Mei Y, Li Y, Xu J, Luo L, Quan X (2018) Comparison of T1 mapping and T1rho values with conventional diffusion-weighted imaging to assess fibrosis in a rat model of unilateral ureteral obstruction. Acad Radiol 26(1):22–29. https://doi.org/10.1016/j.acra.2018.03.023

30. Gao Y, Chen Y, Ma D, Jiang Y, Herrmann KA, Vincent JA, Dell KM, Drumm ML, Brady-Kalnay SM, Griswold MA, Flask CA, Lu L (2015) Preclinical MR fingerprinting (MRF) at 7 T: effective quantitative imaging for rodent disease models. NMR Biomed 28(3):384–394. https://doi.org/10.1002/nbm.3262

6

Noninvasive Renal Perfusion Measurement Using Arterial Spin Labeling (ASL) MRI: Basic Concept

Min-Chi Ku, María A. Fernández-Seara, Frank Kober, and Thoralf Niendorf

Abstract

The kidney is a complex organ involved in the excretion of metabolic products as well as the regulation of body fluids, osmolarity, and homeostatic status. These functions are influenced in large part by alterations in the regional distribution of blood flow between the renal cortex and medulla. Renal perfusion is therefore a key determinant of glomerular filtration. Therefore the quantification of regional renal perfusion could provide important insights into renal function and renal (patho)physiology. Arterial spin labeling (ASL) based perfusion MRI techniques, can offer a noninvasive and reproducible way of measuring renal perfusion in animal models. This chapter addresses the basic concept of ASL-MRI.

This chapter is based upon work from the COST Action PARENCHIMA, a community-driven network funded by the European Cooperation in Science and Technology (COST) program of the European Union, which aims to improve the reproducibility and standardization of renal MRI biomarkers. This introduction chapter is complemented by two separate chapters describing the experimental procedure and data analysis.

Key words Magnetic resonance imaging (MRI), Renal, Perfusion, Arterial spin labeling (ASL), Kidney, Mice, Rats

1 Introduction

Kidneys are highly perfused organs in the body as they receive 20–25% blood of the resting cardiac output. High blood flow to the kidneys ensures adequate delivery of plasma to be filtered by the glomeruli, a physiological process necessary for the regulation of homeostasis. Therefore, the changes in renal blood flow (RBF) will also change the glomerular filtration rate (GFR) and, consequently, the volume and composition of body fluids. Thus, even a slight change in renal perfusion that exceeds renal autoregulation can have a significant impact on the kidney function. The complex interaction between RBF, renal oxygen delivery, renal oxygen consumption, and GFR made measuring of renal perfusion an

Andreas Pohlmann and Thoralf Niendorf (eds.), *Preclinical MRI of the Kidney: Methods and Protocols*, Methods in Molecular Biology, vol. 2216, https://doi.org/10.1007/978-1-0716-0978-1_13,

attractive target to understand the regulation and homeostasis of renal tissue in health and disease.

Renal perfusion, defined as the blood flow that passes through a unit mass of renal tissue within a given time (mL/min/g) that is also a key determinant of glomerular filtration. A unique aspect of the renal perfusion is that the blood flow is regionally specific. Due to the lack of a reliable technic which allowed to precisely measure the regional RBF, it is roughly estimated that 80–85% of the total renal blood flow supplies renal cortex, 10–15% outer medulla and only 1–5% inner medulla [1].The cortical blood flow is tightly regulated by well-documented mechanisms. Conversely, medullary blood flow regulation is less understood and difficult to measure [2]. The capillary density and surface area is higher in the medulla than in the cortex at least in the mice. It is very challenging to measure the medulla renal perfusion because of the complexity of the microcirculation and its tight connection of arterioles from the cortex. Although inner renal medulla receives less than 1–5% of the total renal blood flow, but changes in this region can still have major effect on electros and water homeostasis and control of arterial blood pressure [3]. Regardless, to understand the physiological regulation of renal perfusion and the role of its dysregulation in separate regions will require methods that allow quantification of renal perfusion both at the whole organ level and at the local tissue level. Most of the imaging techniques for assessing renal perfusion that have been used in humans and animals have significant limitations (Table 1) and by far there is still no gold-standard technique available. For instance, renal perfusion can be measured with dynamic contrast-enhanced MRI (DCE-MRI). However, the major drawback of DCE-MRI is the involvement of contrast media for the measurement of perfusion. The contrast media are easily filtered by renal glomeruli and hence it is difficult to obtain absolute quantification. Other known side effects, such as the development of nephrogenic systemic fibrosis, also limit their application to patients with renal deficits.

A noninvasive, practical, robust, and reproducible method to measure renal perfusion is of great interest but remains elusive, both in the clinic and basic research. The Arterial spin labeling (ASL) MRI technique introduced three decades ago for quantifying tissue perfusion [6, 7], is potentially the only available technique to meet all these needs. ASL is a MRI method generating endogenous contrast specifically related to capillary blood flow. It is therefore free of exogenous contrast media. By magnetically labeling arterial blood proton spins with inversion or saturation as a freely diffusible endogenous tracer, ASL allows for the measurement of RBF. Originally developed for measuring cerebral perfusion, the use of endogenous blood signal to obtain tissue perfusion information is particularly relevant for multiple and longitudinal imaging of patients. This attribute is also important for preclinical

Table 1
Overview of methods for monitoring renal blood flow [4, 5]

Invasive	Noninvasive
Scintigraphy	Doppler ultrasound
Positron-emission tomography (PET)	Cine phase-contrast MRI
Multidetector computed tomography (CT)	Arterial spin labeling (ASL) MRI
Contrast-enhanced ultrasound (Sonography)	
Dynamic contrast-enhanced MRI (DCE-MRI)	

imaging applications, as multiple tail-vein injections and/or catheterizations can cause local inflammation and necrosis resulting in reduced access to veins. The mature and reliable animal models combined with reproducible imaging techniques are an indispensable part of scientifically designed kidney disease studies, and play an important role in resolving the general bottleneck in renal disease treatment that is usually delayed due to difficulties in imaging disease progression.

The ASL approach has been rigorously studied in various preclinical applications including correlating the degree of acute rejection and renal cortical blood flow in rat allograft model [8], comparison of imaging results with histologic examination in ischemia-induced acute kidney injury (AKI) [9], early detection of antiangiogenic treatment responses in a mouse xenograft tumor model [10] and validation of the pathophysiological process of contrast-induced acute kidney injury in rats [11]. In this chapter, we address the basic concept and the developments of renal ASL with the emphasis on kidney disease models in rodents.

This introduction chapter is complemented by two separate chapters describing the experimental procedure and data analysis, which are part of this book.

This chapter is part of the book Pohlmann A, Niendorf T (eds) (2020) Preclinical MRI of the Kidney—Methods and Protocols. Springer, New York.

2 Measurement Concept

2.1 Basic Concept of ASL-MRI

ASL provides quantitative parametric images of tissue perfusion. It uses a modified proton magnetization of arterial blood as an endogenous, freely diffusible contrast medium which determines the delivery rate of oxygen and nutrients to the capillary bed and is expressed as the volume of blood traveling through a gram of tissue per minute (mL 100 g^{-1} min^{-1}). The basic ASL experiment collects two image types, referred to as the "label" (or tag) and "control" (or nonlabeled) image respectively. The label is applied

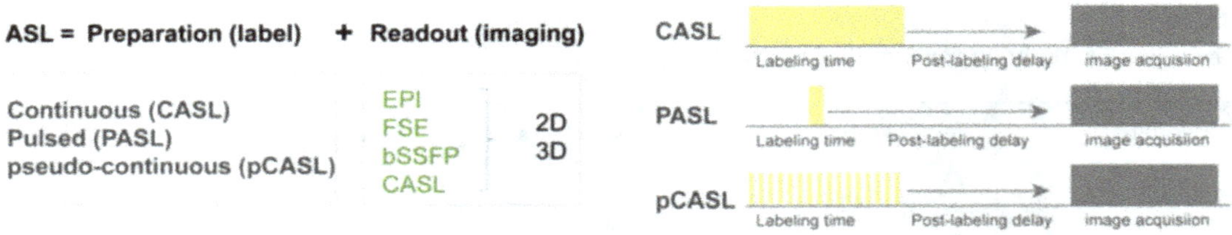

Fig. 1 Left: All ASL pulse sequences consist of two modules: a preparation module to magnetically label flowing blood, and a readout module to generate paired images. Right: Schematic showing different labeling modules. A single or a train of radiofrequency pulse for labeling followed by a postlabel delay before the image is acquired within one TR.

using radiofrequency (RF) pulses to alter the longitudinal magnetization of protons in the arterial blood before it enters the desired imaging plane, and an image is collected after a time delay. The control image is acquired at the same time delay without labeling the arterial blood protons. Provided that the inverted magnetization of the inflowing blood is the only difference between the control and label images, a simple subtraction of the label from the control image yields a perfusion-weighted image in which signal intensity is proportional to perfusion. All ASL pulse sequences consist of two components: (1) a preparation module to magnetically label inflowing blood, and (2) an imaging readout scheme to generate paired images of the target tissue under "control" and "tagged" conditions. ASL methods may be classified as to how each of these modules is constructed (Fig. 1).

2.2 Labeling Methods and Strategies for Kidney perfusion Measurement in Rodents

There are two main labeling strategies that have been developed: pulsed ASL (PASL) [12] and continuous ASL (CASL) (Fig. 1, left). Pulsed and continuous ASL labeling methods differ fundamentally in both the spatial extent and the duration of the labeling (Fig. 1, right), and these differences give rise to the strengths and weaknesses of each approach [13]. PASL uses a single short pulse or a limited number of pulses, to invert a thick slab of arterial water spins. It can be further divided into those that label spins asymmetrically with respect to the plane of imaging (Signal Targeting by Alternating Radiofrequency pulses; **STAR** [14] and Proximal Inversion with Control of Off-Resonance Effects; **PICORE** [15] or symmetrically (Flow-sensitive Alternating Inversion Recovery; **FAIR**) [16]. In contrast, CASL techniques use a continuous radiofrequency wave in a plane upstream of the imaging volume for generating a flow-driven inversion of arterial blood flowing through that plane. Later, a modified form called pseudo-continuous arterial spin labeling (pCASL) has been developed, that uses a long series of short RF-pulses together with a strong slice-selection gradient, also resulting in a flow-driven inversion of upstream blood proton spins. pCASL thus combines favorable features of CASL (high signal-to-noise) with those of PASL

Table 2
Overview of renal ASL studies in rodents

Reference	Scanner	ASL labeling	Image readout	Animal model
[9]	7.0 T (Bruker)	FAIR	EPI	Mouse
[10, 17]	7.0 T (Bruker)	FAIR	SE-EPI	Mouse
[18]	11.5 T (Bruker)	FAIR	SE-EPI	Mouse
[19]	11.5 T (Bruker)	pCASL	bSSFP	Mouse
[20]	7.0 T (Bruker)	FAIR	bSSFP	Mouse
[21]	3.0 T clinical whole body (Siemens)	FAIR	bSSFP	Rat
[22]	3.0 T clinical whole body (Siemens)	FAIR	bSSFP	Rat
[23]	3.0 T clinical whole body (Siemens)	FAIR	bSSFP	Rat

(lower energy deposition). Today most commercially available ASL products are based on pCASL or a PASL variant. Table 2 shows examples of preclinical studies using ASL for measuring RBF in animal models and list each of the labeling and readout methods.

2.2.1 Pulsed ASL (PASL)

The PASL variant (FAIR) is the major method used for measuring renal perfusion in rodents due to its ease of implementation. FAIR uses a single long-duration RF pulse which is applied to invert the arterial magnetization as blood flows through the labeling plane while a gradient is applied in the direction of arterial flow. In FAIR ASL the magnetization is usually prepared using a global inversion which is referred to as the "labeling" and a slice selective inversion which is referred to as "control." The sequence begins with a spatially selective inversion pulse limited to a small region in and around the imaged slice. In the standard labeling scheme the selective inversion slice (control) is in the same plane as the imaging slice with a thickness of 1.5–5 times the thickness of the imaging slice. The inversion pulse is usually slightly wider than the imaging slice to minimize artifacts and ensure uniform inversion. For the "labeling," the same inversion pulse is applied but without the slice-selection gradient. This causes an inversion of spins within the entire sensitive volume of the RF coil (Fig. 2a). By subtracting the control image from the labeling image, a perfusion-weighted image (PWI) is formed, which with the appropriate modeling can be quantified using a perfusion map in units of mL/100 g/min. In various preclinical MRI situations, for instance with dedicated small brain birdcage transmit/receive (TX/RX) resonators, the transmit coil used may not be long enough to provide a sufficiently global inversion for FAIR perfusion measurements.

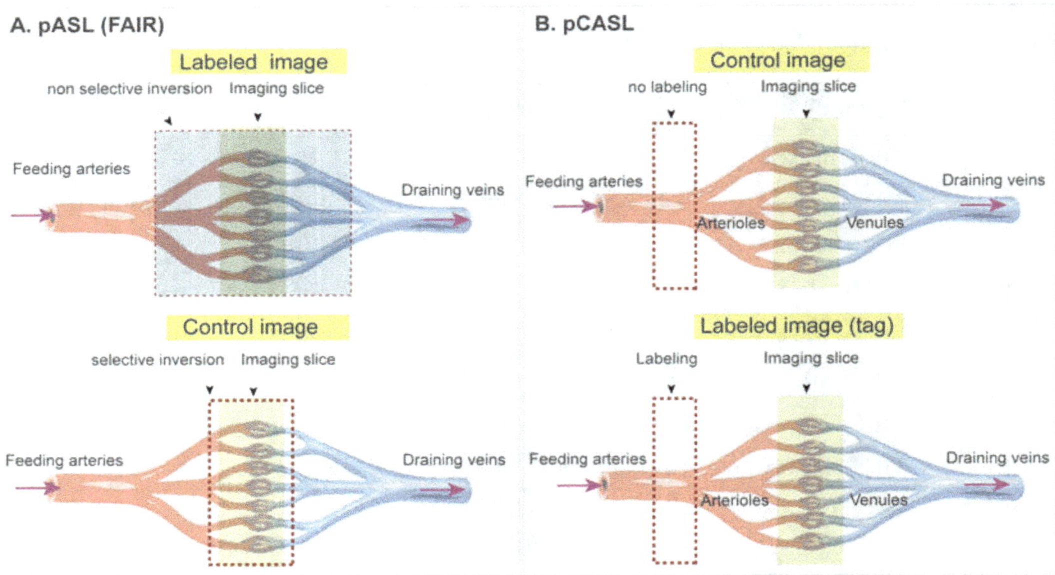

Fig. 2 Basic principle of arterial spin labeling (ASL) acquisition. It consists of a differential technique during which two acquisitions are carried out: one with the labeling of arterial protons (label image) and a control image. Arterial blood is labelled by inverting its magnetization. After an inflow time (inversion time), which allows the labeled blood to flow into the tissue of interest, an image is acquired with an appropriate readout sequence. (**a**) FAIR uses a nonselective inversion pulse for the labeled images that becomes selective with the addition of a slice selection gradient for the control. (**b**) The magnetic labeling of arterial protons is carried out upstream from the volume of interest, by radiofrequency pulses. The labeled protons then migrate via the arterial vessels toward the tissue where they pass from the capillary compartment to the extravascular compartment (example shown: pCASL)

2.2.2 Continuous ASL (CASL) and Pseudo-Continuous ASL (pCASL)

CASL uses a continuous flow-driven radiofrequency inversion of blood upstream of the imaging volume. The radiofrequency wave is transmitted either by a dedicated, separate labeling coil or by the volume transmit coil that is also used for imaging. The latter approach has the advantage that no special hardware components are required but the disadvantage of depositing high amounts of RF energy leading to magnetization transfer contrast that has to be properly corrected. One drawback of CASL labeling approach is the consequently high transmitter duty-cycle requirement.

The pCASL technique has evolved from the original CASL technique in both, brain and kidney applications [24]. pCASL uses series of short and high-power RF and gradient pulses instead of the long RF pulses used in CASL to generate a flow-driven inversion. Compared to FAIR, pseudo-continuous ASL (pCASL) provides significant advantages such as increased SNR and better definition of the labeling bolus. FAIR (pulsed ASL) may be attractive for renal imaging because it can label closer to the tissue, but pCASL offers the potential advantage of high SNR of the kidneys and the whole abdomen, which would be desirable in some specific applications (e.g., metastatic). An earlier study compared the performances of FAIR and pCASL in terms of sensitivity, absolute quantification, reproducibility, and flexibility of implementation using healthy mice [18]. It was reported that the application of pCASL at 11.75 T scanner had higher sensitivity compared to FAIR (> Þ20%). Finally, since pCASL can be straightforwardly used in multislice mode and in any imaging orientation, it may be considered as a method of choice for mouse kidney perfusion studies.

2.3 Imaging Readout

A typical ASL MRI acquisition combines an ASL magnetization preparation module (labeling methods) followed by a subsequent rapid imaging module (readouts) to capture the blood flow–weighted contrast. These two aspects of the acquisition are independent of each other. It is important to note that the majority of the ASL imaging developments has focused on the optimization of preparation module of the ASL acquisition [20].

An important prerequisite for successful kidney imaging is the ability to get fast imaging to limit the sensitivity to motion [19]. As such, ASL has been implemented with a wide variety of fast image readout techniques, which in turn can be optimized according to a specific application. The fast image readout techniques can be broadly classified as two-dimensional (2D) or 3D acquisition schemes. Whereas 3D readouts are generally recommended for brain ASL, a consensus of the optimal readout module for renal applications has yet to be established. This consideration has been recently achieved to recommend a 2D readout in humans (unpublished by PARENCHIMA ASL expert panel).

With respect to 2D readouts, to determine the optimal readout for renal ASL, a number of factors should be considered. The optimal readout should have a short echo time (TE) in order to provide the highest image signal-to-noise ratio (SNR), and to reduce the amount of signal dephasing and distortion. At longer TEs, the short tissue intrinsic T_2 and T_2* in the abdomen leads to rapid signal drop and the loss of perfusion signal. The ideal readout should be collected in a short shot length to enable multiple slices through the kidney to be acquired prior to the decay of the ASL label, thus enabling whole-kidney perfusion assessment [25]. Many ASL MRI studies have utilized either echo-planar imaging (EPI) or true fast imaging with steady-state free precession (bSSFP; True FISP) readouts [20] though the readout of ASL can be measured with any method. Both EPI and bSSFP readouts are prone to off-resonance artifacts on high field MRI scanners [20] where the majority of animal studies are done by using such high field or ultra-high field (> = 7 T) scanners. Specifically, B0 inhomogeneity results in increased distortion / ghosting and banding artifacts from EPI and True FISP imaging readouts. These artifacts are particularly problematic for abdominal imaging applications such as kidney where cardiac and respiratory motions well as adipose tissue can make precise shimming difficult. In addition, the increase in T1 relaxation times which is proportional with the field strength can result in spoiled gradient echo images with a lower signal-to-noise ratio (SNR) relative to these other imaging readouts. The low SNR is specifically problematic for ASL MRI techniques as the differential blood flow signal is typically less than 10% of the mean tissue signal.

Though the optimization of EPI acquisitions allow for whole-kidney coverage but nevertheless provide sub-optimal and slice-dependent perfusion-weighted SNR and is susceptible to off-resonance conditions mentioned above. There is an urgent need to develop a rapid and robust ASL MRI imaging readout that is balanced on blood flow labeling from the ASL labeling module and also avoid B0 inhomogeneities and motion artifacts on high field preclinical MRI scanners.

While several groups independently optimize the bSSFP image readout and shown the advantage over EPI readouts [25], more advanced methods now provide alternative readouts, such as 3D gradient and spin echo (GRASE) [26, 27]. 3D GRASE has superior SNR compared to 2D acquisitions. An alternative to 3D GRASE is 3D rapid acquisition with relaxation enhancement (RARE) combined with a spiral readout trajectory (shorter echo times and superior SNR), but can introduce through-plane blurring due to long readout times.

3 Overview of Applications

3.1 ASL for Measuring Kidney Perfusion in Animal Models

The encouraging results using ASL for measuring human renal perfusion mandate further validation of renal ASL measurements using animal models. For example, in vivo interventional swine model has been used with FAIR-ASL technique to track cortical perfusion changes during pharmacologic and physiologic alterations in renal blood flow [28]. For measuring renal hemodynamics and oxygenation in X-ray contrast agent induced acute kidney injury (CIAKI), a rat model was used. Rats were injected with contrast media and followed by ASL measurements [29]. Other models, for instance ischemia induced AKI in mice, was done by transient unilateral clamping of the renal pedicle for either 35 min for moderate AKI or 45 min for severe AKI. Using ASL, renal perfusion impairment was found more pronounced in severe compared to moderate AKI, with severe AKI causing a 33% reduction in renal perfusion [9]. In addition, ASL can be useful for longitudinal assessment of renal perfusion impairment due to acute and chronic renal allograft rejection in translational mouse models [30]. By combining with the histological assessment, perfusion impairment can be validated and revealed its relationship to the severity of

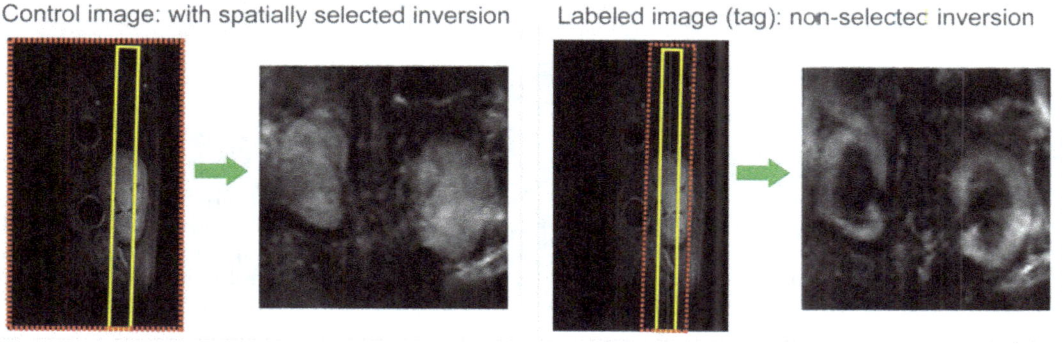

Fig. 3 An example of arterial spin labeling (ASL) acquisition using FAIR-EPI

vascular changes and renal damage. Other applications such as exploring the renoprotective efficacy of drug treatment in ischemia-induced AKI or in renal allograft recipients revealed that the renoprotective effect of the drug was associated with improved renal perfusion [22]. Thus, noninvasive perfusion imaging might provide insights into the underlying disease mechanisms in acute and chronic renal allograft rejection and might facilitate monitoring of novel treatment strategies. Similar approach can be applied to monitor kidney function of most common kidney diseases, such as CIAKI, diabetic nephropathy, and kidney transplant. In addition, ASL techniques can also be used to monitor the therapeutic responses of treatments to common renal hypoxia disease. Figure 3 is an example of ASL measurement using FAIR for labeling and EPI for image readout in a healthy mouse. Table 2 lists all examples of preclinical studies using ASL for measuring RBF in rodent models.

Acknowledgments

This work was funded in part (Thoralf Niendorf, Sonia Waiczies, Andreas Pohlmann, and Joao Periquito) by the German Research Foundation (Gefoerdert durch die Deutsche Forschungsgemeinschaft (DFG), Projektnummer 394046635, SFB 1365, RENOPROTECTION. Funded by the Deutsche Forschungsgemeinschaft (DFG, German Research Foundation), Project number 394046635, SFB 1365, RENOPROTECTION).

This chapter is based upon work from COST Action PARENCHIMA, supported by European Cooperation in Science and Technology (COST). COST (www.cost.eu) is a funding agency for research and innovation networks. COST Actions help connect research initiatives across Europe and enable scientists to enrich their ideas by sharing them with their peers. This boosts their research, career, and innovation.

PARENCHIMA (renalmri.org) is a community-driven Action in the COST program of the European Union, which unites more than 200 experts in renal MRI from 30 countries with the aim to improve the reproducibility and standardization of renal MRI biomarkers.

References

1. Wentland AL, Artz NS, Fain SB, Grist TM, Djamali A, Sadowski EA (2012) MR measures of renal perfusion, oxygen bioavailability and total renal blood flow in a porcine model: non-invasive regional assessment of renal function. Nephrol Dial Transplant 27:128–135
2. Kennedy-Lydon TM, Crawford C, Wildman SS, Peppiatt-Wildman CM (2013) Renal pericytes: regulators of medullary blood flow. Acta Physiol 207:212–225
3. Cowley AW Jr, Mattson DL, Lu S, Roman RJ (1995) The renal medulla and hypertension. Hypertension 25:663–673
4. Schneider AG, Goodwin MD, Bellomo R (2013) Measurement of kidney perfusion in critically ill patients. Crit Care 17:220
5. Lemoine S, Papillard M, Belloi A, Rognant N, Fouque D, Laville M, Rouviere O, Juillard L (2011) Renal perfusion: noninvasive measurement with multidetector CT versus fluorescent microspheres in a pig model. Radiology 260:414–420
6. Detre JA, Leigh JS, Williams DS, Koretsky AP (1992) Perfusion imaging. Magn Reson Med 23:37–45
7. Williams DS, Detre JA, Leigh JS, Koretsky AP (1992) Magnetic resonance imaging of perfusion using spin inversion of arterial water. Proc Natl Acad Sci U S A 89:212–216
8. Wang JJ, Hendrich KS, Jackson EK, Ildstad ST, Williams DS, Ho C (1998) Perfusion quantitation in transplanted rat kidney by MRI with arterial spin labeling. Kidney Int 53:1783–1791
9. Hueper K, Gutberlet M, Rong S, Hartung D, Mengel M, Lu X, Haller H, Wacker F, Meier M, Gueler F (2014) Acute kidney injury: arterial spin labeling to monitor renal perfusion impairment in mice-comparison with histopathologic results and renal function. Radiology 270:117–124
10. Rajendran R, Huang W, Tang AM, Liang JM, Choo S, Reese T, Hentze H, van Boxtel S, Cliffe A, Rogers K, Henry B, Chuang KH (2014) Early detection of antiangiogenic treatment responses in a mouse xenograft tumor model using quantitative perfusion MRI. Cancer Med 3:47–60
11. Liang L, Chen WB, Chan KW, Li YG, Zhang B, Liang CH, Liu GS, Zhang SX (2016) Using intravoxel incoherent motion MR imaging to study the renal pathophysiological process of contrast-induced acute kidney injury in rats: comparison with conventional DWI and arterial spin labelling. Eur Radiol 26:1597–1605
12. Kwong KK, Belliveau JW, Chesler DA, Goldberg IE, Weisskoff RM, Poncelet BP, Kennedy DN, Hoppel BE, Cohen MS, Turner R et al (1992) Dynamic magnetic resonance imaging of human brain activity during primary sensory stimulation. Proc Natl Acad Sci U S A 89:5675–5679
13. Nery F, Gordon I, Thomas DL (2018) Non-invasive renal perfusion imaging using arterial spin labeling MRI: challenges and opportunities. Diagnostics 8:2
14. Edelman RR, Siewert B, Adamis M, Gaa J, Laub G, Wielopolski P (1994) Signal targeting with alternating radiofrequency (STAR) sequences: application to MR angiography. Magn Reson Med 31:233–238
15. Wong EC, Buxton RB, Frank LR (1997) Implementation of quantitative perfusion imaging techniques for functional brain mapping using pulsed arterial spin labeling. NMR Biomed 10:237–249
16. Kim SG (1995) Quantification of relative cerebral blood flow change by flow-sensitive alternating inversion recovery (FAIR) technique: application to functional mapping. Magn Reson Med 34:293–301
17. Rajendran R, Lew SK, Yong CX, Tan J, Wang DJ, Chuang KH (2013) Quantitative mouse renal perfusion using arterial spin labeling. NMR Biomed 26:1225–1232
18. Duhamel G, Prevost V, Girard OM, Callot V, Cozzone PJ (2014) High-resolution mouse kidney perfusion imaging by pseudo-continuous arterial spin labeling at 11.75T. Magn Reson Med 71:1186–1196
19. Prevost VH, Girard OM, Callot V, Cozzone PJ, Duhamel G (2015) Fast imaging strategies for mouse kidney perfusion measurement with pseudocontinuous arterial spin labeling (pCASL) at ultra high magnetic field (11.75 tesla). J Magn Reson Imaging 42:999–1008
20. Gao Y, Goodnough CL, Erokwu BO, Farr GW, Darrah R, Lu L, Dell KM, Yu X, Flask CA (2014) Arterial spin labeling-fast imaging with steady-state free precession (ASL-FISP): a

rapid and quantitative perfusion technique for high-field MRI. NMR Biomed 27:996–1004

21. Zimmer F, Zollner FG, Hoeger S, Klotz S, Tsagogiorgas C, Kramer BK, Schad LR (2013) Quantitative renal perfusion measurements in a rat model of acute kidney injury at 3T: testing inter- and intramethodical significance of ASL and DCE-MRI. PLoS One 8: e53849
22. Klotz S, Pallavi P, Tsagogiorgas C, Zimmer F, Zollner FG, Binzen U, Greffrath W, Treede RD, Walter J, Harmsen MC, Kramer BK, Hafner M, Yard BA, Hoeger S (2016) N-octanoyl dopamine treatment exerts renoprotective properties in acute kidney injury but not in renal allograft recipients. Nephrol Dial Transplant 31:564–573
23. Tan H, Thacker J, Franklin T, Prasad PV (2015) Sensitivity of arterial spin labeling perfusion MRI to pharmacologically induced perfusion changes in rat kidneys. J Magn Reson Imaging 41:1124–1128
24. Roberts DA, Detre JA, Bolinger L, Insko EK, Lenkinski RE, Pentecost MJ, Leigh JS Jr (1995) Renal perfusion in humans: MR imaging with spin tagging of arterial water. Radiology 196:281–286
25. Buchanan CE, Cox EF, Francis ST (2018) Evaluation of 2D imaging schemes for pulsed arterial spin labeling of the human kidney cortex. Diagnostics 8:43
26. Robson PM, Madhuranthakam AJ, Smith MP, Sun MR, Dai W, Rofsky NM, Pedrosa I, Alsop DC (2016) Volumetric arterial spin-labeled perfusion imaging of the kidneys with a three-dimensional fast spin echo acquisition. Acad Radiol 23:144–154
27. Cutajar M, Thomas DL, Banks T, Clark CA, Golay X, Gordon I (2012) Repeatability of renal arterial spin labelling MRI in healthy subjects. MAGMA 25:145–153
28. Artz NS, Wentland AL, Sadowski EA, Djamali A, Grist TM, Seo S, Fain SB (2011) Comparing kidney perfusion using noncontrast arterial spin labeling MRI and microsphere methods in an interventional swine model. Investig Radiol 46:124–131
29. Chen WB, Liang L, Zhang B, Liu CL, Liu HJ, Luo HY, Zeng QX, Liang CH, Liu GS, Zhang SX (2015) To evaluate the damage of renal function in CIAKI rats at 3T: using ASL and BOLD MRI. Biomed Res Int 2015:593060
30. Hueper K, Schmidbauer M, Thorenz A, Brasen JH, Gutberlet M, Mengel M, Hartung D, Chen R, Meier M, Haller H, Wacker F, Rong S, Gueler F (2017) Longitudinal evaluation of perfusion changes in acute and chronic renal allograft rejection using arterial spin labeling in translational mouse models. J Magn Reson Imaging 46:1664–1672

7

Hardware Considerations for Preclinical Magnetic Resonance of the Kidney

Paula Ramos Delgado, Ekkehard Küstermann, André Kühne, Jason M. Millward, Thoralf Niendorf, Andreas Pohlmann, and Martin Meier

Abstract

Magnetic resonance imaging (MRI) is a noninvasive imaging technology that offers unparalleled anatomical and functional detail, along with diagnostic sensitivity. MRI is suitable for longitudinal studies due to the lack of exposure to ionizing radiation. Before undertaking preclinical MRI investigations of the kidney, the appropriate MRI hardware should be carefully chosen to balance the competing demands of image quality, spatial resolution, and imaging speed, tailored to the specific scientific objectives of the investigation. Here we describe the equipment needed to perform renal MRI in rodents, with the aim to guide the appropriate hardware selection to meet the needs of renal MRI applications.

This publication is based upon work from the COST Action PARENCHIMA, a community-driven network funded by the European Cooperation in Science and Technology (COST) program of the European Union, which aims to improve the reproducibility and standardization of renal MRI biomarkers. This chapter on hardware considerations for renal MRI in small animals is complemented by two separate publications describing the experimental procedure and data analysis.

Key words Magnetic Resonance Imaging (MRI), Kidney, Mice, Rats, Hardware, RF coils, Renal MRI

1 Introduction

The detection, staging, and monitoring of kidney diseases (KD) using measurements of renal function and structure is critical in clinical nephrology. The use of animal models in kidney research promotes the understanding of disease and therapy mechanisms. While current imaging modalities such as computed tomography or ultrasound can provide some information on structural changes in the kidney, these approaches offer limited insights into functional changes.

Magnetic resonance imaging (MRI) is a noninvasive imaging technology that offers an unparalleled level of anatomical and functional detail, along with diagnostic sensitivity. MRI is suitable

Andreas Pohlmann and Thoralf Niendorf (eds.), *Preclinical MRI of the Kidney: Methods and Protocols*, Methods in Molecular Biology, vol. 2216, https://doi.org/10.1007/978-1-0716-0978-1_8,

for longitudinal studies due to the lack of exposure to ionizing radiation. Together with established imaging techniques, novel approaches such as dynamic contrast-enhanced MRI (DCE-MRI), arterial spin labeling (ASL), blood oxygen level dependent MRI (BOLD), and diffusion-weighted imaging (DWI) can provide a broad characterization of the kidney, including renal vascular perfusion, oxygenation, and glomerular filtration rate.

For performing dedicated MR measurements of the kidney, the appropriate MRI hardware should be carefully chosen to balance the competing demands of image quality, spatial resolution and imaging speed, tailored to the specific scientific objectives of the investigation. This chapter is intended to outline the key hardware components of an MRI scanner and to provide an overview of currently established technologies, with the goal to guide the appropriate hardware selection that meets the needs of preclinical MRI of the kidney.

This chapter on hardware considerations for renal MRI in small animals is part of the book Pohlmann A, Niendorf T (eds) (2020) Preclinical MRI of the Kidney–Methods and Protocols. Springer, New York.

2 Static Magnetic Field Strength (B_0)

A superconducting magnet that generates a constant homogeneous magnetic field is the core hardware component of an MRI scanner. This strength of this static magnetic field (B_0) is proportional to the net polarization produced within the sample. The detected MR signal on a receive RF coil depends on B_0^2, whereas the noise increases linearly with B_0 [1]. B_0 governs the signal-to-noise ratio (SNR), which is the currency for MR image quality. This provides strong motivation and momentum to move to increasingly higher magnetic field strengths for preclinical and clinical renal MRI applications [2–4]. The proportionality of SNR with B_0 is linear in the quasi-static regime, as demonstrated theoretically [5, 6] and experimentally [7]. For higher magnetic field strengths, wave propagation and the increasing resonance frequencies must be considered [2]. Additionally, an experimental study on intrinsic SNR behaviour with increasing B_0 field strengths (3.0, 7.0, and 9.4 T) in the human brain reported a superlinear increase in SNR ($SNR \propto B_0^{1.65}$) [7]. This observation was also confirmed in a simulation study [8].

Relaxation time constants of biological tissues also change with the magnetic field strength, thus influencing the SNR as well as the contrast-to-noise ratio (CNR), which ultimately has an impact on the image quality. The longitudinal relaxation time (T_1) increases nonlinearly with increasing B_0 [1, 9–11]. The transversal relaxation (T_2) and T_2* decrease at different slopes linearly [1, 9, 12–14]. These dependencies on B_0 are responsible for the reduced

T_1-weighted contrast and increased BOLD effect at higher magnetic field strengths (*see* **Note 1**). MRI methods based on T_2*-weighting (e.g., susceptibility weighted imaging, BOLD) will benefit from the T_2* shortening, and thus increase in sensitivity at high magnetic field strengths, which underlies their broad application in renal MRI. An example of renal T_2*-mapping ($R_2^* = 1/T_2^*$) is the study of oxygenation and haemodynamics in renal disorders (for a review *see* [15]). MR spectroscopy also benefits from the enhanced signal dispersion achieved at higher magnetic field strengths, which results in better resolved spectra, and permits improved accuracy of metabolite identification and quantification [1, 16].

However, MRI at high magnetic field strengths is susceptible to more severe B_0 and B_1 inhomogeneities, compared to lower field strengths. These inhomogeneities are primarily due to differences in the magnetic susceptibility at tissue interfaces. Susceptibility artifacts present themselves as T_2*-induced signal losses (or even signal voids) in areas with very high B_0 gradients, low phase-encoding bandwidth-related image distortion and off-resonance effects caused by ΔB_0-induced frequency dispersions. MRI of the kidney poses additional challenges due to the anatomical context. The kidneys are adjacent to bowels, in close proximity to skin/fat/muscle boundaries (e.g., perirenal fat) or in areas containing cavities might be particularly prone to susceptibility artifacts.

Artifacts are visible as signal losses at interfaces between fat and tissue or air and tissue (susceptibility artifacts), image blurring, image distortion, and broadening of spectral lines in MRS, which interferes with the reliable differentiation of metabolites. B_0 inhomogeneities can be mitigated using B_0 shimming (*see* Subheading 3).

B_1 inhomogeneities lead to variations in the flip angle driven by the RF pulse excitation. B_1 inhomogeneities affect tissue contrast and SNR, appearing as signal intensity variations or losses across the field of view. Nonuniformities in B_1 are caused by the RF coil (e.g., surface RF coil, *see* Subheading 4) or by the creation of standing waves and constructive/destructive interferences within the object under investigation, due to the reduction of the effective wavelength which at higher field strengths becomes shorter, and can approach the dimensions of the specific anatomical structures under study [17]. While the RF wavelength inside tissue at 3.0 T (~128 MHz) is about 30 cm, at 7.0 T (~300 MHz) it is reduced to about 13 cm [18] and to 6.5 cm at 14.0 T (~600 MHz). In preclinical renal MRI, this is not a major concern, as the size of the abdomen in small animals is typically much smaller than the RF wavelength.

RF power requirements for spin excitation increase quadratically with B_0. This imposes major concerns, especially for human applications, since the RF power deposition can easily reach the regulatory limits specified by IEC guidelines for the specific absorption rate (SAR) [16]. This constraint can be adressed by modification and adaptation of MR pulse sequences, acquisition strategies, and RF coils [18, 19]. In the case of preclinical studies, these issues have received less attention since there are no enforced SAR guidelines for small animals. Nevertheless, the physiological effects of tissue heating due to heavy RF deposition in experimental animals could be a serious confounding factor in preclinical studies that should not be ignored.

2.1 SNR Comparison for Magnetic Field Strength

The SNR gains resulting from increasing B_0, field have been computationally estimated for brain MRI to range from $B_0^{1.2}$ (close to the brain surface) up to $B_0^{2.1}$ (at the center of the head) [8]. Pohmann et al. [7] investigated the field dependence of SNR for magnetic field strengths ranging between 3.0 T and 9.4 T using gradient echo techniques, and reported that SNR increases superlinearly ($B_0^{1.65}$). Using this relationship, the calculated relative SNR (normalized for the typical case of a 3.0 T scanner) and resolution gains (in μm, in-plane resolution 1 mm) corresponding to all static magnetic field strengths from 1.5 T to 21.1 T are shown in Table 1.

The increase in SNR provided by higher magnetic field strengths can be invested in enhanced spatial resolution or improvements in imaging speed. The triad of B_0, spatial resolution, and imaging speed form the so-called SNR conundrum in which the competing constraints of SNR, CNR, spatial resolution, and imaging speed govern the image quality. For example, increasing the matrix size for a certain field of view will increase the spatial resolution—which will permit the visualization of more subtle anatomical structures in the kidney—but at a cost of reducing the SNR, or signal intensity per pixel/voxel. Although resolution in the frequency-encoding direction can be conveniently enhanced by increasing the matrix size without major scan time penalty, increasing spatial resolution along the phase-encoding direction substantially prolongs the scan time. Boosting the SNR is also possible by modifying the size of the field of view or the slice thickness: the larger these parameters are, the more signal is acquired. Another way to further increase SNR is signal averaging, which reduces the noise but comes at the cost longer scan times. Depending on the individual experimental context, longer scan times may be a reasonable price to pay (especially for ex vivo studies). For in vivo studies, animal welfare considerations call for the minimum scan time possible to achieve the scientific objective, and shorter scans promote higher throughput of individual animals to improve the experimental sample size.

Additional strategies to gain SNR include the use of SNR-promoting rapid imaging techniques such as RARE imaging, and dedicated RF coil technology, including cryogenically cooled RF coils (*see* Subheading 4).

Table 1
Relative SNR and resolution gain with increasing static magnetic field strength

Magnetic field, B_0 (T)	Relative SNR gain	Resolution gain (in-plane 1 mm) (μm^2)
1.5	0.3	(1550 × 1550)
3.0	1.0	(495 × 495)
4.7	2.1	(235 × 235)
7.0	4.0	(122 × 122)
9.4	6.6	(75 × 75)
11.7	9.4	(52 × 52)
14.0	12.7	(39 × 39)
16.4	16.5	(30 × 30)
17.6	18.5	(27 × 27)
21.1	25.0	(20 × 20)

SNR values were computed as proportional to $B^{1.65}$. The relative SNR gain was calculated relative to that of 3.0 T

2.2 Magnetic Field Strengths Used in Recently Published Studies

To provide guidance as to which B_0 is necessary or sufficient for preclinical MRI of the kidney, a total of 121 publications published over the past 10 years were reviewed. Of these, 66 publications reported on renal MRI in rats, and 55 in mice. Figure 1 shows the number of publications found per magnetic field strength for renal MRI in rats and mice. In rats, a total of 25 publications (38%) were performed at 3.0 T, closely followed by 9.4 T with 20 papers (30%). In mice the preferred magnetic field strength was 7.0 T (25 publications, 46%). The magnetic field strengths of 9.4 T (8 papers, 15%), 3.0 T (7 papers, 13%), and 11.7 T (6 publications, 11%) were also used for MRI studies of mouse kidney.

Figure 2 illustrates the number of publications per magnetic field strength, listed by year for rats and mice. In rats, the number of studies performed at 3.0 and 9.4 T was quite stable for the last 7 years. Studies at 4.7 T (7 papers, 11%) were also widely reported, as shown in the trends displayed since 2009. The use of field strengths of 1.5 and 7.0 T (7 and 6 publications, respectively) varied during the period under investigation. In contrast, 7.0 T was established as the typical magnetic field strength for preclinical MRI of the kidney in mice during this period. In the last few years, 11.7 T and 16.4 T have also emerged as MR systems suitable for the study of the mouse kidney.

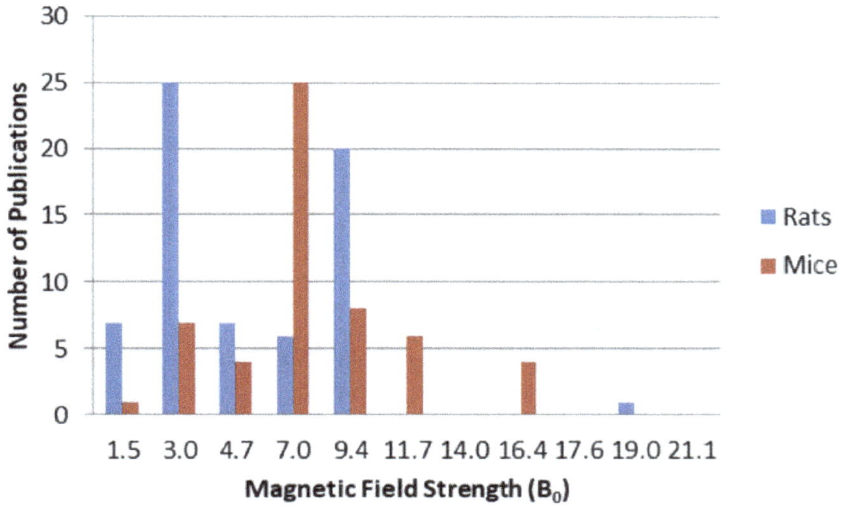

Fig. 1 Number of publications per magnetic field strength for renal MRI in rats and mice, within a total of 121 reports on preclinical renal MRI published in the past 10 years

3 Gradient Systems

To enable the spatial localisation of the MR signal, magnetic field gradients are used, which are provided by gradient coils. Gradient coils produce a linear variation of the magnetic field as a function of the spatial position (X-, Y-, and Z-direction) modifying the resonance frequency for spatial encoding of the MR signal.

Typical parameters governing the performance of the gradient system are the peak gradient strength, the rise time, and the slew rate. The peak gradient strength is the maximum achievable gradient strength (in mT/m). Typical peak gradient amplitudes in preclinical scanners are in the range of 200–1000 mT/m. Clinical scanners used for preclinical MRI of the kidney provide maximum gradient amplitudes ranging between 45 mT/m and 82 mT/m. The gradient rise time is the time needed to change the gradient field from zero to the peak amplitude (in ms). The gradient slew rate is the most important parameter, and refers to the speed at which a gradient can be switched. It is defined as the peak gradient strength divided by the gradient rise time (in T/m/s). This defines the maximum scanning speed, since it influences the minimum achievable repetition time (TR) and echo time (TE), as well as the echo spacing in fast imaging techniques such as RARE or EPI (*see* **Note 2**). Typical slew rates in preclinical scanners are in the range of 640–9000 T/m/s. Clinical scanners used for preclinical MRI of the kidney offer slew rates ranging between 150 T/m/s and 200 T/m/s. Gradient coils can be driven in two modes: (a) constant rise time, in which the slew rate is adapted for each gradient amplitude and (b) maximum slew rate, where the rise is adjusted for each gradient amplitude.

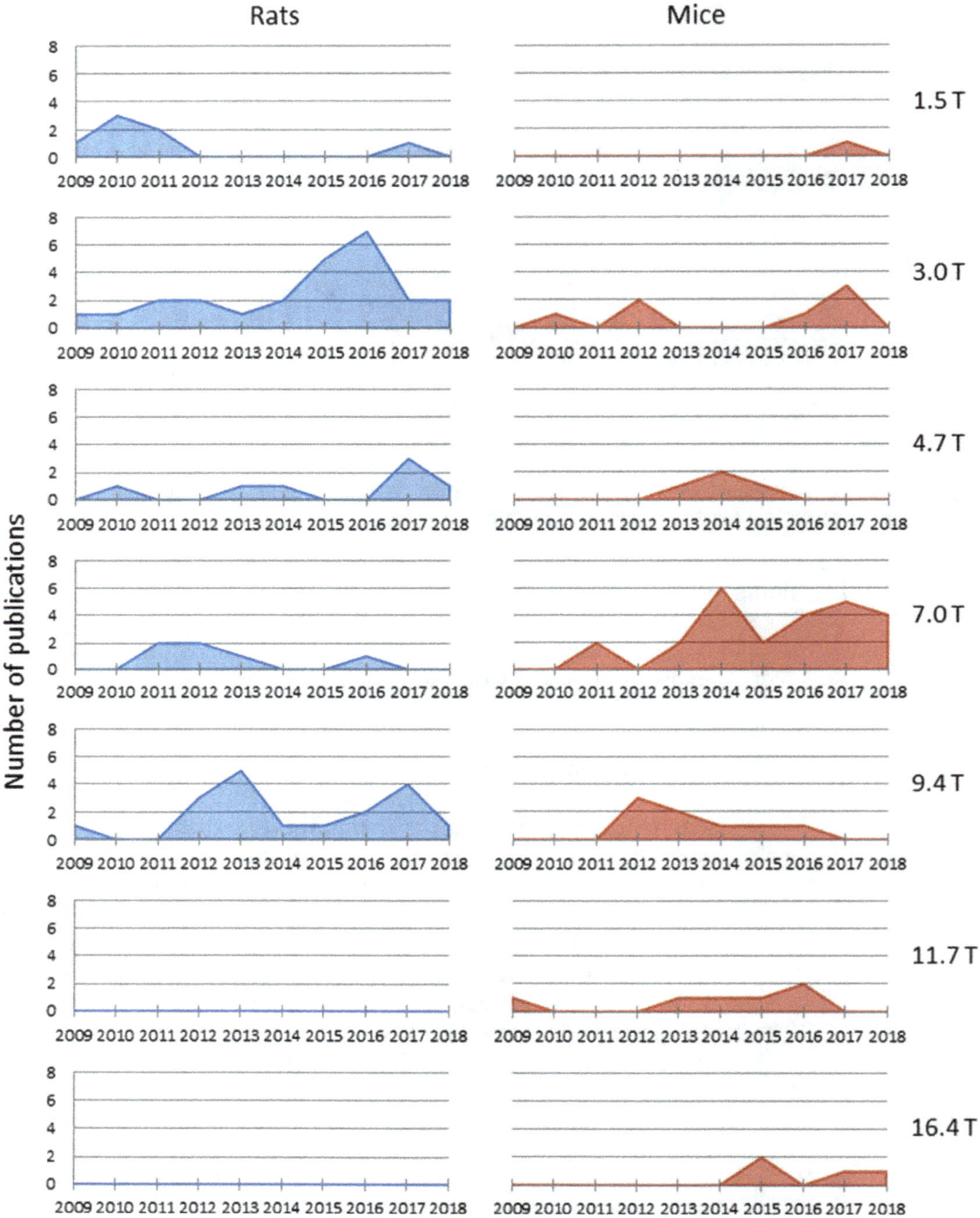

Fig. 2 Number of selected publications ordered by magnetic field strength and year, within a total of 121 reports published in the past 10 years (2009–2018) for preclinical renal MRI in rats and mice

The duty cycle defines the amount of time during which the gradient system can be run at maximum power amplitude (in % time). This parameter depends not only on the gradient system specifications mentioned above but also on the specific MR imaging technique used. Typical duty cycles in existing preclinical scanners can reach almost 100%. For this purpose, gradient coils are water-cooled to ensure proper heat dissipation and temperature management.

The accuracy of the spatial representation depends on the quality of the linear magnetic field gradients and on the homogeneity of the static magnetic field (typically given in parts per million, ppm). Any deviation will appear as object distortion in the image, and thus a correction procedure called "shimming" is typically performed. During system installation, the manufacturer places small metal plates inside the scanner bore to improve the uniformity of the main magnetic field in a static and permanent manner—this is "passive" shimming. The distribution of these ferromagnetic pieces is adjusted over several iterations until the achieved magnetic field uniformity meets the vendor's specification. In addition to passive shimming, resistive shim coils are used for B_0 homogenization. These adjustments are performed with a shim calibration tool on an empty magnet, and therefore the B_0 homogeneity becomes impaired as soon as a sample or subject (human or animal) is placed inside the magnet bore.

An "active" shimming procedure can be conducted during measurement adjustments with every MR scan. This is crucial for techniques such as fat suppression or MR spectroscopy, since the introduction of any matter—an object or animal—inevitably introduces local magnetic field perturbations of the main static magnetic field, which then must be actively compensated for. Especially at the boundaries between tissue and air-filled areas, where magnetic field distortions are pronounced due to the different magnetic susceptibility which can cause severe signal losses and image distortions. Corrective magnetic fields produced by electrical RF coils, designated as shim gradients [20] which are superimposed upon the main magnetic field. Typically, the shim gradient system contains a set of first-order gradients which impose linear field changes in the X-, Y-, and Z-directions, and some second order gradients, which create spherical harmonics in the Z^2, ZX, ZY X^2-Y^2, and XY directions [21]. Some MR systems are also equipped with more sophisticated shim gradients which provide third and fourth order correction terms [22].

Depending on the specific pulse sequence and imaging technique used, the scientist has to adjust these magnetic field corrections to meet certain quality prequisites. Especially with T_2*-weighted sequences (e.g., gradient-echo or EPI sequences) the image quality improves with improved B_0 homogeneity. MR spectroscopic methods are even more demanding [23]. Usually, state-of-the-art MR systems provide automated methods to perform the B_0 shimming task, but the user still needs to check the performance and correct the shim settings manually if necessary.

For B_0 shimming a global approach covering the entire FOV, or a localized shim covering a target area can be used. In general, the smaller the region of interest the better the achievable B_0 homogeneity. In the case of renal MRI, the B_0 homogeneity achieved after shimming across one kidney will be better than that for the whole abdomen, with air-filled lungs and gut. In the case of tissues that are moving due to respiration, cardiac activity or peristaltic motion, the magnetic field distortions change over time, which require different strategies. The time-averaged global shim would be the fastest and easiest solution, if this is sufficient. Alternatively, shimming—and also data acquisition—would be performed in synchrony with the breathing by using a trigger signal from a physiological monitor [24].

4 Radio Frequency (RF) Coils

Besides the static magnetic field and the spatial encoding with the gradient system, MRI requires transmission of RF pulses and reception of the MR signal from the sample or subject.

For signal excitation, the RF transmit resonator, or RF coil, sends RF pulses with a particular frequency, bandwidth, shape, duration, amplitude, and phase modulation to tilt the net magnetization vector oriented in parallel with the main magnetic field during equilibrium. B_0 (typically assigned as the Z-direction), is tilted into the perpendicular transverse (X-Y) plane by a given flip angle α. After excitation, the magnetization precesses back to equilibrium and induces a signal in the RF receive coil (for a comprehensive review *see* [25]).

Depending on the transmission and reception capabilities, three general types of RF coils are commonly used: (1) transmit-receive (Tx/Rx) or transceiver RF coils, (2) transmit-only (Tx) RF coils, and (3) receive-only (Rx) RF coils. These generally have two types of geometry: (1) volume RF coils and (2) surface RF coils. Both RF coil types and geometries determine the amount of tissue or organ coverage and sensitivity to the MR signal.

Volume RF resonators are designed to produce a uniform RF field over a large field-of-view (FOV), and are typically used as transmit-receive RF coils or transmit RF coils (using a surface RF coil for reception). The most widely used type of volume RF coils in both human and preclinical MRI are birdcage resonators [26, 27] driven in quadrature mode. This means that two spatially orthogonal RF channels are used for RF transmission as well as signal reception. This RF coil configuration provides a 41.4% SNR gain over simple single channel or "linear" RF coils, due to the coherent signal increases which scale linearly with the number of channels, while the incoherent noise increases with the square root of the number of channels. For example, Chang et al. [28] used this RF coil setup in a renal hypoxia study in a mouse model after myocardial infarction of different sizes using BOLD MRI. Other types of volume resonators include saddle RF coils, Helmholtz RF coils, and the transverse electromagnetic (TEM) resonators, among others.

Smaller anatomical coverage and FOVs, but enhanced SNR, are provided by surface RF coils. Due to the principle of reciprocity, the closer the position of the RF coil is to the tissue of interest, the higher is the attainable SNR. However, the sensitivity drops with increasing distance to the RF coil surface, which thus results in a reduced FOV, and an inhomogeneous sensitivity profile [29]. Within a short distance of typically up to ~1 cm, a surface RF coil outperforms a volume RF coil in terms of sensitivity. Since the kidneys are located beneath the skin, surface RF coils positioned directly above are used for optimal signal reception in renal MRI. This is advantageous not only for X-nuclei MR imaging (*see* Subheading 5) but also for other applications with low SNR, such as perfusion or diffusion-weighted imaging.

Surface RF coils may be used as transmit/receive devices or as receive-only RF coils in conjunction with a volume RF coil used for homogeneous RF transmission. The first option is technically very simple since only one RF coil is necessary, which occupies less space. In the case of small animal imaging, it is most likely a simple single-turn loop with at least two tunable capacitances for tuning and matching. Images will show a strong spatially varying SNR decay, due to the addition of the inhomogeneous excitation and reception profiles [30]. This effect may be mitigated, for example, by using adiabatic excitation RF pulses [31].

The second option involves the use of two RF coils (Tx: volume RF coil, Rx: surface RF coil) which are tuned to the same resonant frequency. To avoid RF coupling between both coils, the surface RF coil must be detuned during transmission while the volume RF coil must be detuned during reception. Thus, both RF coils must include an option, using active and passive diodes, to allow for tuning and detuning during the MR experiment. This is the most common setup, since it improves the SNR in comparison with a Tx/Rx volume RF coil, while still maintaining a homogeneous B_1. For example, Hüper et al. [32] used a four-element quadrature surface receive RF coil in combination with a transmit volume RF coil to investigate renal perfusion in acute and chronic renal allograft rejection in translational mouse models. The use of the surface RF coil improved the SNR from 15 (with a standard transceive volume RF coil) to 35.

Further SNR gains in small animal MRI are achieved with arrays of surface RF coils for signal reception [33], which are typically used together with a volume RF coil for signal excitation (*see* **Notes 3** and **4**). The use of RF coil arrays for brain imaging is especially widespread, and these are routinely offered by manufacturers. State-of-the-art small-animal MRI systems are usually equipped with 4–16 Rx channels, to which custom-tailored RF coils may be connected. Less popular are metamaterial-inspired RF coils, which have been developed for superficial tissue imaging in order to provide the best compromise of high SNR over a large FOV, while using only one receive channel [34].

Depending on the size of the sample and the RF coil, and their corresponding temperatures and resistances, their noise electronic contribution varies [35–37]. This factor is even more crucial in preclinical applications where the noise contribution of the RF coil, capacitors, sample, shield, receive electronics, and transmission lines are important [26]. This fact is exploited in small-animal imaging by the use of cryogenically cooled (cryo-cooled) RF coils. By lowering the temperature of the receiver chain, the noise contributions corresponding to temperatures and resistances can be reduced [38–40], thus achieving a significant increase in SNR, which has been reported in the literature (for a review *see* [15]). Unfortunately, only negligible effects are achieved in human MR [15, 41]. With increasing size of the sample, the relative contribution to the noise increases, and eventually becomes the dominating noise source—this is the default situation for human MR. Thus, only small animal MR applications will benefit from this cooling approach, since the noise contributions from the sample and RF coil are in the same order of magnitude. The SNR gain achieved with such cryo-cooled RF coils is higher at lower static magnetic fields [15, 26, 42]. A recognized limitation of cryo-cooled surface RF coils is that only transceive capabilities are supported, resulting in nonuniform excitation and reception profiles, which might hamper quantitative measurements.

Another option for the small-animal MR imaging of the kidney is the use of clinical scanners together with RF coils tailored for the human hand/wrist or knee. These are typically 8- to 16-element RF coil arrays which provide quasi-homogeneous excitation and reception profiles. Although these RF coils have a small size, they are not optimized for small-animal imaging and are not designed with matching/tuning capabilities. Moreover, RF coils tailored for rodent imaging are designed for a broad range of loadings (i.e., from almost empty to full loading, with a typical frequency-diameter product in the range 2–30 MHz · m [26]), in comparison to the clinical setups. Therefore, these clinical RF coils will achieve a lower efficiency than that of dedicated RF coils designed for preclinical MR systems. Alternatively, RF coils tailored for renal MRI of small rodents provided by RF coil manufactures can be connected with clinical MR scanners to enhance the fill factor and SNR.

In the following subsections, examples of possible RF coil setups are shown from different vendors. A list of the available MR system and RF coil vendors can be found in Table 2.

4.1 Commercially Available RF Coils Suitable for Kidney MRI in Rats

Due to the considerable anatomical homology with humans, rats have become one of the most commonly use rodents in animal research, particularly, in preclinical MRI. With a weight of 150–450 g, both clinical and preclinical MR systems and RF coils can be used to perform renal MR experiments:

Clinical MR System

- Tx/Rx wrist RF coil (e.g., Siemens eight-channel wrist RF coil, Fig. 3A).
- Tx/Rx knee RF coil (e.g., Siemens 15-channel knee RF coil, Fig. 3B).

Preclinical MR System

- Tx/Rx volume resonator (e.g., Bruker Biospin, Ettlingen, Germany, quadrature rat body RF coil with inner diameter (ID) = 72 mm (Fig. 3C), 82 mm or 86 mm; RAPID Biomed, Rimpar, Germany 2 × 4-channel volumetric rat array with ID = 72 mm).
- Tx/Rx quadrature volume resonator (e.g., MRI.TOOLS GmbH, Berlin, Germany, supporting an ID ranging from 54 mm to 86 mm and magnetic field strengths of 3.0 T, 4.7 T, 7.0 T, 9.4 T, and 11.T (Fig. 3D).
- Rx surface RF coil (e.g., 2 × 2 RAPID Biomed, Rimpar, Germany) rat cardiac surface array RF coil; 4 × 1 element (e.g., Bruker Biospin, Ettlingen, Germany) rat cardiac surface array RF coil, Fig. 3E) in combination with Tx volume resonator (e.g., Bruker rat body RF coils with ID 72 mm (Fig. 3F), 82 mm or 86 mm).

4.2 Commercially Available RF Coils Suitable for Kidney MRI in Mice

Mice are the most commonly used rodent in biomedical research. Their genetic similarity to humans has made them extremely useful, allowing the development of mouse models of many human diseases. Mice have an average weight of 15–40 g, making them too small for standard human RF coils:

Clinical System

- There are no standard human RF coils that are small enough to be suitable for mice MRI. Alternatively, a Tx/Rx quadrature volume resonator (MRI.TOOLS GmbH, Berlin, Germany), supporting an ID ranging from 30 mm to 45 mm and magnetic field strengths of 3.0 and 7.0 T can be used for renal MRI with clinical MR scanners (Fig. 4A).

Table 2
List of vendors of MR equipment and RF coils

	Vendor	Website
Clinical MRI	Canon Medical Systems	us.medical.canon
	General Electric Medical Systems Inc.	www.gehealthcare.com
	MRI Devices Corp.	www.allmri.com
	MR Instruments Inc.	www.mrinstruments.com
	MRI.TOOLS GmbH	www.mritools.de
	NOVA Medical Inc.	www.novamedical.com
	RAPID Biomedical GmbH	www.rapidbiomed.de
	Philips Medical Systems	www.medical.philips.com
	ScanMed	www.scanmed.com
	Siemens Medical Systems	www.siemens-healthineers.com
	Tesla Engineering Limited	www.tesla.co.uk
Preclinical MRI	Bruker BioSpin MRI GmbH	www.bruker.com
	Doty Scientific, Inc.	www.dotynmr.com
	MR Solutions	www.mrsolutions.com
	MRI.TOOLS GmbH	www.mritools.de
	RAPID Biomedical GmbH	www.rapidbiomed.de

Preclinical System

- Tx/Rx volume resonator (Bruker Biospin, Ettlingen, Germany) quadrature mouse body RF coil with ID = 35 mm, Fig. 4B); 2 × 4 -channel volumetric mouse array (RAPID Biomed, Rimpar, Germany) with 35 mm ID.
- Tx/Rx quadrature volume resonator (MRI.TOOLS GmbH, Berlin, Germany, supporting an ID ranging from 30 mm to 45 mm and magnetic field strengths of 3.0 T, 4.7 T, 7.0 T, 9.4 T, and 11.T (Fig. 4A).
- Rx surface RF coil (e.g., RAPID Biomed, Rimpar, Germany) 2 × 2 mouse cardiac surface array RF coil; 2 × 2 element mouse cardiac surface array RF coil (e.g., Bruker Biospin, Ettlingen, Germany, Fig. 4B) in combination with Tx volume resonator (e.g., Bruker Biospin, Ettlingen, Germany) quadrature mouse body RF coils with ID 72 mm (as shown in Fig. 4E), 82 mm or 86 mm).
- Tx/Rx 2 × 2 element array rat/mouse CryoProbe (e.g., Bruker Biospin, Ettlingen, Germany, Fig. 4C).

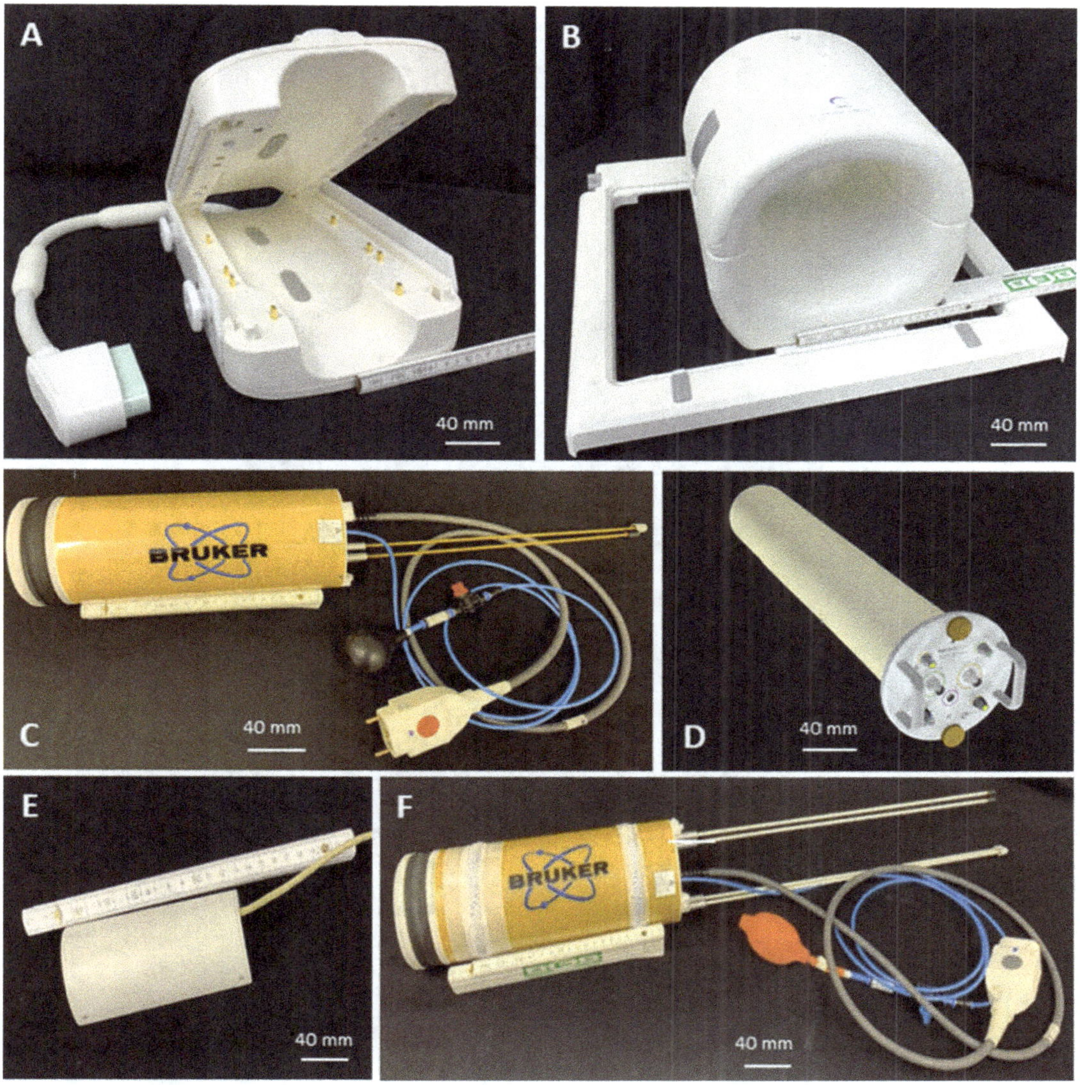

Fig. 3 Example RF coils suitable for kidney MRI of the rat. (**a**) Siemens 8-channel wrist RF coil, (**b**) Siemens 15-channel knee RF coil, (**c**) Bruker quadrature rat body RF coil with inner diameter (ID) 72 mm, (**d**) MRI.TOOLS GmbH quadrature rat body RF coil with ID of 72 mm, (**e**) 4 × 1 element Bruker rat cardiac Rx surface array RF coil, (**f**) Bruker rat body Tx volume resonator with ID 72 mm.

5 Multinuclear Imaging

The most frequent MRI method in biomedical research is proton (^{1}H) imaging. Hydrogen is the most abundant nucleus in living organisms. It also is the nucleus which is the most sensitive to interactions with an external magnetic field, due to its high gyromagnetic ratio ($\gamma = 42.576$ MHz/T).

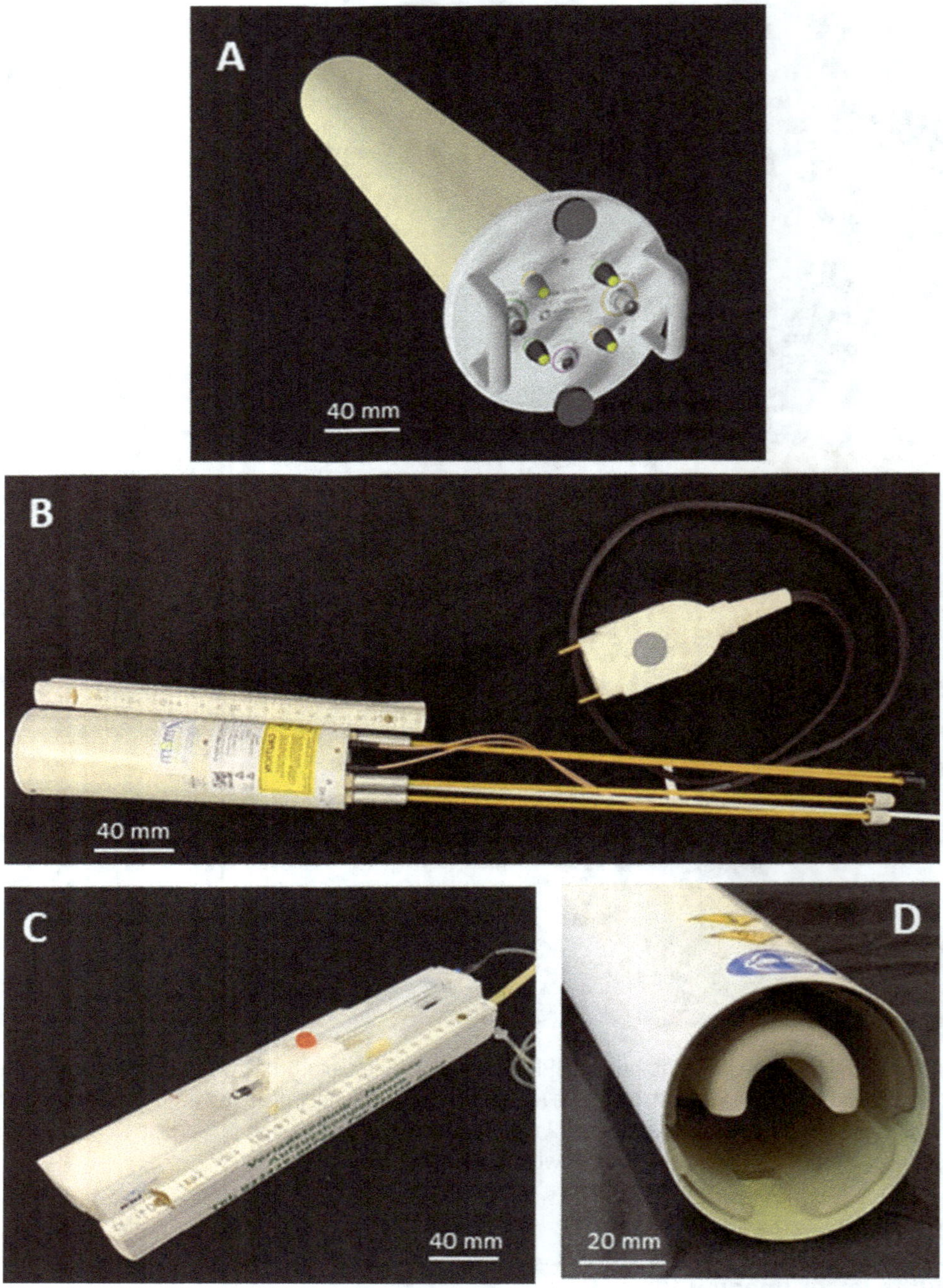

Fig. 4 Example RF coils suitable for kidney MRI of the mouse. (**a**) MRI.TOOLS GmbH quadrature mouse body RF coil with an ID = 42 mm, (**b**) Bruker quadrature mouse body RF coil with 35 mm ID, (**c**) Bruker 2 × 2 element mouse cardiac surface array RF coil, (**d**) Tx/Rx quadrature surface RF coil with cryo-cooling technology (CryoProbe)

In preclinical renal MRI, structural and functional information is typically investigated using in vivo ^{1}H MR imaging of the kidney. Techniques such as T_2/T_2* mapping, arterial spin labeling (ASL), dynamic contrast-enhanced imaging (DCE-MRI) or diffusion-weighted imaging (DWI) are performed in order to study the oxygenation, perfusion, clearance rate, and water and metabolite motion within the kidneys.

Physiometabolic probing is supported by imaging and spectroscopic applications of other nuclei such as ^{13}C, ^{17}O, ^{23}Na, ^{35}Cl, ^{39}K, ^{31}P, and ^{19}F [43]. The detection of X-nuclei is challenging because of the low intrinsic SNR due to the smaller γ, compared to ^{1}H, and by the lower abundance of these nuclei in biological tissues.

Increasing B_0 is the most effective way to increase sensitivity—the benefits of higher B_0 are unique metabolic and functional information, as well as outstanding anatomical detail [44–47]. X-nuclei MR also benefits from the increase in SNR achieved with cryo-cooled transceive surface RF coils, which are currently available for ^{13}C, ^{31}P, ^{19}F, and ^{1}H [48, 49].

Changes in the biodistribution of endogenous metabolites that can be detected with ^{23}Na- or ^{31}P-MR have been demonstrated to be markers of renal disease [50–53]. For more details on preclinical ^{23}Na-MRI protocols, see the chapters by Grist JT et al. "Sodium (^{23}Na) MRI of the Kidney: Basic Concept" and "Sodium (^{23}Na) MRI of the Kidney: Experimental Protocol." Similarly, renal perfusion, oxygenation, and inflammatory cell infiltration can be investigated using ^{19}F-MRI [54–57]. *See* the chapters by Grist JT et al. "Sodium (^{23}Na) MRI of the Kidney: Basic Concept" and "Sodium (^{23}Na) MRI of the Kidney: Experimental Protocol" on how to perform ^{19}F-MRI renal studies in rodents.

Hyperpolarization techniques have great potential for explorations into renal metabolic diseases (e.g., hyperpolarized ^{13}C-MRI), where SNR is boosted up to a 20,000-fold compared to conventional ^{13}C-MRI [58]. Experimental protocols to perform hyperpolarized ^{13}C-MRI in preclinical studies are provided in the chapters by von Morze C et al. "Hyperpolarized Carbon (^{13}C) MRI of the Kidneys: Basic Concept" and by Laustsen C et al. "Hyperpolarized Carbon (^{13}C) MRI of the Kidney: Experimental Protocol."

6 Physiological Monitoring

A major difference between clinical and preclinical MRI is the need to anesthetize the animals prior to imaging. Since most anaesthetic drugs produce physiological changes (temperature decrease, depression of cardiorespiratory function, etc.), monitoring the anaesthetized animals is a very crucial aspect in preclinical MRI studies. Even in the most simple case, that is, the scanning of spontaneously breathing animals without any further intervention or treatment, respiration and temperature of the animal has to be monitored continuously during the scan in order to guarantee the appropriate anaesthetic status and to avoid hypothermia. In particular, hypothermia is a critical issues in rodent imaging, since mice have a low mass vs. a large surface which promotes heat loss [59, 60]. This problem is less severe in rats due to their larger weight, but it is not negligible [61]. Heating systems must be therefore used to maintain temperature homeostasis.

Physiological monitoring of the animal is even more essential in functional MR imaging, since changes may produce confounding effects on the outcome of the MR experiment [62]. Careful monitoring and recording of physiological data should be performed at all times during the experiment to ensure the validity of the results and their reproducibility. The frequency of physiological monitoring depends on the invasiveness of the experimental procedure as well as the time after induction of anaesthesia. As a rule of thumb, the more invasive the procedure and the longer the time under anaesthesia, the more frequent the physiological monitoring of the animal should be performed. Additionally, the correct positioning of the animals on the animal bed systems, along with careful intubation (if needed) are essential to ensure respiratory and circulatory comfort during imaging, and to promote recovery of the animal after the experiment.

Typical physiological parameters monitored during MR experiments include temperature, heart rate, and respiration rate. Many manufacturers already offer these three monitoring channels, and are ready to use these signals for the purpose of gating or triggering the MR imaging techniques. Additionally, information on blood pressure, blood oxygen saturation, transcutaneous pCO_2, or pH can also be collected. In some cases, invasive withdrawal of blood samples is necessary—this is a very difficult task since the sampling has to be executed using long tubes with considerable dead volumes and very limited visual control.

Finally, all equipment must allow for remote physiological monitoring, and strictly comply with MR safety requirements. Several integrated animal handling solutions for physiological monitoring and anaesthesia are commercially available. Examples are given in Table 3.

7 Practical Points to Consider When Planning a Study

The aim of this chapter is to outline the main hardware components required for preclinical MRI of the kidney and to guide the appropriate hardware selection to meet the individual needs.

This section is intended to provide a summary of the prequisites needed and to help prepare for preclinical renal MR applications:

Table 3
Examples of commercially available equipment for physiological monitoring in preclinical MRI

Physiological parameter (s)	Examples of vendor equipment
Temperature	Omniflex (Neoptix, Inc., Canada) Fiber optic temperature probes (SA Instruments, Inc. Stony Brook, NY, USA) RightTemp (Kent Scientific Corp., Torrington, CT, USA) MultiSens (Opsens Solutions, Canada)
Respiration rate/ECG and gating	BioVet (m2m imaging, Cleveland, OH, USA) Model 1030 Monitoring & Gating system (Small Animall Instruments, Inc. Stony Brook, NY, USA)
Blood pressure	CODA monitor (Kent Scientific Corp., Torrington, CT, USA)
Blood oxygen saturation, heart rate	Pulse oximeter (SA Instruments, Inc. Stony Brook, NY, USA) MouseOx (STARR Life Sciences Corp., USA)
Transcutateous pCO_2	Capnograph (SA Instruments, Inc. Stony Brook, NY, USA) CapnoScan (Kent Scientific Corp., Torrington, CT, USA)
Several	PhysioSuite (Kent Scientific Corp., Torrington, CT, USA) PLUGSYS (Harvard Apparatus, Holliston, MA, USA)

7.1 MRI System

7.1.1 Clinical or Preclinical?

With a 3.0 T clinical MR system, renal MRI of rats is feasible with acceptable image quality and spatial resolution. However, if possible, we recommend to use a dedicated ultrahigh field MR system tailored for small-animal imaging with a magnetic field strength of 7.0 or 9.4 T. The reason is that the SNR gain achieved with preclinical MR scanners compared to that at lower B_0 is instrumental for achieving good spatial and temporal resolution, as well as for reducing the scan times needed to perform MR examinations.

7.1.2 Should I Consider Moving to a High Magnetic Field Strength?

As discussed above (*see* Subheading 2), the use of a higher magnetic field strength results in an increase in SNR proportional to B_0 ($SNR \propto B_0^{1.65}$). This means that renal MR images will achieve greater SNR that can be traded off for to achieve higher spatial resolution or reduced scan time as needed (*see* Table 1). Also, higher B_0 increases the BOLD effect. In general, all methods based on T_2*-weighting will benefit from an increase in the magnetic field strength. MR spectroscopy applications also profit from the increased B_0. Therefore, we strongly recommend the use of a high B_0 for these MR applications. However, not all facilities have such high field MR scanners readily available, in which case it might be advisable to perform the experiments using a lower magnetic field system, as opposed to moving animals, equipment, and personnel to another facility.

7.1.3 Higher Magnetic Fields Are All Rainbows and Unicorns, and Should Always Be Used, Right?

Not necessarily! Be aware that higher magnetic field strengths suffer from greater B_0 and B_1 inhomogeneities than lower field strengths, which must be corrected in order to fully benefit from the boost in SNR. Also, due to the B_0-dependent changes of the relaxation properties, the method-specific and protocol-specific imaging parameters have to be adopted in order to generate similar image contrasts that are comparable to those achieved at lower B_0. If the focus is the transfer of MR methods from preclinical models to clinical applications, use of the same static magnetic field strength is advisable. The "loss" of SNR may be partially compensated for by the use of cryo-cooled RF coils, which would be more cost-effective than the procurement of a high field small animal MR scanner.

7.1.4 OK, But ... Which B_0 Is Everyone Else Using?

The move to higher magnetic field strengths is supported by a large body of literature (see Figs. 1 and 2) which reports the most typical magnetic field strengths for rats to be 3.0 and 9.4 T and for mice to be 7.0 and 9.4 T. The continued use of 3.0 T scanners for rats is mainly due to the use of readily available clinical MR systems, which are then adapted for rat MR experiments. However, these are typically performed using hand/wrist or knee RF coils tailored for clinical applications in humans, and are not optimized for animal imaging, with the main disadvantages being a loss of signal due to incorrect loading, and the inability to match and tune the RF coil.

7.1.5 What About the Gradient System?

Depending on the MR application of your choice, a high gradient slew rate might be needed. Fast imaging techniques need fast gradient switching speeds, since this parameter influences the minimum achievable repetition time (TR), echo time (TE), and the echo spacing. However, a higher slew rate means a greater monetary investment will be needed at the acquisition of a new MR scanner. Equally, the duty cycle is a crucial parameter in hardware-demanding sequences, which generally includes all fast imaging techniques. We recommend the procurement of a gradient system tailored according to the individual experimental needs.

7.2 RF Coil Setup

7.2.1 Which Kind of RF Coil Should I Use to Get the Most Juice from My Clinical MR Scanner?

The best option is to use a hand/wrist RF coil; a knee RF coil is a second-best option. Both of these are RF coil arrays which provide high SNR and full FOV coverage. However, these RF coils are tailored for clinical applications in humans and are not optimized for animal imaging, with the main disadvantages being a loss of signal due to incorrect loading and the inability to match and tune the RF coil. Also, the clinical MR system must be adapted for rat MR experiments (mice are too small and do not provide enough loading in clinical systems). Alternatively, dedicated RF coils provided by RF coil vendors which are customized for renal MRI of rats can be connected to the clinical MR scanner.

7.2.2 Which RF Coil Setups Are the Most Suitable for Renal Applications in My Preclinical MR Scanner?

The anatomical position of the kidneys suggests placement of the RF coil in close proximity to the dorsal skin of the animal. We recommend the use of a surface RF coil for signal reception together with a volume RF coil for excitation. This is the most common setup since it improves the SNR in comparison with a Tx/Rx volume RF coil, while still maintaining a homogeneous B_1. Also, be aware that this setup needs the synchronized detuning of the RF coils in turns in order to avoid RF coupling between the two coils (the surface RF coil must be detuned during transmission while the volume RF coil must be detuned during reception).

7.3 X-Nuclei

7.3.1 What If I Want to Perform X-Nuclei MRI/MRS?

Broadband RF chains, including the transmission path and the receive path, together with RF coils specifically tailored for X-nuclei are needed. Due to the typically low SNR inherent to X-nuclei MR applications, a good option would be the use of a cryo-cooled RF coil. Imaging of a single kidney can be performed in mice using a mouse cryo-cooled RF coil. To image both kidneys simultaneously in mice, a rat cryo-cooled RF coil could be used. However, bear in mind that cryo-cooled RF coils are designed as transceive surface RF antennae, and provide inhomogeneous transmit and sensitivity profiles. Therefore, if your MR application needs exact T_1 contrasts or quantification based on absolute signal intensities, a B_1 correction must be performed.

7.4 Animal Handling and Physiological Monitoring

Please also *see* the chapter by Kaucsar T et al. "Preparation and Monitoring of Small Animals in Renal MRI."

7.4.1 How Should I Position the Rodent in the Animal Bed Prior to the Experiment?

This depends on the kind of RF coil being used. Typically, the kidneys are measured from the dorsal side using a combination of a volume RF coil for RF pulse transmission and a surface RF coil to receive the MR signal. The volume RF coil will be placed inside the bore and fixed, while the surface RF coil is typically displaceable or is fixed on the animal bed. The position of the animal will then be adapted according to this setup.

7.4.2 What Is the Essential Physiological Monitoring that Should Be Performed During Small-Animal Renal MR Experiments?

The essential physiological monitoring includes respiration, which is also used for triggering, and body temperature, which should be maintained at a normal level.

7.4.3 What Other Physiological Parameters Can I Measure, and Which Equipment Should I Use?

A wide variety of MR compatible equipment exists in the market that allows for measurement of temperature, respiration rate, blood pressure, blood oxygen saturation and respiration rate, and transcutaneous pCO_2, among others. *See* Table 3 for exemples of commercially available equipment for physiological monitoring in preclinical MRI.

7.5 Image Acquisition

7.5.1 Should I Perform B_0 Shimming in Every MR Study?

Preferably, yes. Active shimming protocols homogenize the B_0 field in a small region of interest, and help to improve the performance of T_2*-weighted MR protocols such as EPI. For performing MRS of the kidney (or any other organ), shimming should always be completed during the MR study adjustments. In general, we recommend to always perform shimming in every renal MR study.

7.5.2 Should I Always Do Triggering of the Signal? What Are my Options?

Renal MR imaging should be synchronized with animal respiration, preferably triggered to the exhalation phase [32, 63]. If possible, the animals should be allowed to breathe spontaneously under anaesthesia.

8 Notes

1. After the decade of the brain and the (re)discovery of the brain–heart–kidney network, a new era of kidney imaging is expected. The most important brain research tool is fMRI, and it has served as strong motivation for continued technological improvements in hardware development. Similar techniques are valuable for renal imaging. BOLD-based and BV/BF-based techniques greatly benefit from higher magnetic fields, providing a higher SNR, a higher CNR, and better spatial resolution. Nevertheless, the use of higher magnetic fields brings new problems that call for new hardware solutions.
2. Although there is an increased demand on gradient performance, this will exacerbate the problems associated with acoustic noise. New gradient designs should take into account the acoustic noise pressure level as a parameter. Gradient systems that are targeted to the region of interest only may be a solution. The higher gradient performance with increased bandwidth, as well as the increased physiological noise, reduce the gain in the SNR. A limit of the tissue contribution to thermal noise may be found by new RF coil designs.
3. Modern MRI systems come equipped with multiple receiver units allowing parallel acquisition. A combination of small, multielement receive-only RF coils with parallel imaging is a game changer in the way MRI data are acquired. Reducing the RF coil size will allow for the acquisition of data from a small region of interest with higher sensitivity, because of the close proximity of the RF coil to the region, and thus limited noise contribution from tissue. The use of multiple elements, which are decoupled from each other, will help to achieve extended tissue coverage.
4. A problem associated with parallel imaging arises in the storage and processing of large amounts of data. Therefore, considerable effort must be invested into the handling of "Big Data." Boosting the data transfer rate, the use of array processors and the application of renal MRI will push the limits of data science.

Acknowledgments

This work was funded in part (Thoralf Niendorf, Andreas Pohlmann) by the German Research Foundation (Gefoerdert durch die Deutsche Forschungsgemeinschaft (DFG), Projektnummer 394046635, SFB 1365, RENOPROTECTION. Funded by the Deutsche Forschungsgemeinschaft (DFG, German Research Foundation), Project number 394046635, SFB 1365, RENOPROTECTION).

This publication is based upon work from COST Action PARENCHIMA, supported by European Cooperation in Science and Technology (COST). COST (www.cost.eu) is a funding agency for research and innovation networks. COST Actions help connect research initiatives across Europe and enable scientists to enrich their ideas by sharing them with their peers. This boosts their research, career, and innovation.

PARENCHIMA (renalmri.org) is a community-driven Action in the COST program of the European Union, which unites more than 200 experts in renal MRI from 30 countries with the aim to improve the reproducibility and standardization of renal MRI biomarkers.

References

1. de Graaf RA, Brown PB, McIntyre S, Nixon TW, Behar KL, Rothman DL (2006) High magnetic field water and metabolite proton T_1 and T_2 relaxation in rat brain in vivo. Magn Reson Med 56(2):386–394. https://doi.org/10.1002/mrm.20946
2. Ladd ME (2018) The quest for higher sensitivity in MRI through higher magnetic fields. Z Med Phys 28(1):1–3. https://doi.org/10.1016/j.zemedi.2017.12.001
3. Moser E, Laistler E, Schmitt F, Kontaxis G (2017) Ultra-high field NMR and MRI—the role ofmagnet technology to iIncrease sensitivity and specificity. Front Phys 5:33. https://doi.org/10.3389/fphy.2017.00033
4. Niendorf T, Barth M, Kober F, Trattnig S (2016) From ultrahigh to extreme field magnetic resonance: where physics, biology and medicine meet. MAGMA 29(3):309–311. https://doi.org/10.1007/s10334-016-0564-1
5. Hoult DI (2000) Sensitivity and power deposition in a high-field imaging experiment. J Magn Reson Imaging 12:46–67. https://doi.org/10.1002/1522-2586(200007)12:1<46::AID-JMRI6>3.0.CO;2-D
6. Hoult DI, Richards RE (1976) The signal-to-noise ratio of the nuclear magnetic resonance experiment. J Magn Reson 24(1):71–85. https://doi.org/10.1016/0022-2364(76)90233-X
7. Pohmann R, Speck O, Scheffler K (2016) Signal-to-noise ratio and MR tissue parameters in human brain imaging at 3, 7, and 9.4 Tesla using current receive coil array. Magn Reson Med 75:801–809. https://doi.org/10.1002/mrm.25677
8. Guérin B, Villena JF, Polimeridis AG, Adalsteinsson E, Daniel L, White JK, Wald LL (1980) The ultimate signal-to-noise ratio in realistic body models. Magn Reson Med 78:1969–1980. https://doi.org/10.1002/mrm.26564
9. Merkle EM, Dale BM (2005) Abdominal MRI at 3.0 T: the basics revisited. Am J Roentgenol 186(6):1524–1532. https://doi.org/10.2214/AJR.05.0932
10. Rooney WD, Johnson G, Li X, Cohen ER, Kim SG, Ugurbil K, Springer CS (2007) Magnetic field and tissue dependencies of human brain longitudinal ^1H_2O relaxation *in vivo*. Magn Reson Med 57(2):308–318. https://doi.org/10.1002/mrm.21122
11. Seehafer JU, Kalthoff D, Farr TD, Wiedermann D, Hoehm M (2010) No increase of the blood oxygenation level-dependent functional magnetic resonance imaging signal with higher field strength: implications for

brain activation studies. J Neurosci 30 (15):5234–5241. https://doi.org/10.1523/JNEUROSCI.0844-10.2010

12. Schenck JF (1995) Imaging of brain iron by magnetic resonance: T_2 relaxation at different field strengths. J Neurol Sci 134:10–18. https://doi.org/10.1016/0022-510X(95)00203-E
13. Duyn JH (2012) The future of ultra-high field MRI and fMRI for study of the human brain. NeuroImage 62:1241–1248. https://doi.org/10.1016/j.neuroimage.2011.10.065
14. Baldanchani P, Naidich TP (2015) Ultra-high-field MR neuroimaging. Am J Neuroradiol 36 (7):1204–1215. https://doi.org/10.3174/ajnr.A4180
15. Niendorf T, Pohlmann A, Reimann HM, Waiczies H, Peper E, Huelnhagen T, Seeliger E, Schreiber A, Kettritz R, Strobel K, Ku MC, Waiczies S (2015) Advancing cardiovascular, neurovascular, and renal magnetic resonance imaging in small rodents using cryogenic radiofrequency coil technology. Front Pharmacol 6:255. https://doi.org/10.3389/fphar.2015.00255
16. Schick F (2005) Whole-body MRI at high field: technical limits and clinical potential. Eur Radiol 15(5):946–959. https://doi.org/10.1007/s00330-005-2678-0
17. Van de Moortele PF, Akgun C, Adriany G, Moeller S, Ritter J, Collins CM, Smith MB, Vaughan JT, Ugurbil K (2005) B_1 destructive interferences and spatial phase patterns at 7 T with a head transceiver array RF coil. Magn Reson Med 54:1503–1518. https://doi.org/10.1002/mrm.20708
18. Niendorf T, Graessl A, Thalhammer C, Dieringer MA, Kraus O, Santoro D, Fuchs K, Hezel F, Waiczies S, Ittermann B, Winter L (2013) Progress and promises of human cardiac magnetic resonance at ultrahigh fields: a physics perspective. J Magn Reson 229:208–222. https://doi.org/10.1016/j.jmr.2012.11.015
19. Fiedler T, Ladd ME, Bitz AK (2017) SAR simulations & safety. NeuroImage 168:33–58. https://doi.org/10.1016/j.neuroimage.2017.03.035
20. Stockmann JP, Wald LL (2018) In vivo B_0 field shimming methods for MRI at 7T. NeuroImage 168:71–87. https://doi.org/10.1016/j.neuroimage.2017.06.013
21. Juchem C, de Graaf RA (2016) B_0 magnetic field homogeneity and shimming for *in vivo* magnetic resonance spectroscopy. Anal Biochem 529:17–29. https://doi.org/10.1016/j.ab.2016.06.003
22. Pan JW, Lo KM, Hetherington HP (2012) Role of very high order and degree B_0 shimming for spectroscopic imaging of the human brain at 7 Tesla. Magn Reson Med 68 (4):1007–1017. https://doi.org/10.1002/mrm.24122
23. Motyka S, Moser P, Hingerl L, Hangel G, Heckova E, Strasser B, Eckstein K, Robinson SD, Poser BA, Gruber S, Trattnig S, Bogner W (2019) The influence of spatial resolution on the spectral quality and quantification accuracy of whole-brain MRSI at 1.5T, 3T, 7T, and 9.4T. Magn Reson Med 82(2):551–565. https://doi.org/10.1002/mrm.27746
24. Meyer A, Stolz K, Dreher W, Bergemann J, Thimmashetty VH, Lueschen N, Azizi Z, Khobragade V, Maedler K, Kuestermann E (2015) Manganese-mediated MRI signals correlate with functional β-cell mass during diabetes progression. Diabetes 64(6):2138–2147. https://doi.org/10.2337/db14-0864
25. Gruber B, Froeling M, Leiner T, Klomp DWJ (2018) RF coils: a practical guide for nonphysicists. J Magn Reson Imaging 48:590–604. https://doi.org/10.1002/jmri.26187
26. Doty FD, Entzminger G, Kulkarni J, Pamarthy K, Staab JP (2007) Radio frequency coil technology for small-animal MRI. NMR Biomed 20:304–325. https://doi.org/10.1002/nbm.1149
27. Lopez Rios N, Pouliot P, Papoutsis K, Foias A, Stikov N, Lesage F, Dehaes M, Cohen-Adad J (2018) Design and construction of an optimized transmit/receive hybrid birdcage resonator to improve full body images of medium-sized animals in 7T scanner. PLoS One 13(2):e0192035. https://doi.org/10.1371/journal.pone.0192035
28. Chang D, Wang YC, Xu TT, Peng XG, Cai Y, Wang L, Bai YY, Ju S (2017) Noninvasive identification of renal hypoxia in experimental myocardial infarctions of different sizes by using BOLD MR imaging in a mouse model. Radiology 286(1):129–139. https://doi.org/10.1148/radiol.2017161998
29. Wallner BK, Edelman RR, Bajakian RL, Kleefield J, Atkinson DJ, Mattle HP (1990) Signal normalization in surface-RF coil MR imaging. Am J Neuroradiol 11(6):1271–1272
30. Hayes CE, Axel L (1985) Noise performance of surface RF coils for magnetic resonance imaging at 1.5 T. Med Phys 12(5):604–607. https://doi.org/10.1118/1.595682
31. Garwood M, DelaBarre L (2001) The return of the frequency sweep: designing adiabatic pulses for contemporary NMR. J Magn Reson 153 (2):155–177. https://doi.org/10.1006/jmre.2001.2340

32. Hueper K, Schmidbauer M, Thorenz A, Bräsen JH, Gutberlet M, Mengel M, Hartung D, Chen R, Meier M, Haller H, Wacker F, Rong S, Gueler F (2017) Longitudinal evaluation of perfusion changes in acute and chronic renal allograft rejection using arterial spin labeling in translational mouse models. J Magn Reson Imaging 46(6):1664–1672. https://doi.org/10.1002/jmri.25713
33. Gareis D, Wichmann T, Lanz T, Melkus G, Horn M, Jakob PM (2007) Mouse MRI using phased-array RF coils. NMR Biomed 20 (3):326–334. https://doi.org/10.1002/nbm.1156
34. Zubkov M, Hurshkainen AA, Brui EA, Glybovski SB, Gulyaev V, Anisimov NV, Volkov DV, Pirogov YA, Melchakova IV (2018) Small-animal, whole-body imaging with metamaterial-inspired RF coil. NMR Biomed 31:e3952. https://doi.org/10.1002/nbm.3952
35. Hoult DI, Lauterbur PC (1979) The sensitivity of the zeugmatographic experiment involving human sample. J Magn Reson 34(2):425–433. https://doi.org/10.1016/0022-2364(79)90019-2
36. Edelstein WA, Glover GH, Hardy CJ, Redington RW (1986) The intrinsic signal-to-noise ratio in NMR imaging. Magn Reson Med 3 (4):604–618. https://doi.org/10.1002/mrm.1910030413
37. Marques JP, Simonis FFJ, Webb AG (2019) Low-field MRI: an MR physics perspective. J Magn Reson Imaging 49:1528–1542. https://doi.org/10.1002/jmri.26637
38. Kovacs H, Moskau D, Spraul M (2005) Cryogenically cooled probes—a leap in NMR technology. Prog Nucl Magn Reson Spectrosc 46:131–155. https://doi.org/10.1016/j.pnmrs.2005.03.001
39. Ratering D, Baltes C, Nordmeyer-Massner J, Marek D, Rudin M (2008) Performance of a 200-MHz cryogenic RF probe designed for MRI and MRS of the murine brain. Magn Reson Med 59:1440–1447. https://doi.org/10.1002/mrm.21629
40. Baltes C, Radzwill N, Bosshard S, Marek D, Rudin M (2009) Micro MRI of the mouse brain using a novel 400MHz cryogenic quadrature RF probe. NMR Biomed 22:834–842. https://doi.org/10.1002/nbm.1396
41. Xie L, Layton AT, Wang N, Larson PEZ, Zhang JL, Lee VS, Liu C, Johnson GA (2016) Dynamic contrast-enhanced quantitative susceptibility mapping with ultrashort echo time MRI for evaluating renal function. Am J Physiol Ren Physiol 310(2):F174–F182. https://doi.org/10.1152/ajprenal.00351.2015
42. Poirier-Quinot M, Ginefri JC, Girard O, Robert P, Darrasse L (2008) Performance of a miniature high-temperature superconducting (HTS) surface RF coil for in vivo microimaging of the mouse in a standard 1.5T clinical whole-body scanner. Magn Reson Med 60 (4):917–927. https://doi.org/10.1002/mrm.21605
43. Hu R, Kleimaier D, Malzacher M, Hoesl MAU, Paschke NK, Schad LR (2019) X-nuclei imaging: current state, technical challenges, and future directions. J Magn Reson Imaging 51(2):355–376. https://doi.org/10.1002/jmri.26780
44. Nagel AM, Umathum R, Rösler MB, Ladd ME, Litvak I, Gor'kov PL, Brey WW, Schepkin VD (2016) ^{39}K and ^{23}Na relaxation times and MRI of rat head at 21.1T. NMR Biomed 29:759–766. https://doi.org/10.1002/nbm.3528
45. Schepkin VD, Brey WW, Gor'kov PL, Grant SC (2010) Initial *in vivo* rodent sodium and proton MR imaging at 21.1 T. Magn Reson Imaging 28(3):400–407. https://doi.org/10.1016/j.mri.2009.10.002
46. Schepkin VD, Elumalai M, Kitchen JA, Qian C, Gor'kov PL, Brey WW (2014) In vivo chlorine and sodium MRI of rat brain at 21.1 T. MAGMA 27:63–70. https://doi.org/10.1007/s10334-013-0387-2
47. Waiczies S, Rosenberg JT, Kuehne A, Starke L, Ramos Delgado P, Millward JM, Prinz C, Periquito J, Pohlmann A, Niendorf T (2019) Fluorine19 MRI at 21.1 T: enhanced spin–lattice relaxation of perfluoro15crown5ether and sensitivity as demonstrated in *ex vivo* murine neuroinflammation. MAGMA 32:37–49. https://doi.org/10.1007/s10334-018-0710-z
48. Waiczies S, Millward JM, Starke L, Ramos Delgado P, Huelnhagen T, Prinz C, Marek D, Wecker D, Wissmann R, Koch S, Boehm-Sturm P, Waiczies H, Niendorf T, Pohlmann A (2017) Enhanced fluorine-19 MRI sensitivity using a cryogenic radiofrequency probe: technical developments and *ex vivo* demonstration in a mouse model of neuroinflammation. Sci Rep 7:9808. https://doi.org/10.1038/s41598-017-09622-2
49. Sack M, Wetterling F, Sartorius A, Ende G, Weber-Fahr W (2014) Signal-to-noise ratio of a mouse brain ^{13}C CryoProbe™ system in comparison with room temperature coils: spectroscopic phantom and *in vivo* results. NMR Biomed 27:709–715. https://doi.org/10.1002/nbm.3110

50. Boska MD, Meyerhoff DJ, Twieg DB, Karczmar GS, Matson GB, Weiner MW (1990) Image-guided ^{31}P magnetic resonance spectroscopy of normal and transplanted human kidneys. Kidney Int 38:294–300. https://doi.org/10.1038/ki.1990.199

51. Klemm A, Rzanny R, Fünfstück R, Werner W, Schubert J, Kaiser WA, Stein G (1998) ^{31}P-magnetic resonance spectroscopy (^{31}P-MRS) of human allografts after renal transplantation. Nephrol Dial Transplant 13 (12):3147–3152. https://doi.org/10.1093/ndt/13.12.3147

52. Maril N, Margalit R, Mispelter J, Degani H (2004) Functional sodium magnetic resonance imaging of the intact rat kidney. Kidney Int 65:927–935. https://doi.org/10.1111/j.1523-1755.2004.00475.x

53. Kalayciyan R, Wetterling F, Neudecker S, Haneder S, Gretz N, Schad LR (2013) Bilateral kidney sodium-MRI: enabling accurate quantification of renal sodium concentration through a two-element phased array system. J Magn Reson Imaging 38(3). https://doi.org/10.1002/jmri.24024

54. Pohlmann A, Schreiber A, Ku MC, Waiczies H, Kox S, Kettritz R, Waiczies S, Niendorf T (2014) Assessment of renal inflammatory cell infiltration in a murine ANCA-induced glomerulonephritis model by 19F-MRI. In: Joint Annual Meeting ISMRM-ESMRMB 2014, Milan, Italy. https://doi.org/10.13140/RG.2.1.4143.4326

55. Ruiz-Cabello J, Barnett BP, Bottomley PA, Bulte JWM (2011) Fluorine (^{19}F) MRS and MRI in biomedicine. NMR Biomed 24 (2):114–129. https://doi.org/10.1002/nbm.1570

56. Hitchens TK, Ye Q, Eytan DF, Janjic JM, Ahrens ET, Ho C (2011) ^{19}F MRI detection of acute allograft rejection with in vivo perfluorocarbon labeling of immune cells. Magn Reson Med 65(4):1144–1153. https://doi.org/10.1002/mrm.22702

57. Hu L, Chen J, Yang X, Senpan A, Allen JS, Yanaba N, Caruthers SD, Lanza GM, Hammerman MR, Wickline SA (2014) Assessing intrarenal nonperfusion and vascular leakage in acute kidney injury with multinuclear ^{1}H/^{19}F MRI and perfluorocarbon nanoparticles. Magn Reson Med 71:2186–2196. https://doi.org/10.1002/mrm.24851

58. Pedersen M, Ursprung S, Jensen JD, Jespersen B, Gallagher F, Lautsten C (2019) Hyperpolarised ^{13}CMRI metabolic and functional imaging: an emerging renal MR diagnostic modality. MAGMA 33(1):23–32. https://doi.org/10.1007/s10334-019-00801-y

59. Gordon CJ (2017) The mouse thermoregulatory system: its impact on translating biomedical data to humans. Physiol Behav 179:55–66. https://doi.org/10.1016/j.physbeh.2017.05.026

60. Reimann HM, Hentschel J, Marek J, Huelnhagen T, Todiras M, Kox S, Waiczies S, Hodge R, Bader M, Pohlmann A, Niendorf T (2016) Normothermic mouse functional MRI of acute focal thermostimulation for probing nociception. Sci Rep 6:17230. https://doi.org/10.1038/srep17230

61. Hitt BA, Mazze RI, Cook TL, Beppu WJ, Kosek JC (1977) Thermoregulatory defect in rats during anesthesia. Anesth Analg 56 (1):9–15. https://doi.org/10.1213/00000539-197701000-00006

62. Niles DJ, Gordon JW, Fain SB (2016) Effect of anesthesia on renal R_2* measured by blood oxygen level-dependent MRI. NMR Biomed 28(7):811–817. https://doi.org/10.1002/nbm.3314

63. Nikken JJ, Krestin GP (2007) MRI of the kidney-state of the art. Eur Radiol 17 (11):2780–2793. https://doi.org/10.1007/s00330-007-0701-3

8

Recommendations for Preclinical Renal MRI: A Comprehensive Open-Access Protocol Collection to Improve Training, Reproducibility, and Comparability of Studies

Andreas Pohlmann, Susan J. Back, Andrea Fekete, Iris Friedli, Stefanie Hectors, Neil Peter Jerome, Min-Chi Ku, Dario Livio Longo, Martin Meier, Jason M. Millward, João S. Periquito, Erdmann Seeliger, Suraj D. Serai, Sonia Waiczies, Steven Sourbron, Christoffer Laustsen, and Thoralf Niendorf

Abstract

Renal MRI holds incredible promise for making a quantum leap in improving diagnosis and care of patients with a multitude of diseases, by moving beyond the limitations and restrictions of current routine clinical practice. Clinical and preclinical renal MRI is advancing with ever increasing rapidity, and yet, aside from a few examples of renal MRI in routine use, it is still not good enough. Several roadblocks are still delaying the pace of progress, particularly inefficient education of renal MR researchers, and lack of harmonization of approaches that limits the sharing of results among multiple research groups.

Here we aim to address these limitations for preclinical renal MRI (predominantly in small animals), by providing a comprehensive collection of more than 40 publications that will serve as a foundational resource for preclinical renal MRI studies. This includes chapters describing the fundamental principles underlying a variety of renal MRI methods, step-by-step protocols for executing renal MRI studies, and detailed guides for data analysis. This collection will serve as a crucial part of a roadmap toward conducting renal MRI studies in a robust and reproducible way, that will promote the standardization and sharing of data.

This chapter is based upon work from the COST Action PARENCHIMA, a community-driven network funded by the European Cooperation in Science and Technology (COST) program of the European Union, which aims to improve the reproducibility and standardization of renal MRI biomarkers.

Key words Magnetic resonance imaging (MRI), Kidney, Animals, Acute kidney injury, Chronic kidney disease, Training, Standardization

Andreas Pohlmann and Thoralf Niendorf (eds.), *Preclinical MRI of the Kidney: Methods and Protocols*, Methods in Molecular Biology, vol. 2216, https://doi.org/10.1007/978-1-0716-0978-1_1,

1 Who Is Pulling the Brakes in Renal MRI?

1.1 Renal MRI in Clinical Practice—Fantasy, Dream, or Reality?

Magnetic resonance imaging (MRI) of the kidney is not brain surgery—it's better! It can save lives without invasive surgery, noninvasively. This statement—a play on Donald W McRobbie's "MRI is not rocket science, it's better" in *MRI From Picture to Proton*—is one that Dr. Susan Back, radiologist and director of Pediatric Genitourinary Imaging at the Children's Hospital of Philadelphia, would sign on to without hesitation. It's Thursday afternoon and she is just running an MRI scan on a 4-year-old boy with a left kidney urinary tract dilation, which was gradually increasing on ultrasound. This is the last sequence in the MRI protocol: a contrast-enhanced dynamic 3D T_1-weighted GRE sequence with a temporal resolution of ~8 s, used for quantitative functional urography [1]. Before, an anatomic T_2-weighted MR urogram [1] was performed to identify possible anatomic causes of obstruction (Fig. 1), which are difficult to find with ultrasound. These renal MRI data play a key role in the diagnosis and treatment decisions. The configuration of the kidney on the MRI is concerning for an ureteropelvic junction obstruction because there is an abrupt transition from the renal pelvis to the proximal ureter. However, having this anatomic image and the functional information generated

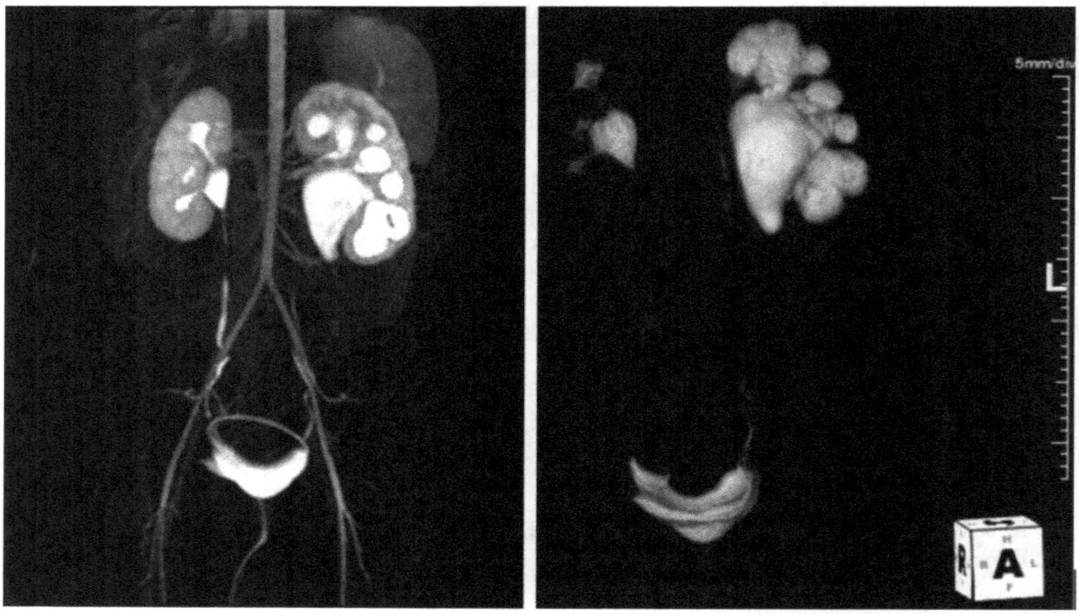

Fig. 1 Renal MRI used for diagnosis and treatment planning of a 4-year-old boy with a left kidney urinary tract dilation. The anatomic portion of the MR urogram study (left: postprocessed image created by superimposing the vascular/parenchymal enhancement phase with the renal excretion phase; right: 3D rendering) depicted the left urinary tract dilation with an abrupt transition in caliper between the dilated renal pelvis and the proximal ureter

using dynamic imaging shows good excretion and proves that the kidney is not obstructed. For the decision on whether to operate, the urologist takes a look at the quantitative functional information. Offline analysis of the dynamic data using the Parametric MRI software package (www.parametricmri.com) [2] provided a wide range of quantitative parameters for assessment of renal function, including renal transit time, calyceal transit time, volumetric differential renal function (vDRF), and Patlak differential renal function (pDRF). The other good news is that the left kidney is functioning similarly to the normal right kidney (vDRF: 48%/52%, pDRF: 49%/51%) so the urologist decides not to operate and the child would be put under observation.

While this scene of renal MRI in clinical routine use vividly illustrates the dream and ambition of many renal MRI researchers—clinicians (nephrologists, urologists, radiologists, surgeons, etc.), clinical scientists, MRI scientists, and basic scientists alike—it may, to the more realistic ones, be perhaps no more than a wild phantasy. However, for the vast majority of kidney patients worldwide, reality couldn't be more different: diagnosis and treatment decisions are predominantly based on plasma and urine parameters, that are known to be insensitive and unspecific. Information on increased serum creatinine is literally too little too late. Currently, the estimated glomerular filtration rate (eGFR; commonly calculated from serum creatinine including variables for age, gender, race) is "the best overall index of kidney function" [3], but it "is an unreliable tool to assess renal function in health and disease, as well as in clinical practice and research" [4]. It is like trying to study the complex bio system of the vast Amazon river basin solely by taking water samples at the mouth of the river.

1.2 Renal MRI, Where Are You?

Renal MRI undoubtedly holds great potential to improve diagnosis and care for millions of patients. The scientific literature reveals hundreds of renal MRI studies, both in patients and animals, aiming to demonstrate its clinical value, and to detail and validate the observed changes in functional and structural parameters. On reading the introductions of these studies we are typically being reminded of the millions of patients suffering from renal disease—acute kidney injuries (AKI) and chronic kidney diseases (CKD)—as well as the steadily growing number of diabetes patients of which many are inevitably en route to diabetic nephropathy. This is usually followed by highlighting the urgent need for more sensitive and specific bio markers, with renal MRI being a prime candidate. Yet renal MRI is still virtually absent from the radar screen of the nephrologist, and patients like those at the Children's Hospital of Philadelphia are a rare exception. What is going wrong?

1.3 Function, Function, Function

If the three most important characteristics that determine the value of a house are often considered to be "location, location, location," then the three most important characteristics of the kidney are "function, function, function"—rather than its structure/morphology. Morphology, however, is what conventional clinical MRI is all about in the vast majority of cases. Radiologists are trained to detect and identify the subtle deviations from "normal" morphology on grayscale images with different T_1 or $T_2(T_2^*)$ weighting. This leads to three challenges for renal MRI: (1) assessing functional images, for example of perfusion or blood oxygenation, requires new training and learning of what "normality" means; (2) almost all renal MRI techniques provide "exotic" pseudocolored parametric maps rather than conventional weighted images; (3) interpreting changes in these MR parameters in the context of the complex renal physiology is anything but trivial—in other words: we don't really know what they mean.

Particularly for the last point, preclinical research is crucial because it enables researchers to obtain from the same organ MRI data together with physiological parameters from invasive probes, as well as histological data. Obvious examples are the comparison of T_1 and ADC with the degree of fibrosis from histology [5], ASL perfusion with invasively measured renal blood flow and local flux, or T_2^* with invasively measured tissue oxygenation [6]. Moreover, in preclinical studies the application of (ir)reversible experimental interventions permits studying the complex relationships between MRI parameters and quantitative physiological parameters in the context of kidney-specific control of hemodynamics and oxygenation (*see* the chapter by Cantow K et al. "Reversible (Patho) Physiologically Relevant Test Interventions: Rationale and Examples"). Clearly, a lot more work needs to be done to establish and translate renal MRI into clinical practice, and preclinical research is an essential part of this process. Shedding some light on where we are with regard to research activity in MRI of the kidney may help us drive forward the development of renal MRI.

1.4 Research Activity in Renal MRI

Renal and cardiac MRI both started as niche applications, with their own unique challenges for clinical translation, ranging from acquisition to analysis and interpretation. Cardiac MRI has already become an established clinical tool, which is supported and driven by a dedicated international society (Society for Cardiovascular Magnetic Resonance (SCMR), scmr.org) and guided by >10 published consensus/position statements (scmr.org/page/guidelines). Renal MRI, on the other hand, is struggling to get off the ground.

Conceivably, this divergence is partially due to the usefulness of morphological MRI, which is rather different for both applications. Unlike cardiac MRI, with its workhorse - cardiac function assessment - being based on (cinematic) morphological images, renal MRI depends on multi-parametric structural and functional information, derived from T1, T2, BOLD, DWI, ASL, etc. A second reason might be the availability of treatment and the nature of the diseases. Due to the still rather limited treatment options for CKD, performing complicated and expensive MRI exams still seems less critical than in cardiac disease where there are more management options. It is expected that the emergence of new CKD treatments will stimulate the interest in renal MRI.

It is interesting to consider exactly how much clinical and preclinical research activity in cardiac and renal MRI there has been, and how it has grown over the years. Using publications listed in PubMed as an indicator, we performed tailored searches with PubMed's *Medical Subject Headings* (MeSH) to obtain lists of literature on renal/cardiac MRI in humans/animals (Fig. 2, upper panels). Additionally we used PubMed's *MeSH Major Topic* to restrict the searches to papers that focus on renal/cardiac MRI while excluding articles that only mention these terms but have another focus (Fig. 2, lower panels) (*see* **Note 1**).

The number of publications in both fields has grown considerably over the years, but at very different rates. Around 1000 cardiac MRI papers per year were published during 2014–2018; the equivalent number for renal MRI papers was only around 200. After restricting the search to papers with a main focus on MRI of the kidney/heart the number of papers per year were 400 and 70, respectively. In other words, a lot more research activity in renal MRI is needed. From the number of publications one can deduce that there is considerably more clinical research than preclinical research in renal MRI. Conceivably, this is partially due to the more limited availability of preclinical MRI systems. However, preclinical renal MRI has recently seen a rapid increase to 37% of all renal MRI publications. This highlights the importance of animal research in renal MRI, considering that only 5% of cardiac MRI papers are preclinical (as of 2018).

The *renal MRI research community* is still rather small. While a recent SCMR meeting attracted more than 1900 attendees [7], international meetings on renal MRI have had approximately 150–200 attendees [8, 9]. Around 200 experts in renal MRI from 30 countries are part of PARENCHIMA (renalmri.org), a community-driven Action in the COST program of the European Union, with the aim to improve the reproducibility and standardization of renal MRI biomarkers. In fact, the number of research groups active in preclinical renal MRI is only 1/5 of those active in clinical renal MRI (*see* **Note 2**). One important conclusion from this is that accelerating the development of renal MRI will require more researchers and institutions to enter the field. We may ask ourselves, "What hurdles are slowing down progress and impeding clinical translation?"

1.5 The Usual Suspects

For a novel MRI technique, the road to routine clinical use is a stony one, involving issues such as reimbursement, available time for MRI, evidence needed that the new method is superior to existing techniques, and availability of hardware/software and trained staff. However, most renal MRI techniques are still at an early phase of development. Here, learning how to correctly

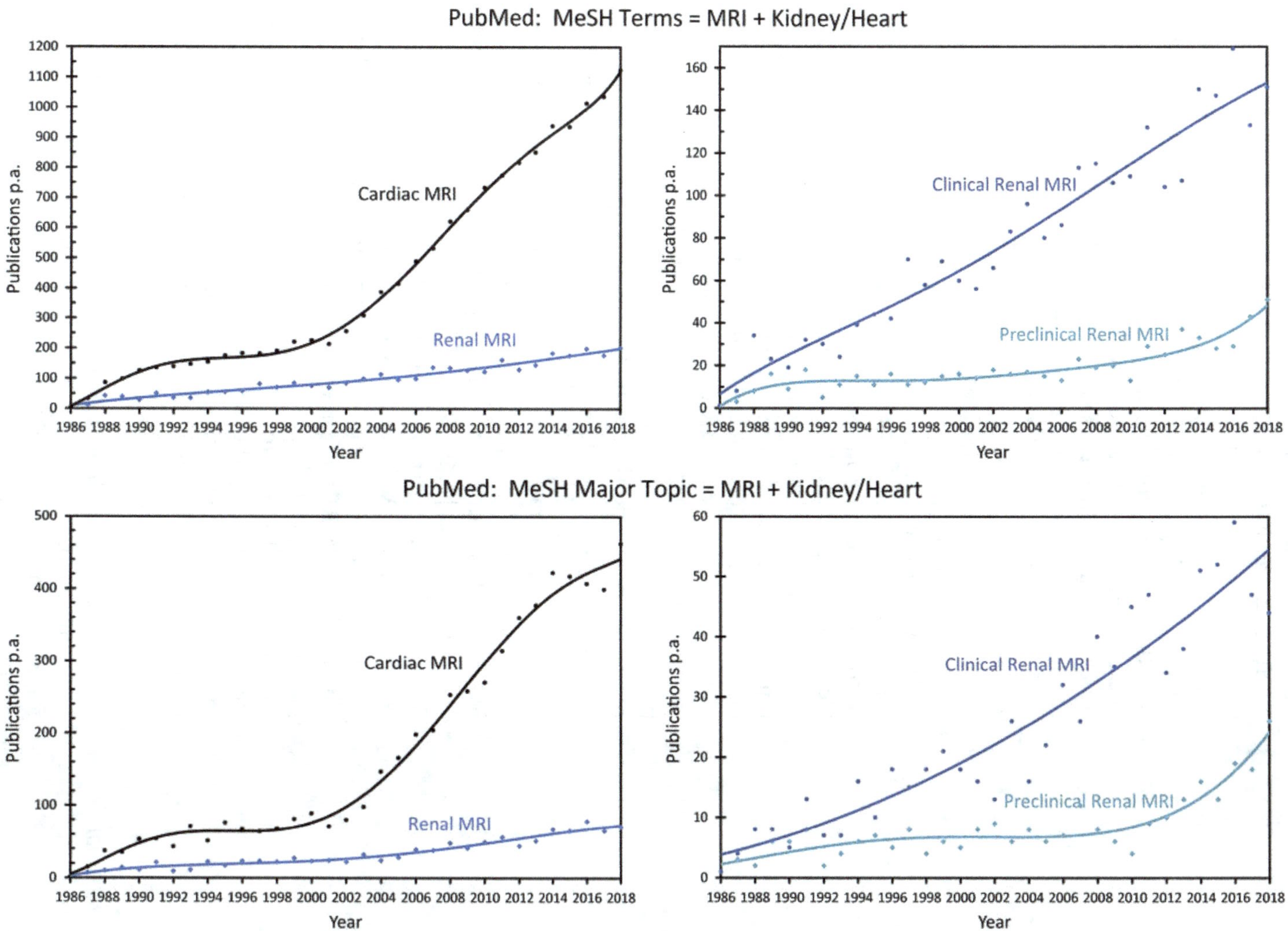

Fig. 2 Number of publications on renal or cardiac MRI over the years. Left panels: (pre)clinical renal MRI versus (pre)clinical cardiac MRI. Right panels: clinical renal MRI versus preclinical renal MRI. Lower panels: Search restricted to publications with the main focus on renal or cardiac MRI

interpret the MRI parameters (T_1, T_2*, ADC, etc.) and establishing normal ranges for these MRI parameters are only two of the items on the to-do list.

When searching for the culprits for the slow development of renal MRI, we also encounter the usual suspects: lack of training and standardization. This will sound familiar to most academic researchers. The workforce of academic research consists primarily of PhD students, who typically start their MRI research lacking the most relevant knowledge, and thus spend half or even more of their 3- to 4-year project learning the necessary theory, skills, hands-on experience and the many "secret tricks" that are essential for performing successful studies but are not found in the usual literature. This is problem #1: inefficient learning.

When designing a study, researchers encounter a further difficulty. Puzzled by the great variety of protocols (and diversity of equipment) in the literature, and often lacking an explanation for the choice of parameters, they are forced to design their study based on their own rationales and gut feelings. This is problem #2: lack of standardization. This not only hampers new researchers in setting up their studies but, even more devastatingly, has a detrimental effect on the comparability and reproducibility of research. This is a major obstacle to fast and efficient research and development.

When researchers finally publish their results, they do so in the usual format of a scientific paper, which focuses on a concise description of the problem, proposed solution, main findings, and a discussion of the meaning and limitations of the study. Important details about the practicalities of actually conducting the experiments are usually omitted. When individuals leave the lab, most of their crucial experience and expertise is lost. The cycle starts again with the next student.

2 How Can Training and Standardization Be Improved?

2.1 A Roadmap for Improved Training and Standardization of Renal MRI

Let's recap: the box of diagnostic tools available to the nephrologists is still rather poorly equipped (mostly insensitive and nonspecific plasma/urine markers), and renal MRI has the potential to be a game changer for the treatment of AKI and CKD. To address the numerous challenges of clinical translation of renal MRI, much more research activity is needed, and the community needs to grow. Among the factors preventing rapid progress are inefficient learning and lack of standardization. To overcome these roadblocks we suggest a roadmap for improving the training and standardization of preclinical and clinical renal MRI (Fig. 3). This combines protocol collections in the *Springer Protocols* book format with consensus-based technical recommendation papers based on the Delphi method.

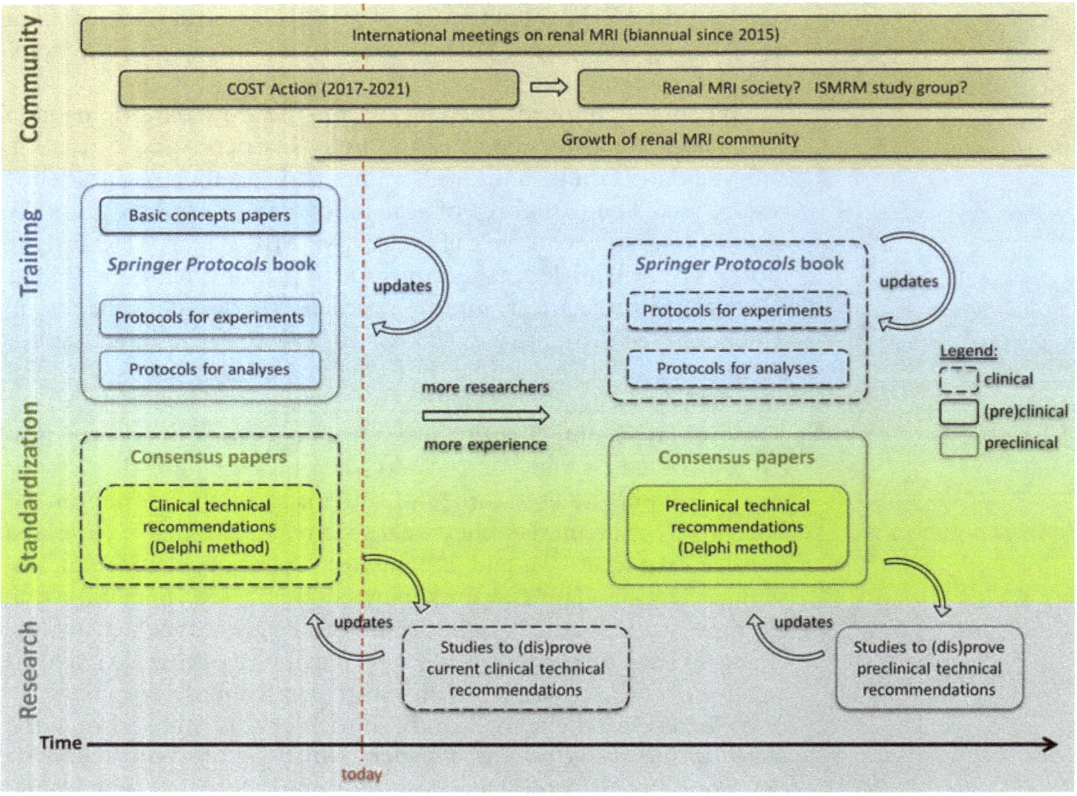

Fig. 3 Suggested roadmap for improving the training and standardization of preclinical and clinical renal MRI. It combines *Springer Protocols* books (excellent for training but also provides working protocols that help to improve comparability/standardization of future studies) with consensus-based technical recommendation papers (established tool to move toward standardization of studies). clinical = human MRI, (pre)-clinical = human and animal MRI, preclinical = animal MRI

Springer Protocols is "the world's largest collection of protocols of biomedical and life sciences," currently with over 58,000 step-by-step experimental protocols in more than 2000 books. The protocols are published individually as electronic publications in the PubMed cited journal *Methods in Molecular Biology* as well as in the form of printed books, with each book representing a collection of protocols for a specific topic. "Each protocol is provided in readily-reproducible step-by-step fashion, opening with an introductory overview, a list of the materials and reagents needed to complete the experiment, and followed by a detailed procedure that is supported with a helpful notes section offering tips and tricks of the trade as well as troubleshooting advice." [10]. This format makes *Springer Protocols* an excellent tool for training, and by providing working protocols, they also help to improve the reproducibility, comparability, and standardization of studies. Researchers are less likely to perform studies with "arbitrary" protocols and parameters when tested and proven protocols are readily available.

An established step toward standardization are consensus-based technical recommendation papers published as articles in technical journals. The process of developing expert consensus on technical aspects is a challenge. Here the Delphi method [11] can help to generate consensus statements: anonymous surveys that ensure all opinions are heard, free from peer pressure, are followed by rounds of face-to-face discussions. This iterative method permits "reaching reliable consensus in practice guidelines on health-care-related issues and on topics where there is little or no definitive evidence and where opinion is important" [12].

Because step-by-step protocols and technical recommendations address different ends of the training-standardization spectrum (Fig. 3), both perfectly complement each other. When deciding which step to take first, one needs to take into account the specific situation, that is, the size of the research community, the amount of hands-on experience available, the range of different equipment in use, the range of different subjects/objects being investigated, and so on. In these aspects clinical and preclinical renal MRI differ significantly. The number of research groups active in clinical renal MRI is five times the number of those active in preclinical renal MRI (*see* Subheading 1.4). In the clinical setting the range of setups (RF coils, field strengths) and subjects is much smaller than in preclinical settings. Even though we highlighted pediatric renal MRI in the introduction, the vast majority of renal MRI studies are performed on adult subjects at 1.5 or 3.0T. In preclinical renal MRI predominantly two species of very different size—mice and rats—are investigated at fields strengths of 3.0T, 4.7T, 7.0T, 9.4T, 11.7T, and 16.4T, with a wide range of RF coils ranging from human wrist coils to RX surface array + TX volume resonator combinations tailored for mouse or rat cardiac MRI, to cryogenically cooled TX/RX surface coils. These variations in setup influence numerous factors, including the achievable signal-to-noise ratio, the spatial resolution, and the relaxation times (T_1, T_2, T_2*), thus leading to substantially different MRI protocols. Both the great technical variety and the small size of the preclinical renal MRI community make reaching consensus-based technical recommendations particularly challenging, because many different sets of recommendations would be needed to address all commonly used study setups. Therefore, while consensus-based technical recommendations may be the natural first step for clinical renal MRI, for preclinical MRI we decided to focus instead on creating a comprehensive *Springer Protocols* collection to improve training and comparability of studies.

Both, consensus-based recommendations papers and protocols collections, can only be fully effective if they are made openly accessible. Therefore, we are very glad that it was possible to make these publications open-access thanks to support from the COST Action PARENCHIMA (renalmri.org).

2.2 Driving on the Road to more Efficient Renal MRI Research: Are We There Yet?

The answer is, of course, "not yet," as there is still some distance left to drive. But a giant leap has been made already, thanks to the COST Action PARENCHIMA (renalmri.org), which unites more than 200 experts in renal MRI from 30 countries, and the time, effort, and energy invested by more than 100 authors. After recent clinical position papers (https://academic.oup.com/ndt/issue/33/suppl_2) confirmed the demand, two projects have been implemented: The consensus-based technical recommendations for clinical translation of renal MRI (described in [12]) and the *Springer Protocols* book on preclinical renal MRI (described in Subheading 3).

Four papers present the results of applying the Delphi method to clinical renal MRI: arterial spin labeling (ASL) perfusion, blood oxygenation level dependent (BOLD) MRI, diffusion-weighed imaging (DWI), and mapping of renal T_1/T_2 [13–16]. This process generated over 160 consensus statements but also flagged topics where experts were currently unable to agree on a recommendation. These first ever technical recommendations for renal MRI should spark research into their appropriateness, with the aim to either prove or disprove specific recommendations. The findings of these future studies should then be fed back into updated and revised versions of the technical recommendations papers (Fig. 3). We hope that this approach will gradually lead to an alignment of the methods for measuring renal MRI biomarkers. It goes without saying that also the spectrum of methods covered must be extended in the future.

In the roadmap (Fig. 3), we propose to supplement these fresh off the press, already existing publications with the respective other parts, so that there will be step-by-step protocols as well as consensus-based technical recommendations available for both clinical and preclinical renal MRI. Here, the *Springer Protocols* for clinical MRI of the kidney are a placeholder for any type of protocol style journal, that is, *Methods in Molecular Biology (Springer Protocols)*, *Nature Protocols*, *Protocol Exchange*, *Journal of Visualized Experiments (JoVE)*, and so on. In contrast to the *Springer Protocols*, the latter permits independent publications on specific methods, which could be advantageous for clinical renal MRI, as it would not be necessary to publish protocols for many methods simultaneously. Needless to say, regularly updating all protocols and recommendations will be a challenging but, nevertheless, very important part of advancing the progress of renal MRI.

3 The Springer Protocols Book on Preclinical Renal MRI

Since Douglas Adams's *The Hitchhiker's Guide to the Galaxy* was first published in 1979, the number "42" has been claimed to be the answer to the question of "life, the universe, everything." After more than 2 years of hard work by 90 authors, the answer to the question, "How can we improve the training and standardization of preclinical renal MRI?" resulted in the 42 (other) chapters of this *Springer Protocols* book Pohlmann A, Niendorf T (eds) (2020) "Preclinical MRI of the Kidney—Methods and Protocols," Springer, New York. In the following subsections we describe the tailored concept of the book and the topics covered by the chapters.

3.1 Concept and Special Features of the Book

When we started to think about the structure and content of this book on preclinical renal MRI (with main focus on small animals), it immediately became clear that a simple collection of independent chapters would not suffice, for a multitude of reasons. First, there are many important aspects involved in renal MRI that are relevant to any MRI method: it does not make sense that for every individual method the protocol would include considerations and instructions regarding the MRI hardware, animal preparation, physiological monitoring, or image slice planning and shimming. Second, due to the complexity of MRI it is very challenging to include all the information about a method in a single chapter. If the book was to become a one-stop-shop for learning renal MRI in small animals, a concept was needed. In the following we describe its concept and special features.

3.1.1 Provide all the Necessary Information for each Method

With a few exceptions, we included three chapters for each renal MRI method:

1. There is one chapter describing the **basic concepts** of the method. We believe a sound understanding of the measurement concept is essential when planning, performing, analyzing, and interpreting a study. This is complemented by a brief **overview of the preclinical renal applications**, in order to illustrate for what kind of questions and applications each technique is useful for.
2. A **step-by-step experimental protocol**, which we know from the many existing *Springer Protocols* books. These protocols are the core of the book. For less complex methods they include also instructions for data analysis.
3. Detailed **step-by-step protocols for data analysis**.

3.1.2 Generalize Protocols by Peer Review

Although we trusted that each author had extensive experience and described the protocols correctly and in an understandable manner, we endeavored to make sure these were free from lab specific techniques, assumptions and limitations, which could be due, for example, to the (un)availability of equipment or traditions. Because these **protocols should also serve to move toward the harmonization of studies**, we felt it was important to ensure that the protocols were as universal as possible and would work in many labs and settings. For this reason we implemented a coauthor peer review process, that is, every chapter had to have one or several external coauthors from other laboratories. The roles of these coauthors are as follows:

1. To check whether the protocol would be applicable in other settings,
2. To check whether the steps and parameters are reasonable and their rationale clear and correct,
3. To add example protocols for additional lab settings.

3.1.3 Avoid Magic Numbers

Magic numbers—that is, numbers which are not explained and whose choice appears to be arbitrary—are not only a bad idea for software program codes but also for lab protocols. How often have we all read scientific publications and just could not figure out why the authors chose that particular set of measurement parameters! Was there a clever rationale behind their choice that sadly we didn't know, a lab tradition which might be reasonable but perhaps not applicable to our setting, or just a gut feeling of a student that didn't know how to make sense of all the different examples in the literature?

In any case, we wanted to reduce the magic numbers in our protocols to a minimum, so all authors were instructed to explain the rationales for their parameter choices in generic terms. If possible, advice for adapting them to other settings (other species, other field strengths) was to be given in the Notes section. Of course, example parameter sets are very valuable because they may allow readers to start straight away with a running protocol. They are also important in terms of harmonization, as mentioned. Therefore, examples of parameter sets for specific settings were requested, but separately in the Notes section, for example parameter sets for mice in a 7T MRI system and rats in a 9.4T system. For some techniques parameter sets for rats in a clinical 3T MRI system were also included.

3.1.4 Describe the Pragmatic Way for Data Analyses

It was important to us to dedicate separate chapters to the analyses because data analysis is an essential part of each study, but it is very rarely described in adequate detail. Statements like "T_2* was calculated by pixel-wise exponential fitting to the data using an in-house developed software written in MATLAB®" don't really help anyone who wants to learn how to analyze the data correctly. We are sure many of us have used similar statements in previous journal publications, but the fault is not always entirely ours: often there is simply no space (word limits!) and time to give a detailed description. Here, we wanted to make sure there was space (by having an entire chapter solely for the analysis) and time (by rewarding the effort and time spent in the detailed description with a first authorship).

It was key to present the most pragmatic approach to data analysis. What is the point in describing how to do your own code if there is established software available? So if analysis software existed, authors should describe how to get it and how to use it. Otherwise, the step-by-step instructions should focus on how to write a software program. Including pseudo code was encouraged, as well as providing downloadable code examples via GitHub or similar.

Finally, we asked to provide the readers with ideas on how to validate that their analyses give correct results. This could include for example a table of reference values or using synthetic test data.

3.1.5 Prevent Tunnel Vision—A Successful Study Needs More Than an MRI Protocol

Indeed, performing the actual MRI study is only part of the story. One must not forget that physiological MRI also requires consideration of many factors that are less important in anatomical imaging. Considerations about physiological monitoring, choosing the right animal model, measuring at the right time of the day, and using the most suitable anesthesia all have important implications.

For this reason, the first part of the book was dedicated to topics like animal models, preparation, monitoring and physiological interventions. We also questioned the need to always perform in vivo experiments on animals for training, development, and testing. Hence, one chapter provides a step-by-step protocol for the preparation of ex vivo rodent phantoms.

3.1.6 Embrace Competition—There Are Other Great Techniques Besides MRI

There are numerous questions for which it makes sense to go multimodal. Not only ultrasound and photoacoustic imaging but also invasive probes that provide quantitative physiological measurements are extremely valuable complements. Therefore, this book includes more than just MRI.

3.1.7 Make Access to This Information Free of Charge

Thanks to support from the COST Action PARENCHIMA (renalmri.org) it was possible to make all chapters open access!

3.2 Content of the Book

An overview of topics covered by the *Springer Protocols* book on preclinical renal MRI is shown in Fig. 4. Part II contains four chapters about animal models, preparation, monitoring, physiological interventions, and rodent phantoms. In Part III there are 13 chapters describing the basic concepts of the techniques, followed by Part IV with 14 step-by-step protocols for conducting experiments. Finally, Part V contains ten chapters that address data analysis; this includes the subsegmentation of the kidney into morphology-based regions of interest or concentric objects, as well as image denoising using nonlocal means (NLM) filtering.

More detailed information on the book structure and chapters is provided below by listing all chapters in the format [chapter

Topics	Part I	Part II	Part III	Part IV	Part V
Recommendations for Preclinical Renal MRI	Intro				
Animal Models of Renal Pathophysiology and Disease		Animals			
Preparation & Monitoring of Animals		Animals			
Reversible (Patho)physiological Test Interventions		Animals			
Ex Vivo Rodent Phantoms for Testing and Training		Animals			
Quantitative Physiological Measurements by Invasive Probes			Concept	Exp. Prot.	
Ultrasound & Photoacoustic Imaging			Concept		
MRI Hardware Considerations			Concept		
Essential Practical Steps (Slice Planning, Shimming)				Exp. Prot.	
Kidney Volume Measurement				Exp. Prot.	
T_1 Mapping			Concept	Exp. Prot.	Analysis
T_2 and T_2* Mapping (BOLD)			Concept	Exp. Prot.	Analysis
Diffusion (DWI, ADC, IVIM)			Concept	Exp. Prot.	Analysis
Dynamic Contrast-Enhanced (DCE)-derived Perfusion & Filtration			Concept	Exp. Prot.	Analysis
Arterial Spin Labelling (ASL) for Perfusion Measurement			Concept	Exp. Prot.	Analysis
pH Imaging by Chemical Exchange Saturation Transfer (CEST)			Concept	Exp. Prot.	Analysis
Sodium (^{23}Na) MRI			Concept	Exp. Prot.	Analysis
Hyperpolarized Carbon (^{13}C) MR			Concept	Exp. Prot.	Analysis
Fluorine (^{19}F) MR Methods for Functional Imaging			Concept		Analysis
Inflammatory Cell Assessment by Fluorine MRI				Exp. Prot.	
Oxygen Tension & Blood Volume Measurment with Fluorine MRI				Exp. Prot.	
MR Elastography			Concept	Exp. Prot.	
Subsegmentation of the Kidney (ROIs, concentric objects)					Analysis
Image Denoising for Improved Parametric Mapping					Analysis
	1	4	13	14	11

Fig. 4 Overview of topics covered by the *Springer Protocols* book on preclinical renal MRI. There are 4 chapters about animal models, preparation, monitoring, physiological interventions, and rodent phantoms; 13 chapters describing the basic concepts of the techniques; 14 chapters with step-by-step protocols for experiments, and 11 data analysis protocols

number] [chapter title] [author list]. Each chapter is PubMed-listed as an entry in *Methods Mol Biol.*

3.2.1 Part I—Introduction

1. *Recommendations for Preclinical Renal MRI: A Comprehensive Open-Access Protocol Collection to Improve Training, Reproducibility, and Comparability of Studies* (Andreas Pohlmann, Susan J. Back, Andrea Fekete, Iris Friedli, Stefanie Hectors, Neil Peter Jerome, Min-Chi Ku, Dario Livio Longo, Martin Meier, Jason M. Millward, João S. Periquito, Erdmann Seeliger, Suraj D. Serai, Sonia Waiczies, Steven Sourbron, Christoffer Laustsen, and Thoralf Niendorf).

3.2.2 Part II—Animal Models, Preparation, Monitoring, and Physiological Interventions

1. *Animal Models of Renal Pathophysiology and Disease* (Adam Hosszu, Tamas Kaucsar, Erdmann Seeliger, and Andrea Fekete).
2. *Preparation and Monitoring of Small Animals in Renal MRI* (Tamas Kaucsar, Adam Hosszu, Erdmann Seeliger, Henning M Reimann, and Andrea Fekete).

3. *Reversible (Patho)physiologically Relevant Test Interventions: Rationale and Examples* (Kathleen Cantow, Mechthild Ladwig-Wiegard, Bert Flemming, Andrea Fekete, Adam Hosszu, and Erdmann Seeliger).
4. *Preparation of Ex Vivo Rodent Phantoms for Developing, Testing, and Training MR Imaging of the Kidney and Other Organs* (Jason M. Millward, Joao Periquito, Paula Ramos Delgado, Christian Prinz, Thoralf Niendorf, and Sonia Waiczies).

3.2.3 Part III—Basic Concepts of Measurement Techniques

5. *Quantitative Assessment of Renal Perfusion and Oxygenation by Invasive Probes: Basic Concepts* (Kathleen Cantow, Roger G. Evans, Dirk Grosenick, Thomas Gladytz, Thoralf Niendorf, Bert Flemming, and Erdmann Seeliger).
6. *Ultrasound and Photoacoustic Imaging of the Kidney: Basic Concepts and Protocols* (Sandra Meyer and Dieter Fuchs Martin Meier).
7. *Hardware Considerations for Preclinical Magnetic Resonance of the Kidney* (Paula Ramos Delgado, Ekkehard Küstermann, André Kühne, Thoralf Niendorf, Andreas Pohlmann, and Martin Meier).
8. *MRI Mapping of Renal T_1: Basic Concepts* (Stefanie Hectors, Sabrina Doblas, Philippe Garteiser, Gwenaël Pagé, Bernard E. Van Beers, John C Waterton, and Octavia Bane).
9. *MRI Mapping of the Blood Oxygenation Sensitive Parameter T_2* in the Kidney: Basic Concepts* (Lu-Ping Li, Bradley Hack, Erdmann Seeliger, and Pottumarthi V. Prasad).
10. *Renal Diffusion Weighted Imaging (DWI) for Apparent Diffusion Coefficient (ADC), Intravoxel Incoherent Motion (IVIM), and Diffusion Tensor Imaging (DTI): Basic Concepts* (Neil Peter Jerome, Anna Caroli, and Alexandra Ljimani).
11. *Dynamic Contrast Enhancement (DCE) MRI–Derived Renal Perfusion and Filtration: Basic Concepts* (Michael Pedersen, Pietro Irrera, Walter Dastrù, Frank G Zöllner, Kevin M Bennett, Scott C Beeman, G Larry Bretthorst, Joel R Garbow, and Dario Livio Longo).
12. *Noninvasive Renal Perfusion Measurement Using Arterial Spin Labeling (ASL) MRI: Basic Concepts* (Min-Chi Ku, María A Fernández-Seara, Frank Kober, and Thoralf Niendorf).
13. *Renal pH Imaging Using Chemical Exchange Saturation Transfer (CEST)-MRI: Basic Concepts* (Dario Livio Longo, Pietro Irrera, Lorena Consolino, Phillip Zhe Sun, and Michael T. McMahon).
14. *Sodium (^{23}Na) MRI of the Kidney: Basic Concepts* (James T. Grist, Esben Søvsø Hansen, Frank G. Zöllner, and Christoffer Laustsen).

15. *Hyperpolarized Carbon (^{13}C) MRI of the Kidneys: Basic Concepts* (Cornelius von Morze, Galen D. Reed, Zhen J. Wang, Michael A. Ohliger, and Christoffer Laustsen).
16. *Functional Imaging Using Fluorine (^{19}F) MR Methods: Basic Concepts* (Sonia Waiczies, Christian Prinz, Ludger Starke, Jason M. Millward, Paula Ramos Delgado, Jens Rosenberg, Marc Nazaré, Helmar Waiczies, Andreas Pohlmann, and Thoralf Niendorf).
17. *MR Elastography of the Abdomen: Basic Concepts* (Suraj D. Serai and Meng Yin).

3.2.4 Part IV—Experimental Protocols

18. *Monitoring Renal Hemodynamics and Oxygenation by Invasive Probes: Experimental Protocol* (Kathleen Cantow, Mechthild Ladwig-Wiegard, Bert Flemming, Andreas Pohlmann, Thoralf Niendorf, and Erdmann Seeliger).
19. *Essential Practical Steps for MRI of the Kidney in Experimental Research* (Andreas Pohlmann, João dos Santos Periquito, and Thoralf Niendorf).
20. *Assessment of Renal Volume with MRI: Experimental Protocol* (Andreas Müller and Martin Meier).
21. *Experimental Protocols for MRI Mapping of Renal T_1* (Philippe Garteiser, Octavia Bane, Sabrina Doblas, Iris Friedli, Stefanie Hectors, Gwenaël Pagé, Bernard E. Van Beers, and John C. Waterton).
22. *Experimental Protocols for Mapping of Renal T_2* and T_2* (Andreas Pohlmann, Kaixuan Zhao, Sean B. Fain, Pottumarthi V. Prasad, and Thoralf Niendorf).
23. *Renal MRI Diffusion: Experimental Protocol* (João S. Periquito, Martin Meier, Thoralf Niendorf, Andreas Pohlmann, and Neil Peter Jerome).
24. *Dynamic Contrast Enhanced (DCE) MRI–Derived Renal Perfusion and Filtration: Experimental Protocol* (Pietro Irrera, Lorena Consolino, Walter Dastrù, Michael Pedersen, Frank G. Zöllner, and Dario Livio Longo).
25. *Renal Blood Flow Using Arterial Spin Labeling (ASL) MRI: Experimental Protocol and Principles* (Kai-Hsiang Chuang, Martin Meier, María A Fernández-Seara, Frank Kober, and Min-Chi Ku).
26. *Renal pH Mapping Using Chemical Exchange Saturation Transfer (CEST) MRI: Experimental Protocol* (Kowsalya Devi Pavuluri, Lorena Consolino, Dario Livio Longo, Pietro Irrera, Phillip Zhe Sun, and Michael T. McMahon).

27. *Sodium (^{23}Na) MRI of the Kidney: Experimental Protocol* (James T. Grist, Esben Søvsø Hansen, Frank G. Zöllner, and Christoffer Laustsen).
28. *Hyperpolarized Carbon (^{13}C) MRI of the Kidney: Experimental Protocol* (Christoffer Laustsen, Cornelius von Morze, and Galen Reed).
29. *Fluorine (^{19}F) MRI for Assessing Inflammatory Cells in the Kidney: Experimental Protocol* (Min-Chi Ku, Adrian Schreiber, Paula Ramos Delgado, Philipp Boehm-Sturm, Ralph Kettritz, Thoralf Niendorf, Andreas Pohlmann, and Sonia Waiczies).
30. *Fluorine (^{19}F) MRI to Measure Renal Oxygen Tension and Blood Volume: Experimental Protocol* (Lingzhi Hu, Hua Pan, and Samuel A. Wickline).
31. *MR Elastography of the Abdomen: Experimental Protocols* (Suraj D. Serai and Meng Yin).

3.2.5 Part V—Protocols for Advanced Analyses

32. *Subsegmentation of the Kidney in Experimental MR Images Using Morphology-Based Regions of Interest or Multiple-Layer Concentric Objects* (Leili Riazy, Bastien Milani, João S. Periquito, Kathleen Cantow, Thoralf Niendorf, Menno Pruijm, Erdmann Seeliger, and Andreas Pohlmann).
33. *Denoising for Improved Parametric MRI of the Kidney: Protocol for Nonlocal Means Filtering* (Ludger Starke, Karsten Tabelow, Thoralf Niendorf, and Andreas Pohlmann).
34. *Analysis Protocols for MRI Mapping of Renal T_1* (Philippe Garteiser, Gwenaël Pagé, Sabrina Doblas, Octavia Bane, Stefanie Hectors, Iris Friedli, Bernard E. Van Beers, and John C. Waterton).
35. *Analysis Protocols for MRI Mapping of the Blood Oxygenation Sensitive Parameters T_2* and T_2 in the Kidney* (João S. Periquito, Ludger Starke, Carlota M. Santos, Andreia C. Freitas, Nuno Loução, Pablo García Polo, Rita G. Nunes, Thoralf Niendorf, and Andreas Pohlmann).
36. *Analysis of Renal Diffusion Weighted Imaging (DWI) Using Apparent Diffusion Coefficient (ADC) and Intravoxel Incoherent Motion (IVIM) Models* (Neil Peter Jerome and João S. Periquito).
37. *Analysis Protocol for Dynamic Contrast Enhanced (DCE) MRI of Renal Perfusion and Filtration* (Frank G. Zöllner, Walter Dastrù, Pietro Irrera, Dario Livio Longo, Kevin M Bennett, Scott C. Beeman, G. Larry Bretthorst, and Joel R. Garbow).
38. *Quantitative Analysis of Renal Perfusion by Arterial Spin Labeling* (Kai-Hsiang Chuang, Frank Kober, and Min-Chi Ku).

39. *Analysis Protocol for the Quantification of Renal pH Using Chemical Exchange Saturation Transfer (CEST) MRI* (Hahnsung Kim, Yin Wu, Daisy Villano, Dario Livio Longo, Michael T. McMahon, and Phillip Zhe Sun).
40. *Analysis Protocol for Renal Sodium (^{23}Na) MR Imaging* (James T. Grist, Esben Søvsø Hansen, Frank G. Zöllner, and Christoffer Laustsen).
41. *Analysis Methods for Hyperpolarized Carbon (^{13}C) MRI of the Kidney* (Galen D. Reed, Natalie J. Korn, Christoffer Laustsen, and Cornelius von Morze).
42. *Data Preparation Protocol for Low Signal-to-Noise Ratio Fluorine-19 MRI* (Ludger Starke, Thoralf Niendorf, and Sonia Waiczies).

3.3 Mission and Vision

The mission of this book was to bring together in one collection a comprehensive assortment of protocols, methods, techniques, and recommendations that can form a cornerstone of preclinical renal MR. This collection will serve as an excellent starting point for new researchers interested in breaking into the renal MR field. Expanding the number of researchers is absolutely critical for realizing the full potential of renal MR. By providing a set of carefully constructed protocols, we can avoid the waste of time, money and resources by no longer "re-inventing the wheel." This collection will also greatly facilitate the harmonization of studies, and promote the sharing of data and results across multiple research groups, by getting everyone onto the "same page." These efforts will help us break through those bottlenecks of inefficient learning and lack of standardization. The road ahead to fully realize the scientific and clinical possibilities of renal MR remains long, but the end result will be well worth the effort.

4 Notes

1. The search string for clinical renal MRI was as follows: `((("magnetic resonance imaging"[MeSH Terms]) AND "kidney"[MeSH Terms]) AND "humans "[MeSH Terms])`. For preclinical renal MRI the last AND term was replaced with `AND "animals"[MeSH Terms]) NOT "humans"[MeSH Terms]`. For cardiac MRI the word "`kidney`" was replaced with the word "`heart`." For restricting the search to papers with a main focus on MRI of the kidney/heart `MeSH Terms` was replaced with `MeSH Major Topic`: `((("magnetic resonance imaging"[MeSH Major Topic]) AND "kidney"[-MeSH Major Topic]))` .... We used PubMed's MeSH terms rather than free text search in the title/abstract to reduce the number of false positive/negative search results. However, a

drawback of using MeSH terms is that the indexing process takes rather long (several studies reported average delays of 100–150 days), but it may take significantly longer in some cases. For example, we found that several of our publications from 2017 and after were not yet MeSH indexed. Hence, the presented publication statistics can only be rough estimates of the true numbers of publications. Data for the year 2019 was excluded, because most PubMed listed publications on renal MRI had not been indexed with MeSH Terms yet.

2. We further exploited the publication lists obtained from the above PubMed's searches. We defined *active researchers* as anyone who published on renal MRI since 2015. After exporting the date-restricted publications lists from PubMed in XML format, we used an in-house developed software to extract the affiliations of the first and last authors—these research groups (departments of hospitals and academic institutions were counted individually) were considered to be *active players in renal MRI.* Duplicates were removed automatically (using Matlab's *unique()* function) and manually. The limitations mentioned in **Note 1** also apply here: due to the incomplete MeSH indexing the derived statistics are only rough estimates and data of 2019 could not be included.

Acknowledgments

This work was funded, in part (Thoralf Niendorf, Sonia Waiczies, Andreas Pohlmann, Erdmann Seeliger and Joao Periquito), by the German Research Foundation (Gefoerdert durch die Deutsche Forschungsgemeinschaft (DFG), Projektnummer 394046635, SFB 1365, RENOPROTECTION. Funded by the Deutsche Forschungsgemeinschaft (DFG, German Research Foundation), Project number 394046635, SFB 1365, RENOPROTECTION).

This chapter is based upon the work from COST Action PAR ENCHIMA, supported by European Cooperation in Science and Technology (COST). COST (www.cost.eu) is a funding agency for research and innovation networks. COST Actions help connect research initiatives across Europe and enable scientists to enrich their ideas by sharing them with their peers. This boosts their research, career, and innovation.

PARENCHIMA (renalmri.org) is a community-driven Action in the COST program of the European Union, which unites more than 200 experts in renal MRI from 30 countries with the aim to improve the reproducibility and standardization of renal MRI biomarkers.

References

1. Dickerson EC, Dillman JR, Smith EA, DiPietro MA, Lebowitz RL, Darge K (2015) Pediatric MR urography: indications, techniques, and approach to review. Radiographics 35 (4):1208–1230. https://doi.org/10.1148/rg.2015140223
2. Khrichenko D, Darge K (2010) Functional analysis in MR urography—made simple. Pediatr Radiol 40(2):182–199. https://doi.org/10.1007/s00247-009-1458-4
3. National Kidney Foundation NY, USA. https://www.kidney.org/professionals/kdoqi/gfr_calculator. Accessed 07 Jan 2020
4. Porrini E, Ruggenenti P, Luis-Lima S, Carrara F, Jimenez A, de Vries APJ, Torres A, Gaspari F, Remuzzi G (2019) Estimated GFR: time for a critical appraisal. Nat Rev Nephrol 15(3):177–190. https://doi.org/10.1038/s41581-018-0080-9
5. Friedli I, Crowe LA, Berchtold L, Moll S, Hadaya K, de Perrot T, Vesin C, Martin PY, de Seigneux S, Vallee JP (2016) New magnetic resonance imaging index for renal fibrosis assessment: a comparison between diffusion-weighted imaging and T1 mapping with histological validation. Sci Rep 6:30088. https://doi.org/10.1038/srep30088
6. Pohlmann A, Arakelyan K, Hentschel J, Cantow K, Flemming B, Ladwig M, Waiczies S, Seeliger E, Niendorf T (2014) Detailing the relation between renal T2* and renal tissue pO2 using an integrated approach of parametric magnetic resonance imaging and invasive physiological measurements. Investig Radiol 49(8):547–560. https://doi.org/10.1097/RLI.0000000000000054
7. SCMR (2018) The Society for Cardiovascular Magnetic Resonance—News 2018. scmr.org/page/CMR2018news. Accessed 07 Jan 2020
8. Pohlmann A, Seeliger E, Grosenick D, Waiczies S, Cantow K, Persson PB, Niendorf T (2017) 2nd International Scientific Symposium on Functional Renal Imaging: Where Physiology, Nephrology, Radiology and Physics Meet. www.mdc-berlin.de/renal. Accessed 07 Feb 2020
9. Francis S, Taal M, Selby N (2019) 3rd International Symposium on Functional Renal Imaging. www.nottingham.ac.uk/go/3rdrenalmri. Accessed 07 Feb 2020
10. SpringerNature Springer Protocols. www.springernature.com/gp/librarians/products/product-types/database/springerprotocols. Accessed 10 Feb 2020
11. Dalkey N, Helmer O (1963) An experimental application of the DELPHI method to the use of experts. Manag Sci 9(3):458–467. https://doi.org/10.1287/mnsc.9.3.458
12. Mendichovszky I, Pullens P, Dekkers I, Nery F, Bane O, Pohlmann A, de Boer A, Ljimani A, Odudu A, Buchanan C, Sharma K, Laustsen C, Harteveld A, Golay X, Pedrosa I, Alsop D, Fain S, Caroli A, Prasad P, Francis S, Sigmund E, Fernandez-Seara M, Sourbron S (2020) Technical recommendations for clinical translation of renal MRI: a consensus project of the cooperation in science and technology action PARENCHIMA. MAGMA 33 (1):131–140. https://doi.org/10.1007/s10334-019-00784-w
13. Nery F, Buchanan CE, Harteveld AA, Odudu A, Bane O, Cox EF, Derlin K, Gach HM, Golay X, Gutberlet M, Laustsen C, Ljimani A, Madhuranthakam AJ, Pedrosa I, Prasad PV, Robson PM, Sharma K, Sourbron S, Taso M, Thomas DL, Wang DJJ, Zhang JL, Alsop DC, Fain SB, Francis ST, Fernandez-Seara MA (2020) Consensus-based technical recommendations for clinical translation of renal ASL MRI. MAGMA 33 (1):1–21. https://doi.org/10.1007/s10334-019-00800-z
14. Bane O, Mendichovszky IA, Milani B, Dekkers IA, Deux JF, Eckerbom P, Grenier N, Hall ME, Inoue T, Laustsen C, Lerman LO, Liu C, Morrell G, Pedersen M, Pruijm M, Sadowski EA, Seeliger E, Sharma K, Thoeny H, Vermathen P, Wang ZJ, Serafin Z, Zhang JL, Francis ST, Sourbron S, Pohlmann A, Fain SB, Prasad PV (2020) Consensus-based technical recommendations for clinical translation of renal BOLD MRI. MAGMA 33(1):199–215. https://doi.org/10.1007/s10334-019-00802-x
15. Ljimani A, Caroli A, Laustsen C, Francis S, Mendichovszky IA, Bane O, Nery F, Sharma K, Pohlmann A, Dekkers IA, Vallee JP, Derlin K, Notohamiprodjo M, Lim RP, Palmucci S, Serai SD, Periquito J, Wang ZJ, Froeling M, Thoeny HC, Prasad P, Schneider M, Niendorf T, Pullens P, Sourbron S, Sigmund EE (2020) Consensus-based technical recommendations for clinical translation of renal diffusion-weighted MRI.

MAGMA 33(1):177–195. https://doi.org/10.1007/s10334-019-00790-y

16. Dekkers IA, de Boer A, Sharma K, Cox EF, Lamb HJ, Buckley DL, Bane O, Morris DM, Prasad PV, Semple SIK, Gillis KA, Hockings P, Buchanan C, Wolf M, Laustsen C, Leiner T, Haddock B, Hoogduin JM, Pullens P, Sourbron S, Francis S (2020) Consensus-based technical recommendations for clinical translation of renal T1 and T2 mapping MRI. MAGMA 33(1):163–176. https://doi.org/10.1007/s10334-019-00797-5

9

Animal Models of Renal Pathophysiology and Disease

Adam Hosszu, Tamas Kaucsar, Erdmann Seeliger, and Andrea Fekete

Abstract

Renal diseases remain devastating illnesses with unacceptably high rates of mortality and morbidity worldwide. Animal models are essential tools to better understand the pathomechanisms of kidney-related illnesses and to develop new, successful therapeutic strategies. Magnetic resonance imaging (MRI) has been actively explored in the last decades for assessing renal function, perfusion, tissue oxygenation as well as the degree of fibrosis and inflammation. This chapter aims to provide a comprehensive overview of animal models of acute and chronic kidney diseases, highlighting MRI-specific considerations, advantages, and pitfalls, and thus assisting the researcher in experiment planning.

This publication is based upon work from the COST Action PARENCHIMA, a community-driven network funded by the European Cooperation in Science and Technology (COST) program of the European Union, which aims to improve the reproducibility and standardization of renal MRI biomarkers.

Key words Kidney disease, Magnetic resonance imaging (MRI), Animal models, Rodents

1 Introduction

Renal diseases remain devastating illnesses with unacceptably high rates of mortality and morbidity worldwide. The prevalence of end stage kidney disease is currently between 8% and 16% and is rapidly increasing; the number of patients increased tenfold in the last four decades [1].

Kidney diseases generate a major drain on health and productivity-related resources for healthcare systems; thus, prevention and early treatment would have an enormous social and economic impact.

Understanding the pathologic mechanisms of renal injury is essential for finding new targets for intervention and developing effective treatments for patients with kidney disease [2]. Landmark publications have outlined key areas in which progress is necessary, specifically highlighting the need for superior diagnostic tools [3].

At present, diagnosis of kidney disease is difficult and often involves invasive procedures such as biopsy. Conventional markers of renal function such as serum creatinine and blood urea nitrogen

Andreas Pohlmann and Thoralf Niendorf (eds.), *Preclinical MRI of the Kidney: Methods and Protocols*,
Methods in Molecular Biology, vol. 2216, https://doi.org/10.1007/978-1-0716-0978-1_2, © The Author(s) 2021

are poorly sensitive and poorly selective. The levels of these biomarkers can take several hours or days to reach a new steady state and thus represent a delayed indication of functional change that lags behind structural deterioration during the early stage of acute kidney injury (AKI). In addition, the imbalance between oxygen supply and demand in kidney tissue is the initiating step in the pathophysiology of renal ischemia–reperfusion injury (IRI), and a pivotal early element in the pathophysiology of AKI of other origins. Currently kidney biopsy is the only available method to assess renal microstructure, but it has several disadvantages, including its invasive nature and susceptibility to sampling bias. Thus, noninvasive, in vivo imaging methods such as MRI are indispensable for the adequate assessment of kidney function, oxygenation, and structure in both preclinical and clinical setups. Importantly, several novel techniques are available to generate MRI data by measuring tissue properties linked to filtration, tissue oxygenation, perfusion, fibrosis, inflammation, or tissue edema that can be used as biomarkers of renal disease [4]. MRI affords full kidney coverage, soft tissue contrast that helps to differentiate the renal layers, second-to-minute temporal resolution, support of longitudinal studies, and high anatomical detail without the use of ionizing radiation [5, 6].

Drug discovery is a time-consuming, expensive, and high-risk process. In order to develop one FDA approved drug in the preclinical phase thousands of compounds have to be tested from which only dozens end up in clinical trials [7]. Conducting studies on animal models is a valuable strategy in the preparation for clinical trials because of the high similarity between some animals and humans in their genetics, physiology, diseases, and diagnostic tools. Without doubt the translatability of results obtained in animal models to humans has numerous limitations, but often they represent an indispensable approach for trying to predict the effects of a drug in the complex human system, and also for deciding on an appropriate dose regime for the clinical trial(s) that balances efficacy and safety. Many mechanistic questions can be answered only through invasive procedures or extreme exposures possible only in animals. Moreover, due to the fact that decades may elapse between the onset and clinical manifestations of renal diseases in humans (e.g., diabetic kidney disease), rodent models offer a more feasible means of experimentation because the timeline of pathogeneses are typically much shorter (either naturally or due to tailored disease induction).

An ideal disease model accurately mimics the human condition genetically, experimentally and/or physiologically, but unfortunately such models do not exist. One reason for the poor outcomes in clinical trials is that most animal models do not fully recapitulate the pathological mechanisms underlying human diseases. Human diseases are very complex, but specific factors of a disease are relatively easy to model, which is an advantage and disadvantage at the same time. All of the widely used animal models have their particular limitations; therefore, the model used should be appropriate for the question being addressed [8].

The present chapter summarizes animal models of renal diseases highlighting MRI-specific considerations, advantages, and pitfalls with an aim to assist the researcher in planning an experiment and choosing the best species/strain/model to address the question being asked.

This chapter is part of the book Pohlmann A, Niendorf T (eds) (2020) Preclinical MRI of the Kidney—Methods and Protocols. Springer, New York.

2 Ethical Issues

A wide range of positions exist on the debate over the ethics of animal experiments. On one end of the spectrum people argue that an animal should have as much right to live out a full life, free of suffering as a human and thus all animal experimentation should end. Others argue that while the unnecessary abuse of animals is clearly wrong, animal experimentation must continue because of the enormous scientific resource that animal models provide. A detailed discussion of the growing scholarly literature in animal research ethics is beyond the scope of this chapter; however, the authors feel obliged to provide some fundamental guidelines for conduct of ethical research. The authors of this chapter believe that biomedical animal research is founded on a pivotal ethical principle: "*It is among the most noble and indeed imperative of human endeavors to employ scientific research to prevent, alleviate, and cure the pain, suffering, distress, fear, anxiety, disability, infirmity and death associated with human disease*" [9]. Because the use of animal models to understand human disease is motivated by such a high ethical ideal, we must aim to adhere to the highest ethical standards when conducting research.

When designing a study applying the principles of 3Rs: replacement, reduction, and refinement is advised to provide a framework for performing the most humane animal research possible. *Replacement* means the substitution of animals with alternative techniques or avoid the use of animals altogether. Alternative methods such as cell cultures or novel approaches such as stem cell technologies, tissue engineering, or modeling using artificial intelligence show promise for replacing animals in many areas of research but often give limited information about what happens in the whole living animal. *Reduction* means to obtain information of given amount and precision from fewer animals or more information from the same number of animals. Proper experimental design and statistical analysis of the proposed project is pivotal in using the optimal number of animals. If more animals are used than is necessary for obtaining reliable results, then animal lives are wasted. On the other hand, if too few animals are used then the results can be unreliable and the experiment has to be repeated, using more animals in total. *Refinement* means minimizing the incidence or severity of procedures that result in distress or suffering of animals which still have to be used. Refinement can also improve the quality of research by reducing stress in animals. By law, any suffering or pain to an animal must be minimized. Animals must be anaesthetized for surgery, and, if necessary, analgesics must be administered afterward, which will be discussed in detail in the chapter by Kaucsar T et al. "Preparation and Monitoring of Small Animals in Renal MRI."

3 General Guidelines for Choosing an Animal Model

3.1 Rat or Mouse?

The first major decision when designing a study using an animal model is to choose the most suitable species. Rodent models are the most popular to resemble human disease for a number of reasons: 90% of genes are orthologous in the rat, murine, and human genomes, small size and fast reproduction of rodents facilitates high-throughput studies, and a very good genetic/molecular tool box is available.

Differences within rodents must not be underestimated when designing experiments. Inbred mouse strains are more stable, uniform, repeatable, and better defined than outbred rat strains such as Wistar or Sprague-Dawley where the exact genetic background of each animal is unknown [10].

While rats used to be the preferred rodent in kidney research, this changed with the advent of murine transgenic and knockout technologies in the past decades. Genetically modified mice provide unique opportunities for targeted research of the impact of individual proteins on phenotype and responsiveness to therapeutic interventions. Gene deletion or overexpression generally results in very predictable and precise phenotypes in mice. Furthermore, due to their small size many more mice can be housed in a small space than rats and are therefore cheaper to maintain; they have a short reproductive cycle and accelerated life span.

Murine models of kidney disease do have some limitations and disadvantages that are worth considering. Surgical procedures such as ureteric obstruction, renal ischemia, or kidney transplantation are widely used to model human disease. Surgical manipulations and micropuncture studies are technically much easier to perform in larger animals such as rats.

Moreover, the pathophysiology in rat models is often not replicated in mice. For example, while humans and rats have only one copy of the renin gene, mice either have a single gene or two copies at the renin locus. This may be an important confounding variable considering the central role of the renin–angiotensin–aldosterone system in renal disease and that the plasma renin activity of mice with two renin genes is tenfold higher than their single-gene counterparts [11].

Hypertension is a leading cause of kidney failure; thus, noninvasive blood pressure measurements are a crucial component of studies in the field. While the technique is fairly routine in rats, it has been proven to be rather challenging in mice [12].

Finally, the smaller size of mice means smaller amounts of experimental material to work with. The fundamental limitation in MRI is signal-to-noise ratio, which is in direct correlation with the volume of the subject. Acquiring high-resolution images of relatively small mouse kidneys could be challenging using lower field strength MRI machines. Furthermore, concurrent measurement of multiple variables such as RNA expression, protein levels, histology, and metabolic processes from individual animals can be challenging.

3.2 Which Strain?

The choice of the right strain is essential since disease phenotypes in rodents are strongly influenced by species and strain. For example, there are distinct differences in the susceptibility to ischemic AKI among various mouse strains or even different colonies of the same strain. 129/Sv and National Institute of Health Swiss mice have been shown to be less sensitive to ischemic injury than C57BL/6 or BALB/c mice [13, 14]. Most transgenic models are described to have comparable genetic background with wild-type strains such as C57BL/6 after at least five generations of backcross; however, the wild-type mice from the same transgenic models may differ significantly from ordinary C57BL/6 mice. Similarly, Brown-Norway rats have been found to be almost completely protected against several manifestations of IRI when compared with the commonly used Sprague-Dawley rat model [15]. In conclusion, pilot experiments always have to be performed to determine the appropriate duration of ischemia for a new strain to be studied.

The C57BL/6 mouse strain is also relatively resistant to the development of diabetic kidney disease (DKD). C57BL/6 mice develop significantly less albuminuria and renal histopathological changes than DBA/2J and KK/HIJ mice [16]. Sprague-Dawley rats are far more sensitive to streptozotocin-induced diabetes than nude rats [17].

The remnant kidney model or 5/6 nephrectomy model has been used extensively in rats to study the pathogenesis of glomerulosclerosis. In contrast, mouse strains such as C57BL/6 and C57BLX Swiss-Webster mice do not develop significant glomerulosclerosis or increased systolic blood pressure and proteinuria in this model. C57BL/6 mice and Wistar rats are less susceptible to deoxycorticosterone acetate (DOCA) salt-induced hypertension than 129/Sv mice or Sprague-Dawley rats respectively [18, 19]. Thus, the more susceptible 129/Sv strain is recommended to study hypertension-associated glomerulosclerosis in mice [20].

3.3 Sex

The anatomical structure of the healthy kidney is different in the two sexes. Females have more glomeruli in the kidneys, higher renovascular resistance, lower absolute GFR, and lower renal plasma flow. There are differences on the cellular level as well: males have larger mitochondria and more lysosomes and ribosomes in their proximal tubular cells. Although estrogen and androgen receptors are found in renal tissue in both sexes, animal experimental models (e.g., castration, ovariectomy) suggest that sex hormones are involved in the sexual dimorphism of the kidney [21].

Female sex is a protective factor in several renal diseases which disappear after menopause. Not only the outcome of AKI is better in females [22, 23], but the progression of renal function deterioration during the aging process [24] as well as other chronic renal diseases [25] is also slower in females compared to males. Some studies support the protective role of female hormones (17-β-estradiol, progesterone) [26–28]. Others highlight the negative effect of testosterone: Park et al. found more severe renal injury after testosterone therapy in female, ovariectomized, and castrated male mice [29].

For the aforementioned reasons the use of female rodents is only advised if the study specifically aims to investigate sex differences or the role of sex hormones. Duration of the estrous cycle is 4–5 days in both rats and mice; a vaginal smear has to be obtained and stages of the estrous cycle have to be identified before starting an experiment. C. Caligioni provides a detailed description of assessing the reproductive status of mice [30].

3.4 Other Species

Some nonrodent species are also used, although less frequently. In theory, nonhuman primates are the most similar to human biology, but the heterogeneity is huge among species. Close approximation of genetic, structural, and functional features of nonhuman primates to humans make them ideal experimental models; however, specific ethical considerations are essential [31]. These animals are likely to sense pain, distress, and social relationships in the same way as humans. Moreover, they are expensive to obtain and house, may transmit diseases to humans, and can be difficult to handle due to their strength and intelligence. Experiments with nonhuman primates are limited to a very small number of animals compared to rodents; thus, their statistical value can be doubtful.

Work using dogs played an enormous role in the early advancement of dialysis and transplantation techniques, or the use of azathioprine in immunosuppression, and others [32]. However, ethical considerations and strong feelings of the public have substantially limited the use of companion animals for research purposes.

Farm animals such as pigs are fairly similar to humans in renal anatomy, size, and metabolism. Pigs are the subject of extensive research especially as a potential source of kidneys for xenotransplantation [33]. The size of fully grown pigs limits routine laboratory use; moreover, potential virus or prion transmission from pigs to humans will possibly reduce their use as xenograft sources.

4 Models of AKI

4.1 Ischemia–Reperfusion Injury

Renal IRI is the most common cause of AKI in patients and temporary occlusion of renal blood flow is unavoidable during kidney transplantation. Therefore, models that accurately and reproducibly replicate renal IRI are indispensable for investigating the pathomechanism of AKI and for the development of novel therapeutic agents. There are three commonly used models of IRI: (1) bilateral clamping of renal arteries and veins; (2) unilateral clamping; and (3) unilateral clamping with contralateral nephrectomy [34]. The bilateral model is regularly used because it is considered most relevant to human pathology where blood supply is typically affected in both kidneys. Some studies performed decapsulation prior to renal ischemia that may have renoprotective effects, as reported earlier [35]. However, decapsulation was not conducted in the majority of published studies. Unilateral IRI models without contralateral nephrectomy leave animals with a healthy kidney which takes over the excretory function. Consequently, this model allows for the study of the effect of prolonged ischemia times without excessive postprocedure lethal outcomes. On the other hand, this model does not allow the study of filtration and excretory function of the affected kidney after IRI because of the compensation achieved by the unaffected healthy kidney. In the third model right nephrectomy is performed at the time of left kidney IRI. Tissue from the removed right kidney can be used as highly valuable control in studies where pretreatment that induces or suppresses specific gene or protein expression is involved. Thus, changes in the molecule of interest can be confirmed and quantified in each individual animal used in the experiment. This model is most useful when the researcher aims to test the effect of drugs or compounds administered prior to the induction of IRI, furthermore overall survival is more reliable than with bilateral clamping and this model closely mimics the situation occurring in renal transplantation. Several studies suggest the protective potential of contralateral nephrectomy against IRI by increasing blood flow and other beneficial pleotropic effects (e.g., antiapoptotic, proliferative, vasodilatory) in the remaining kidney [36], which should be taken into consideration when designing an experiment.

The pathological consequences of renal IRI are proportional to the period of ischemia which has to be determined for the individual species, strain, sex, and age. Shorter ischemia causes subclinical AKI, with minor histologic change and without any functional deterioration as assessed by serum creatinine and BUN [37]. As ischemia duration increases clinical AKI develops with moderate renal damage accompanied by renal failure. If the extent of injury is mild, then the full recovery of renal function can be expected. However, longer ischemia generally leads to lethal kidney damage, with continuously deteriorating kidney function and the animals die due to uremia [38]. As a guide, 30–50 min and 20–35 min of occlusion respectively is generally used in rats and mice. Clamping time, maintenance of body temperature, and the type of anesthesia are key parameters to be standardized for reproducibility.

4.2 Renal Transplantation

Renal transplantation is predominantly performed in rats due to the challenging microsurgical techniques involved. Depending on the aim of the study various combinations of inbred and outbred strains model various complications of kidney transplantation such as IRI, acute rejection, or chronic allograft nephropathy [39]. Autotransplantation models are ideal for the study of alloantigen-independent mechanisms such as IRI or the effect of cold storage on the organ. Fisher and Lewis rat strains differ at the major histocompatibility loci I and II which results in chronic allograft nephropathy if no immunosuppression is applied. Thus, transplantation from a Fisher donor to a Lewis recipient is the most commonly used model of chronic allograft nephropathy [40]. Other strains—both as donor and recipient—include outbred strains: Sprague-Dawley, Wistar, and Long-Evans; or inbred strains: Lewis, Brown-Norway, and Dark Agouti [41–43].

A large number of different surgical techniques have been reported, probably due to the technical difficulties associated with rat renal transplantation. Detailed procedures are available in an excellent review by Schumacher et al. which describes all technical aspects, different techniques of vascular anastomosis, strain selection, and more [44].

4.3 Sepsis-Induced AKI

Sepsis is a complex disease that involves at least two stages, which should ideally be reproduced in animal models. An initial proinflammatory burst resulting in hypodynamic circulation with hypotension and organ dysfunction is followed by compensatory immune depression, with hyperdynamic circulation, but these can overlap. There are three types of sepsis animal models: exogenous toxin (e.g., LPS)-induced; alteration of endogenous protective barriers (e.g., cecal ligation and puncture (CLP) or colon ascendens stent peritonitis (CASP)); or exogenous bacteria-induced. The LPS model is predominantly used in rodents as the standard CLP model does not develop AKI, while bacterial infusion models are established mainly in larger animals such as dogs and sheep. C. N. May's group established a model of hyperdynamic sepsis in conscious sheep. In this model sepsis is induced by intravenous infusion of live *Escherichia coli* and is characterized by hypotension, tachycardia, peripheral vasodilation, and AKI [45].

Advantages of LPS injection are that its simple, sterile, and induces systemic inflammation that has many similarities with hypodynamic sepsis pathophysiology in humans. The disadvantage is that early and transient proinflammatory mediator production is more intense than in humans. LPS causes decreased GFR, increased BUN levels, and neutrophil infiltration in the kidney [46]. LPS dose can be titrated to mimic different aspects of sepsis: typical LPS doses cause systemic hypotension and decreased glomerular perfusion, while lower doses do not cause systemic hypotension but decrease glomerular perfusion [47].

4.4 Toxin-Induced AKI

4.4.1 Cisplatin

Cisplatin is a widely used anticancer drug; however, high doses have significant toxic effects on proximal tubules. Cisplatin treatment leads to inflammation and interstitial fibrosis, moreover renal blood flow is also altered. Most studies use a single *i.p.* injection of 6–20 mg/kg cisplatin in rats, which induces AKI within 72 h and both pathology and recovery phase are comparable to those of humans [48]. Higher doses are also used, albeit less frequently [49, 50].

4.4.2 Contrast-Induced AKI (CIAKI)

Intravascular administration of iodinated X-ray contrast media (CM) for computer tomography, MRI or angiography can induce AKI characterized by renal tissue hypoxia due to reduced renal blood flow and consequent oxidative stress [51]. Incidence varies between 3% and 25% depending on several factors. Firstly, the potential to cause CIAKI is less when CM are given intravenously (typically in lower doses, e.g., for computed tomography or urography) than intra-arterially (often in higher doses, e.g., for cardiac procedures), because the renal first-pass concentration is higher for the latter route of administration. Secondly, physicochemical properties of CM solutions such as osmolality and viscosity impinge on their different safety profiles. Thirdly, hydration status of the patient plays an important role. Finally, preexisting conditions such as endothelial dysfunction, for example related to diabetes mellitus, and impaired renal function increase the risk of CIAKI [51].

There are a number of models that reliably induce CIAKI in otherwise healthy animals. The clinical setting of cardiac procedures is emulated by a model, in which a 1.5 mL bolus of a high viscous CM (iodixanol 320 mg iodine/mL) is injected into the thoracic aorta of naïve rats [52–54]. A high dose of intravenously administered iodixanol (rat: 4 g iodine/kg body weight; rabbit: 5 g iodine/kg body weight) also induces CIAKI [55, 56].

In order to emulate conditions of patients who are at increased risk for CIAKI, several animal models employing a combination of contrast agent injection and other injuries (e.g., vasodilator inhibition, dehydration, IRI, diabetes) have been studied. Vasoconstriction induced by inhibition of nitric oxide synthase (e.g., L-NAME, 10 mg/kg body weight) combined with prostaglandin synthesis inhibition (indomethacin, 10 mg/kg body weight) prior to CM administration (iohexol, 1 g iodine/kg body weight) has been employed in rats and mice [57]. Another reliable murine model of CIAKI includes 30 min bilateral renal ischemia and CM administration 24 h after reperfusion [58].

4.4.3 Aristolochic Acid and Folic Acid

Both models are useful to study AKI to chronic kidney disease (CKD) transition. Aristolochic acid nephropathy is characterized by proximal tubular injury, necrosis and oxidative stress resulting in progressive interstitial fibrosis [59]. Aristolochic acid is the underlying cause of Balkan nephropathy and Chinese Herb nephropathy [60].

In folic acid nephropathy folic acid crystal deposits appear in the tubular lumen resulting in obstruction and subsequent acute tubular necrosis, tubular dilatation and cast formation. Mitochondrial dysfunction and early renal fibrosis are typical features of folic acid nephropathy as well.

4.4.4 Glycerol

In rhabdomyolysis skeletal muscle breakdown leads to the release of intracellular proteins and toxic compounds into circulation. AKI is a recurrent complication of rhabdomyolysis, mainly caused by inflammation and oxidative stress. Human symptoms are reproduced in rodents by water deprivation for 24 h followed by glycerol administration into the hindlimb muscle [61]. Elevated BUN and serum creatinine levels in this model are not exclusively the result of declined renal function, but rhabdomyolysis as well, thus GFR or creatinine clearance measurement should be preferred.

5 Models of CKD

5.1 Unilateral Ureteral Obstruction (UUO)

Renal fibrosis is the hallmark of progressive kidney disease that involves glomerular sclerosis tubulointerstitial fibrosis and atherosclerosis. UUO in rodents can be experimentally manipulated with respect to timing, severity and duration, while reversal of the obstruction allows the study of recovery. Complete UUO results in reduced renal blood flow and GFR within 24 h, followed by hydronephrosis, inflammation and tubular cell death within days. In 1–2 weeks severe hydronephrosis and severe fibrosis develops. The surgical procedure is relatively straightforward. Animals undergo a midline incision, the left ureter is located and then ligated [62]. Because clinical congenital obstructive nephropathy involves only partial obstruction, models of partial UUO have been developed in neonatal mice or rats. These models are, however, technically challenging and meticulous technique is essential. In one method a piece of silicone tubing is slit and longitudinally fitted around the ureter forming a sleeve. Another recommended technique involves placement of a fine stainless-steel wire parallel to the ureter. After ligation the wire is pulled out leaving a partial obstruction. The ligature can then be removed at various time points to study recovery mechanisms. Due to functional and cellular compensatory mechanisms we recommend using sham-operated animals as controls instead of the contralateral kidney (unless comparing a therapeutic intervention on the obstructed kidney).

5.2 5/6 Nephrectomy

The 5/6 nephrectomy model mimics progressive renal failure after loss of renal mass in humans. The recommended approach is removal of the right kidney and resection of the upper and lower poles of the left kidney (2/3 of the kidney) [63]. The approach where branches of the renal artery are ligated is not feasible in mice due to their limited renal artery branching. Remnant kidneys develop glomerulosclerosis, tubulointerstitial fibrosis, renal atrophy and proteinuria. Susceptibility to renal injury in the 5/6 nephrectomy model is highly variable between different strains. C57BL/6 mice are resistant compared to 129/Sv or Swiss Webster mice.

5.3 Models of DKD

DKD is the leading cause of end-stage kidney disease worldwide. Unfortunately, animal models that replicate all important functional, structural and molecular features of human DKD are lacking. In both mice and rats, type 1 diabetes mellitus (T1DM) can be induced by streptozotocin, which is transported by GLUT2 transporter and destroys pancreatic beta cells. Renal and hepatic cells also express GLUT2, thus streptozotocin has additional direct nephrotoxic and hepatotoxic effects apart from the injury induced by diabetes [64]. Genetic models of T1DM such as Akita and OVE26 mice are also available [65]. T1DM can be induced by streptozotocin injection in DBA/2J mice, which are susceptible to nephropathy [16]. Streptozotocin induces T1DM with hyperlipidemia in ApoE$^{-/-}$ mice [66].

Models of type 2 diabetes mellitus (T2DM) utilize genetically obese rodents such as ob/ob mice, db/db mice, or Zucker rats [67, 68]. These animals are either leptin deficient or have inactivating mutations in the leptin receptor. High-fat diet can be useful to investigate the mechanisms of insulin resistance, even though the animals do not exhibit classical features of human DKD, they rarely become hyperglycemic and high-fat diet alone may cause renal injury. MKR mice can be used in a nonobese model of T2DM because the insulin receptor is dysfunctional resulting in insulin resistance, hyperglycemia and hyperlipidemia [69].

5.4 Models of Polycystic Kidney Disease

Polycystic kidney disease (PKD) is a genetic disorder associated with cystic bile ducts, bile duct proliferation, and cystic pancreatic ducts. There are two types of PKD in humans: the autosomal dominant PKD (ADPKD) caused by mutations in the PKD1 or PKD2 gene, and autosomal recessive PKD (ARPKD) caused by a mutation in the PKHD1 gene. In ADPKD the renal parenchyma is replaced by cysts originating from all segments of the nephron, collecting tubules, and ducts. In ARPKD cysts originate only from dilated collecting tubules and ducts.

In spontaneous hereditary models of PKD animals have obvious PKD phenotypes, but the responsible genes are not necessarily orthologous with the human genes. Examples of such models are Han:SPRD-Cy rats [70], PCK rats [71], Pcy mice [72], and Jck mice [73].

Transgenic mouse models have also been developed. Thivierge et al. produced a model with a bacterial artificial chromosome in which PKD1 gene expression is increased in the kidney, heart and liver, and the gene product PC1 is overexpressed in renal cysts [74]. Several transgenic models have been developed by deletion of human orthologous genes *Pkd1* [75], *Pkd2* [76] or *Pkhd1* [77]. Nagao et al. published a detailed review of PKD models [78].

5.5 Models of Hypertension

5.5.1 Spontaneously Hypertensive Rats (SHR)

The SHR rat strain was generated by protracted rounds of breeding and selection for high blood pressure. SHR rats develop hypertension at 5–6 weeks of age and systolic blood pressure of 180–200 mmHg by adulthood with high renin levels. Proteinuria increases from 6 weeks of age, GFR decreases by 20% by 15 weeks of age and glomerulosclerosis and tubulointerstitial fibrosis develops at around 50 weeks of age. Progression of hypertensive renal damage in this model mirrors that seen in human hypertension [79]. Unilateral nephrectomy may be required to induce significant renal injury [80].

5.5.2 Deoxycorticosterone Acetate (DOCA)–Salt Hypertension

The subcutaneous implantation of a DOCA pellet, uninephrectomy, and supplementation of 1% NaCl in drinking water or high-salt diet induces moderate-to-severe hypertension with renal injury and low renin levels [81]. Angiotensin II administration can aggravate renal injury. Renal pathological changes include proteinuria, fibrotic alterations, and impaired endothelium-dependent relaxation.

5.6 Podocyte Injury Models

Focal segmental glomerulosclerosis (FSGS) is the primary cause of glomerular diseases, characterized by proteinuria or nephrotic syndrome. Fibrotic lesions in some glomeruli (focal) or in specific parts of a single glomerulus (segmental) are the histological features of the disease.

In animal models FSGS can be induced by podocyte toxins such as puromycin, aminonucleoside or adriamycin [82]. The main disadvantage of drug-induced models is the uncertainty of their similarity to human pathology of the disease as well as a robust variability between rodent strains in susceptibility (e.g., C57BL/6 mice are far more resistant than BALB/c) [83].

Spontaneous FSGS models include the Buffalo/MWF and Munich Wistar Fromter rat models [84, 85]. Excellent transgenic models include the Nep25 mouse model [86], the diphtheria toxin rat model, the Thy-1.1 mouse model [87], and others. Genetically engineered mouse models give valuable insight to protein–protein interactions and their role in the prognosis of FSGS. Yang et al. provide a comprehensive review of FSGS rodent models [88].

6 Humanized Mouse Models

Many elements of mouse biological systems are different from those of humans, especially their immune system. Humanized mice have become important preclinical tools to accurately recapitulate human biological systems. Presently there are three widely used strains of immunodeficient mice: NOD.Cg-Prkdc^{scid}Il2rg^{tm1Wjl} (NSG), NODShi.Cg-Prkdc^{scid}Il2rg^{tm1Sug} (NOG) and C;129S4-Rag2^{tm1Flv}Il2rg^{tm1Flv} (BRG), which lack T, B, and NK cells and have functionally impaired dendritic cells and macrophages. These mice are engrafted with human transplants including peripheral blood mononuclear cells, a combination of bone marrow, liver, and thymus, or hematopoietic stem cells [89]. Humanized mouse models have tremendous potential in the study of the mechanisms of allograft rejection during transplantation or immune-mediated renal diseases such as T1DM [90, 91].

Acknowledgments

This work was funded in part (Erdmann Seeliger) by the German Research Foundation (Gefoerdert durch die Deutsche Forschungsgemeinschaft (DFG), Projektnummer 394046635, SFB 1365, RENOPROTECTION. Funded by the Deutsche Forschungsgemeinschaft (DFG, German Research Foundation), Project number 394046635, SFB 1365, RENOPROTECTION).

This publication is based upon work from COST Action PARENCHIMA, supported by European Cooperation in Science and Technology (COST). COST (www.cost.eu) is a funding agency for research and innovation networks. COST Actions help connect research initiatives across Europe and enable scientists to enrich their ideas by sharing them with their peers. This boosts their research, career, and innovation.

PARENCHIMA (renalmri.org) is a community-driven Action in the COST program of the European Union, which unites more than 200 experts in renal MRI from 30 countries with the aim to improve the reproducibility and standardization of renal MRI biomarkers.

References

1. US Renal Data System Annual Report 2016. (2016). https://www.usrds.org/adr.aspx
2. Liu Y (2006) Renal fibrosis: new insights into the pathogenesis and therapeutics. Kidney Int 69(2):213–217. https://doi.org/10.1038/sj.ki.5000054
3. Levin A, Tonelli M, Bonventre J, Coresh J, Donner JA, Fogo AB, Fox CS, Gansevoort RT, Heerspink HJL, Jardine M, Kasiske B, Kottgen A, Kretzler M, Levey AS, Luyckx VA, Mehta R, Moe O, Obrador G, Pannu N, Parikh CR, Perkovic V, Pollock C, Stenvinkel P, Tuttle KR, Wheeler DC, Eckardt KU (2017) Global kidney health 2017 and beyond: a roadmap for closing gaps in care, research, and policy. Lancet 390(10105):1888–1917. https://doi.org/10.1016/S0140-6736(17)30788-2
4. Selby NM, Blankestijn PJ, Boor P, Combe C, Eckardt KU, Eikefjord E, Garcia-Fernandez N, Golay X, Gordon I, Grenier N, Hockings PD, Jensen JD, Joles JA, Kalra PA, Kramer BK, Mark PB, Mendichovszky IA, Nikolic O, Odudu A, Ong ACM, Ortiz A, Pruijm M, Remuzzi G, Rorvik J, de Seigneux S, Simms RJ, Slatinska J, Summers P, Taal MW, Thoeny HC, Vallee JP, Wolf M, Caroli A, Sourbron S (2018) Magnetic resonance imaging biomarkers for chronic kidney disease: a position paper from the European Cooperation in Science and Technology Action PARENCHIMA. Nephrol Dial Transplant 33(suppl_2):ii4–ii14. https://doi.org/10.1093/ndt/gfy152
5. Prasad PV (2006) Functional MRI of the kidney: tools for translational studies of pathophysiology of renal disease. Am J Physiol Renal Physiol 290(5):F958–F974. https://doi.org/10.1152/ajprenal.00114.2005
6. Haque M, Franklin T, Prasad P (2011) Renal oxygenation changes during water loading as evaluated by BOLD MRI: effect of NOS inhibition. J Magn Reson Imaging 33 (4):898–901. https://doi.org/10.1002/jmri.22509
7. DiMasi JA, Grabowski HG, Hansen RW (2016) Innovation in the pharmaceutical industry: new estimates of R&D costs. J Health Econ 47:20–33. https://doi.org/10.1016/j.jhealeco.2016.01.012
8. Justice MJ, Dhillon P (2016) Using the mouse to model human disease: increasing validity and reproducibility. Dis Model Mech 9 (2):101–103. https://doi.org/10.1242/dmm.024547
9. Tannenbaum J (2017) Ethics in biomedical animal research: the key role of the investigator. In: Conn PM (ed) Animal models for the study of human disease, 2edn edn. Academic Press, Cambridge, Massachusetts, pp 1–44. https://doi.org/10.1016/B978-0-12-809468-6.00001-2
10. Festing MF (2010) Inbred strains should replace outbred stocks in toxicology, safety testing, and drug development. Toxicol Pathol 38(5):681–690. https://doi.org/10.1177/0192623310373776
11. Nishino T, Sasaki N, Nagasaki K, Ahmad Z, Agui T (2010) Genetic background strongly influences the severity of glomerulosclerosis in mice. J Vet Med Sci 72(10):1313–1318. https://doi.org/10.1292/jvms.10-0144
12. Feng M, DiPetrillo K (2009) Non-invasive blood pressure measurement in mice. Methods Mol Biol 573:45–55. https://doi.org/10.1007/978-1-60761-247-6_3
13. Brune S, Pricl S, Wunsch B (2013) Structure of the sigma1 receptor and its ligand binding site. J Med Chem 56(24):9809–9819. https://doi.org/10.1021/jm400660u
14. Lu X, Li N, Shushakova N, Schmitt R, Menne J, Susnik N, Meier M, Leitges M, Haller H, Gueler F, Rong S (2012) C57BL/6 and 129/Sv mice: genetic difference to renal ischemia-reperfusion. J Nephrol 25 (5):738–743. https://doi.org/10.5301/jn.5000053
15. Basile DP, Donohoe D, Cao XIA, Van Why SK (2004) Resistance to ischemic acute renal failure in the Brown Norway rat: a new model to study cytoprotection. Kidney Int 65 (6):2201–2211. https://doi.org/10.1111/j.1523-1755.2004.00637.x
16. Qi Z, Fujita H, Jin J. Davis LS, Wang Y, Fogo AB, Breyer MD (2005) Characterization of susceptibility of inbred mouse strains to diabetic nephropathy. Diabetes 54 (9):2628–2637. https://doi.org/10.2337/diabetes.54.9.2628
17. Mahmoud Abu Abeeleh ZBI, Alzaben KR, Abu-Halaweh SA, Al-Essa MK, Abuabeeleh J, Alsmady MM (2009) Induction of diabetes mellitus in rats using intraperitoneal streptozotocin: a comparison between 2 strains of rats. European J Sci Res 32(3):398–402
18. Hartner A, Cordasic N, Klanke B, Veelken R, Hilgers KF (2003) Strain differences in the development of hypertension and glomerular lesions induced by deoxycorticosterone acetate salt in mice. Nephrol Dial Transplant 18 (10):1999–2004. https://doi.org/10.1093/ndt/gfg299

19. Erdely A, Freshour G, Tain YL, Engels K, Baylis C (2007) DOCA/NaCl-induced chronic kidney disease: a comparison of renal nitric oxide production in resistant and susceptible rat strains. Am J Physiol Renal Physiol 292 (1):F192–F196. https://doi.org/10.1152/ajprenal.00146.2006
20. Ma LJ, Fogo AB (2003) Model of robust induction of glomerulosclerosis in mice: importance of genetic background. Kidney Int 64(1):350–355. https://doi.org/10.1046/j.1523-1755.2003.00058.x
21. Hutchens MP, Dunlap J, Hurn PD, Jarnberg PO (2008) Renal ischemia: does sex matter? Anesth Analg 107(1):239–249. https://doi.org/10.1213/ane.0b013e318178ca42
22. Muller V, Losonczy G, Heemann U, Vannay A, Fekete A, Reusz G, Tulassay T, Szabo AJ (2002) Sexual dimorphism in renal ischemia-reperfusion injury in rats: possible role of endothelin. Kidney Int 62(4):1364–1371. https://doi.org/10.1111/j.1523-1755.2002.kid590.x
23. Mehta RL, Pascual MT, Soroko S, Chertow GM (2002) Diuretics, mortality, and nonrecovery of renal function in acute renal failure. JAMA 288(20):2547–2553
24. Berg UB (2006) Differences in decline in GFR with age between males and females. Reference data on clearances of inulin and PAH in potential kidney donors. Nephrol Dial Transplant 21 (9):2577–2582. https://doi.org/10.1093/ndt/gfl227
25. Kummer S, von Gersdorff G, Kemper MJ, Oh J (2012) The influence of gender and sexual hormones on incidence and outcome of chronic kidney disease. Pediatr Nephrol 27 (8):1213–1219. https://doi.org/10.1007/s00467-011-1963-1
26. Hosszu A, Antal Z, Veres-Szekely A, Lenart L, Balogh DB, Szkibinszkij E, Illesy L, Hodrea J, Banki NF, Wagner L, Vannay A, Szabo AJ, Fekete A (2018) The role of Sigma-1 receptor in sex-specific heat shock response in an experimental rat model of renal ischaemia/reperfusion injury. Transpl Int 31(11):1268–1278. https://doi.org/10.1111/tri.13293
27. Aufhauser DD Jr, Wang Z, Murken DR, Bhatti TR, Wang Y, Ge G, Redfield RR 3rd, Abt PL, Wang L, Svoronos N, Thomasson A, Reese PP, Hancock WW, Levine MH (2016) Improved renal ischemia tolerance in females influences kidney transplantation outcomes. J Clin Invest 126(5):1968–1977. https://doi.org/10.1172/jci84712
28. Satake A, Takaoka M, Nishikawa M, Yuba M, Shibata Y, Okumura K, Kitano K, Tsutsui H, Fujii K, Kobuchi S, Ohkita M, Matsumura Y (2008) Protective effect of 17beta-estradiol on ischemic acute renal failure through the PI3K/Akt/eNOS pathway. Kidney Int 73 (3):308–317. https://doi.org/10.1038/sj.ki.5002690
29. Park KM, Kim JI, Ahn Y, Bonventre AJ, Bonventre JV (2004) Testosterone is responsible for enhanced susceptibility of males to ischemic renal injury. J Biol Chem 279 (50):52282–52292. https://doi.org/10.1074/jbc.M407629200
30. Caligioni CS (2009) Assessing reproductive status/stages in mice. Curr Protoc Neurosci. https://doi.org/10.1002/0471142301.nsa04is48
31. Coors ME, Glover JJ, Juengst ET, Sikela JM (2010) The ethics of using transgenic non-human primates to study what makes us human. Nat Rev Genet 11(9):658–662. https://doi.org/10.1038/nrg2864
32. Yarger WE, Griffith LD (1974) Intrarenal hemodynamics following chronic unilateral ureteral obstruction in the dog. Am J Phys 227(4):816–826. https://doi.org/10.1152/ajplegacy.1974.227.4.816
33. Giraud S, Favreau F, Chatauret N, Thuillier R, Maiga S, Hauet T (2011) Contribution of large pig for renal ischemia-reperfusion and transplantation studies: the preclinical model. J Biomed Biotechnol 2011:532127. https://doi.org/10.1155/2011/532127
34. Wei Q, Dong Z (2012) Mouse model of ischemic acute kidney injury: technical notes and tricks. Am J Physiol Renal Physiol 303(11): F1487–F1494. https://doi.org/10.1152/ajprenal.00352.2012
35. Stone HH, Fulenwider JT (1977) Renal decapsulation in the prevention of post-ischemic oliguria. Ann Surg 186(3):343–355. https://doi.org/10.1097/00000658-197709000-00012
36. Kierulf-Lassen C, Nielsen PM, Qi H, Damgaard M, Laustsen C, Pedersen M, Krag S, Birn H, Norregaard R, Jespersen B (2017) Unilateral nephrectomy diminishes ischemic acute kidney injury through enhanced perfusion and reduced pro-inflammatory and pro-fibrotic responses. PLoS One 12(12): e0190009. https://doi.org/10.1371/journal.pone.0190009
37. Kaucsar T, Godo M, Revesz C, Kovacs M, Mocsai A, Kiss N, Albert M, Krenacs T, Szenasi G, Hamar P (2016) Urine/plasma neutrophil gelatinase associated Lipocalin ratio is a sensitive and specific marker of subclinical acute kidney injury in mice. PLoS One 11(1):e0148043. https://doi.org/10.1371/journal.pone.0148043

38. Kaucsar T, Revesz C, Godo M, Krenacs T, Albert M, Szalay CI, Rosivall L, Benyo Z, Batkai S, Thum T, Szenasi G, Hamar P (2013) Activation of the miR-17 family and miR-21 during murine kidney ischemia-reperfusion injury. Nucleic Acid Ther 23 (5):344–354. https://doi.org/10.1089/nat.2013.0438
39. Shrestha B, Haylor J (2014) Experimental rat models of chronic allograft nephropathy: a review. Int J Nephrol Renovasc Dis 7:315–322. https://doi.org/10.2147/ijnrd.S65604
40. White E, Hildemann WH, Mullen Y (1969) Chronic kidney allograft reactions in rats. Transplantation 8(5):602–617
41. Frodin L, Engberg A (1975) Renal transplantation in the rat. I. Studies concerning the ureteral anastomosis with special reference to the end-to-end technique. Urol Res 3(2):87–90
42. Bramis JP, Schanzer H, Taub RN (1977) Prolongation of rat renal allograft survival by cyclophosphamide and intravenous donor-specific antigens. Eur Surg Res 9(2):140–154. https://doi.org/10.1159/000127934
43. Harvig B, Norlen BJ (1980) A technique for in vivo and in vitro studies on the preserved and transplanted rat kidney. Urol Res 8 (2):107–112
44. Schumacher M, Van Vliet BN, Ferrari P (2003) Kidney transplantation in rats: an appraisal of surgical techniques and outcome. Microsurgery 23(4):387–394. https://doi.org/10.1002/micr.10139
45. Lankadeva YR, Kosaka J, Evans RG, May CN (2018) An ovine model for studying the pathophysiology of septic acute kidney injury. Methods Mol Biol 1717:207–218. https://doi.org/10.1007/978-1-4939-7526-6_16
46. Cunningham PN, Wang Y, Guo R, He G, Quigg RJ (2004) Role of toll-like receptor 4 in endotoxin-induced acute renal failure. J Immunol 172(4):2629–2635. https://doi.org/10.4049/jimmunol.172.4.2629
47. Wang W, Falk SA, Jittikanont S, Gengaro PE, Edelstein CL, Schrier RW (2002) Protective effect of renal denervation on normotensive endotoxemia-induced acute renal failure in mice. Am J Physiol Renal Physiol 283(3): F583–F587. https://doi.org/10.1152/ajprenal.00270.2001
48. Ko JW, Lee IC, Park SH, Moon C, Kang SS, Kim SH, Kim JC (2014) Protective effects of pine bark extract against cisplatin-induced hepatotoxicity and oxidative stress in rats. Lab Anim Res 30(4):174–180. https://doi.org/10.5625/lar.2014.30.4.174
49. Mitazaki S, Kato N, Suto M, Hiraiwa K, Abe S (2009) Interleukin-6 deficiency accelerates cisplatin-induced acute renal failure but not systemic injury. Toxicology 265(3):115–121. https://doi.org/10.1016/j.tox.2009.10.005
50. Zhang J, Rudemiller NP, Patel MB, Wei Q, Karlovich NS, Jeffs AD, Wu M, Sparks MA, Privratsky JR, Herrera M, Gurley SB, Nedospasov SA, Crowley SD (2016) Competing actions of type 1 angiotensin II receptors expressed on T lymphocytes and kidney epithelium during cisplatin-induced AKI. J Am Soc Nephrol 27(8):2257–2264. https://doi.org/10.1681/asn.2015060683
51. Fahling M, Seeliger E, Patzak A, Persson PB (2017) Understanding and preventing contrast-induced acute kidney injury. Nat Rev Nephrol 13(3):169–180. https://doi.org/10.1038/nrneph.2016.196
52. Arakelyan K, Cantow K, Hentschel J, Flemming B, Pohlmann A, Ladwig M, Niendorf T, Seeliger E (2013) Early effects of an x-ray contrast medium on renal T(2) */T (2) MRI as compared to short-term hyperoxia, hypoxia and aortic occlusion in rats. Acta Physiol (Oxf) 208(2):202–213. https://doi.org/10.1111/apha.12094
53. Seeliger E, Becker K, Ladwig M, Wronski T, Persson PB, Flemming B (2010) Up to 50-fold increase in urine viscosity with iso-osmolar contrast media in the rat. Radiology 256 (2):406–414. https://doi.org/10.1148/radiol.10091485
54. Seeliger E, Cantow K, Arakelyan K, Ladwig M, Persson PB, Flemming B (2014) Low-dose nitrite alleviates early effects of an X-ray contrast medium on renal hemodynamics and oxygenation in rats. Investig Radiol 49(2):70–77. https://doi.org/10.1097/RLI.0b013e3182a6fea6
55. Lenhard DC, Frisk AL, Lengsfeld P, Pietsch H, Jost G (2013) The effect of iodinated contrast agent properties on renal kinetics and oxygenation. Investig Radiol 48(4):175–182. https://doi.org/10.1097/RLI.0b013e31827b70f9
56. Lauver DA, Carey EG, Bergin IL, Lucchesi BR, Gurm HS (2014) Sildenafil citrate for prophylaxis of nephropathy in an animal model of contrast-induced acute kidney injury. PLoS One 9(11):e113598. https://doi.org/10.1371/journal.pone.0113598
57. Kiss N, Hamar P (2016) Histopathological evaluation of contrast-induced acute kidney injury rodent models. Biomed Res Int 2016:3763250. https://doi.org/10.1155/2016/3763250
58. Linkermann A, Heller JO, Prokai A, Weinberg JM, De Zen F, Himmerkus N, Szabo AJ,

Brasen JH, Kunzendorf U, Krautwald S (2013) The RIP1-kinase inhibitor necrostatin-1 prevents osmotic nephrosis and contrast-induced AKI in mice. J Am Soc Nephrol 24 (10):1545–1557. https://doi.org/10.1681/asn.2012121169

59. Nortier J, Pozdzik A, Roumeguere T, Vanherweghem JL (2015) Aristolochic acid nephropathy ("Chinese herb nephropathy"). Nephrol Ther 11(7):574–588. https://doi.org/10.1016/j.nephro.2015.10.001
60. De Broe ME (2012) Chinese herbs nephropathy and Balkan endemic nephropathy: toward a single entity, aristolochic acid nephropathy. Kidney Int 81(6):513–515. https://doi.org/10.1038/ki.2011.428
61. Geng Y, Zhang L, Fu B, Zhang J, Hong Q, Hu J, Li D, Luo C, Cui S, Zhu F, Chen X (2014) Mesenchymal stem cells ameliorate rhabdomyolysis-induced acute kidney injury via the activation of M2 macrophages. Stem Cell Res Ther 5(3):80. https://doi.org/10.1186/scrt469
62. Chevalier RL, Forbes MS, Thornhill BA (2009) Ureteral obstruction as a model of renal interstitial fibrosis and obstructive nephropathy. Kidney Int 75(11):1145–1152. https://doi.org/10.1038/ki.2009.86
63. He J, Wang Y, Sun S, Yu M, Wang C, Pei X, Zhu B, Wu J, Zhao W (2012) Bone marrow stem cells-derived microvesicles protect against renal injury in the mouse remnant kidney model. Nephrology (Carlton) 17 (5):493–500. https://doi.org/10.1111/j.1440-1797.2012.01589.x
64. Hewitson TD, Ono T, Becker GJ (2009) Small animal models of kidney disease: a review. Methods Mol Biol 466:41–57. https://doi.org/10.1007/978-1-59745-352-3_4
65. Graham ML, Schuurman HJ (2015) Validity of animal models of type 1 diabetes, and strategies to enhance their utility in translational research. Eur J Pharmacol 759:221–230. https://doi.org/10.1016/j.ejphar.2015.02.054
66. Lassila M, Seah KK, Allen TJ, Thallas V, Thomas MC, Candido R, Burns WC, Forbes JM, Calkin AC, Cooper ME, Jandeleit-Dahm KA (2004) Accelerated nephropathy in diabetic apolipoprotein e-knockout mouse: role of advanced glycation end products. J Am Soc Nephrol 15(8):2125–2138. https://doi.org/10.1097/01.Asn.0000133025.23732.46
67. Chua SC Jr, Chung WK, Wu-Peng XS, Zhang Y, Liu SM, Tartaglia L, Leibel RL (1996) Phenotypes of mouse diabetes and rat fatty due to mutations in the OB (leptin) receptor. Science 271(5251):994–996
68. Zucker LM, Antoniades HN (1972) Insulin and obesity in the Zucker genetically obese rat "fatty". Endocrinology 90(5):1320–1330. https://doi.org/10.1210/endo-90-5-1320
69. Mallipattu SK, Gallagher EJ, LeRoith D, Liu R, Mehrotra A, Horne SJ, Chuang PY, Yang VW, He JC (2014) Diabetic nephropathy in a nonobese mouse model of type 2 diabetes mellitus. Am J Physiol Renal Physiol 306(9):F1008–F1017. https://doi.org/10.1152/ajprenal.00597.2013
70. Kaspareit-Rittinghausen J, Rapp K, Deerberg F, Wcislo A, Messow C (1989) Hereditary polycystic kidney disease associated with osteorenal syndrome in rats. Vet Pathol 26 (3):195–201. https://doi.org/10.1177/030098588902600302
71. Katsuyama M, Masuyama T, Komura I, Hibino T, Takahashi H (2000) Characterization of a novel polycystic kidney rat model with accompanying polycystic liver. Exp Anim 49 (1):51–55. https://doi.org/10.1538/expanim.49.51
72. Takahashi H, Calvet JP, Dittemore-Hoover D, Yoshida K, Grantham JJ, Gattone VH 2nd (1991) A hereditary model of slowly progressive polycystic kidney disease in the mouse. J Am Soc Nephrol 1(7):980–989
73. Atala A, Freeman MR, Mandell J, Beier DR (1993) Juvenile cystic kidneys (jck): a new mouse mutation which causes polycystic kidneys. Kidney Int 43(5):1081–1085
74. Thivierge C, Kurbegovic A, Couillard M, Guillaume R, Cote O, Trudel M (2006) Overexpression of PKD1 causes polycystic kidney disease. Mol Cell Biol 26(4):1538–1548. https://doi.org/10.1128/mcb.26.4.1538-1548.2006
75. Muto S, Aiba A, Saito Y, Nakao K, Nakamura K, Tomita K, Kitamura T, Kurabayashi M, Nagai R, Higashihara E, Harris PC, Katsuki M, Horie S (2002) Pioglitazone improves the phenotype and molecular defects of a targeted Pkd1 mutant. Hum Mol Genet 11 (15):1731–1742. https://doi.org/10.1093/hmg/11.15.1731
76. Wu G, Somlo S (2000) Molecular genetics and mechanism of autosomal dominant polycystic kidney disease. Mol Genet Metab 69(1):1–15. https://doi.org/10.1006/mgme.1999.2943
77. Williams SS, Cobo-Stark P, James LR, Somlo S, Igarashi P (2008) Kidney cysts, pancreatic cysts, and biliary disease in a mouse model of autosomal recessive polycystic kidney disease. Pediatr Nephrol 23(5):733–741. https://doi.org/10.1007/s00467-007-0735-4

78. Nagao S, Kugita M, Yoshihara D, Yamaguchi T (2012) Animal models for human polycystic kidney disease. Exp Anim 61(5):477–488. https://doi.org/10.1538/expanim.61.477
79. Hultstrom M (2012) Development of structural kidney damage in spontaneously hypertensive rats. J Hypertens 30(6):1087–1091. https://doi.org/10.1097/HJH.0b013e328352b89a
80. Zhong F, Mallipattu SK, Estrada C, Menon M, Salem F, Jain MK, Chen H, Wang Y, Lee K, He JC (2016) Reduced Kruppel-like factor 2 aggravates glomerular endothelial cell injury and kidney disease in mice with unilateral nephrectomy. Am J Pathol 186 (8):2021–2031. https://doi.org/10.1016/j.ajpath.2016.03.018
81. Rabe M, Schaefer F (2016) Non-transgenic mouse models of kidney disease. Nephron 133(1):53–61. https://doi.org/10.1159/000445171
82. Grond J, Muller EW, van Goor H, Weening JJ, Elema JD (1988) Differences in puromycin aminonucleoside nephrosis in two rat strains. Kidney Int 33(2):524–529. https://doi.org/10.1038/ki.1988.29
83. LEE VW, HARRIS DC (2011) Adriamycin nephropathy: a model of focal segmental glomerulosclerosis. Nephrology 16(1):30–38. https://doi.org/10.1111/j.1440-1797.2010.01383.x
84. Akiyama K, Morita H, Suetsugu S, Kuraba S, Numata Y, Yamamoto Y, Inui K, Ideura T, Wakisaka N, Nakano K, Oniki H, Takenawa T, Matsuyama M, Yoshimura A (2008) Actin-related protein 3 (Arp3) is mutated in proteinuric BUF/Mna rats. Mamm Genome 19(1):41–50. https://doi.org/10.1007/s00335-007-9078-5
85. Fassi A, Sangalli F, Maffi R, Colombi F, Mohamed E, Brenner BM, Remuzzi G, Remuzzi A (1998) Progressive Glomerular Injury in the MWF Rat is predicted by Inborn Nephron Deficit. J Am Soc Nephrol 9 (8):1399–1406
86. Matsusaka T, Xin J, Niwa S, Kobayashi K, Akatsuka A, Hashizume H, Wang Q-c, Pastan I, Fogo AB, Ichikawa I (2005) Genetic engineering of glomerular sclerosis in the mouse via control of onset and severity of podocyte-specific injury. J Am Soc Nephrol 16(4):1013–1023. https://doi.org/10.1681/asn.2004080720
87. Assmann KJM, Van Son JPHF, Dijkman HBPM, Mentzel S, Wetzels JFM (2002) Antibody-induced albuminuria and accelerated focal glomerulosclerosis in the Thy-1.1 transgenic mouse. Kidney Int 62(1):116–126. https://doi.org/10.1046/j.1523-1755.2002.00428.x
88. Yang JW, Dettmar A, Kronbichler A, Yung Gee H, Saleem M, Heon Kim S, Shin JI (2018) Recent advances of animal model of focal segmental glomerulosclerosis. Clin Exp Nephro 22(4):752–763. https://doi.org/10.1007/s10157-018-1552-8
89. Ito R, Takahashi T, Ito M (2018) Humanized mouse models: application to human diseases. J Cell Physiol 233(5):3723–3728. https://doi.org/10.1002/jcp.26045
90. Kenney LL, Shultz LD, Greiner DL, Brehm MA (2016) Humanized mouse models for transplant immunology. Am J Transplant 16 (2):389–397. https://doi.org/10.1111/ajt.13520
91. Tan S, Li Y, Xia J, Jin CH, Hu Z, Duinkerken G, Li Y, Khosravi Maharlooei M, Chavez E, Nauman G, Danzl N, Nakayama M, Roep BO, Sykes M, Yang YG (2017) Type 1 diabetes induction in humanized mice. Proc Natl Acad Sci U S A 114(41):10954–10959. https://doi.org/10.1073/pnas.1710415114

10

Ultrasound and Photoacoustic Imaging of the Kidney: Basic Concepts and Protocols

Sandra Meyer, Dieter Fuchs, and Martin Meier

Abstract

Noninvasive, robust, and reproducible methods to image kidneys are provided by different imaging modalities. A combination of modalities (multimodality) can give better insight into structure and function and to understand the physiology of the kidney. Magnetic resonance imaging can be complemented by a multimodal imaging approach to obtain additional information or include interventional procedures. In the clinic, renal ultrasound has been essential for the diagnosis and management of kidney disease and for the guidance of invasive procedures for a long time. Adapting ultrasound to preclinical requirements and for translational research, the combination with photoacoustic imaging expands the capabilities to obtain anatomical, functional, and molecular information from animal models. This chapter describes the basic concepts of how to image kidneys using different and most appropriate modalities.

This chapter is based upon work from the COST Action PARENCHIMA, a community-driven network funded by the European Cooperation in Science and Technology (COST) program of the European Union, which aims to improve the reproducibility and standardization of renal MRI biomarkers. This introduction chapter is complemented by two separate chapters describing the experimental procedure and data analysis.

Key words Magnetic resonance imaging (MRI), Kidney, Ultrasound imaging (US), Photoacoustic imaging (PA), Multimodality, Doppler, Contrast, Animals, Rats, Mice

1 Introduction

Magnetic resonance imaging, while very powerful by itself, can be complemented by a multimodal imaging approach to streamline workflow processes, obtain additional information, or include interventional procedures. Ultrasound and computed tomography are modalities of primary choice in renal imaging on patients, with the disadvantage of computed tomography exposing the body to harmful irradiation. Due to its fast, cost-effective, versatile, and nonionizing characteristics, ultrasound imaging is well-established in the clinical practice, often used for first-line diagnostics and follow-ups and as a complementary method to MRI.

Andreas Pohlmann and Thoralf Niendorf (eds.), *Preclinical MRI of the Kidney: Methods and Protocols*, Methods in Molecular Biology, vol. 2216, https://doi.org/10.1007/978-1-0716-0978-1_7,

In the clinic, renal ultrasound has been essential for the diagnosis and management of kidney disease and for the guidance of invasive procedure for decades. Nevertheless, new developments to advance clinical diagnostics and medical treatments are required and strongly rely on appropriate preclinical models. Adapting the ultrasound technology to match preclinical requirements for translational studies and combining it with photoacoustic imaging, expands the researchers' capabilities to obtain anatomical, functional, and molecular information from their animal models.

MRI has the advantage of superior soft-tissue contrast, which facilitates and enables the detection and characterization of renal lesions. This chapter will give an introduction to how detailed kidney images can be created, blood flow visualized and quantified, and capillary as well as renal function assessed in vivo, noninvasively, and in real time using high-frequency ultrasound.

This introduction chapter is complemented by two separate chapters describing the experimental procedure and data analysis, which are part of this book.

This chapter is part of the book Pohlmann A, Niendorf T (eds) (2020) Preclinical MRI of the Kidney—Methods and Protocols. Springer, New York.

2 Measurement Concepts of Ultrasound and Photoacoustics

The basic principle of ultrasound imaging relies on detecting differences in tissue density by using sound waves with frequencies above the range of human hearing—typically in the MHz range. Using piezoelectric elements short, harmless ultrasound pulses are sent into the body. These sound waves are partially reflected back to the transducer by different layers of tissue and the return signals (often referred to as "echo"—hence the term "echography" which is used as a synonym to ultrasound) are recorded. Based on the time it takes for the echo to travel into the tissue and back and the strength of the signal, an image can be computed and displayed in real time. The resulting two-dimensional, grayscale image of an area of interest is referred to as Brightness Mode or B-Mode. Tissue closest to the transducer is displayed at the top and structures further away are shown below; a scale provides depth and size information in real time. With increasing density more echo is recorded resulting in a brighter signal on the screen; therefore, dense structures (e.g., skin) are represented in white and light gray tones, whereas ultrasound gel used for coupling and fluid-filled structures inside the body appear black. Most tissues and organs are displayed in a range of grayscales in between and have a characteristic appearance ("speckle pattern") that aids in their identification. B-Mode is the standard imaging mode on ultrasound systems and worked with the most because it allows for effective visualization of anatomical structures. It can be complemented by additional imaging modes to obtain functional information which are outlined in more detail in Subheading 3.

In ultrasound, the frequency of the sound waves sent into the tissue is of importance as it determines image resolution and penetration depth. In a clinical setting, renal ultrasound scans on adult patients are normally performed with a 3–6 MHz curved array transducer where the term "curved" describes the shape of the transducer surface. Routine measurements include determining the length of the kidney in a sagittal view, the measurement of cortex thickness and of blood flow in the renal and interlobar arteries [1].

By using an appropriate setup and ultrasound imaging system, these parameters and a variety of others can be obtained in preclinical animal models. Dedicated small-animal micro-ultrasound systems provide high spatial resolution down to 30 μm by employing higher frequencies of up to 70 MHz. While early systems for small animal imaging were equipped with mechanical probes, state-of-the-art micro-ultrasound systems are working with digital linear array (flat transducer surface) probes and are suitable for a broad range of applications [2]. In addition to providing higher resolution than clinical machines, ultrasound systems dedicated to preclinical research also:

1. Allow for controlled transducer positioning (Fig. 1a, c) and include a setup for image-guided injections. While clinical ultrasound and also injections are performed handheld, a stationary setup is superior in most preclinical applications.
2. Include an integrated animal handling solution for physiological monitoring and anesthesia. These are crucial components for any kind of imaging focusing on functional analysis (blood flow, perfusion, etc.) and should be controlled and recorded carefully at all times to ensure reproducibility. However, some ultrasound applications to evaluate anatomy can be performed on conscious animals when appropriately restrained or trained.

Since ultrasound relies on the detection of soundwaves, no contrast agent is required to visualize anatomical structures, 3D volumes, or to assess blood flow velocities. It is noteworthy that anatomical structures and volumes measured with dedicated small animal ultrasound match results acquired with dedicated small animal MRI or μCT systems [3].

Above and beyond the capabilities of micro-ultrasound to gather anatomical and functional information, photoacoustic imaging can also be applied in a preclinical setting to add molecular information. Photoacoustic imaging is a hybrid imaging modality that combines the strengths of optical and ultrasound imaging and can be used to monitor endogenous parameters such as blood content or oxygen saturation or various exogenous contrast agents.

In this imaging approach (Fig. 2), short (a few nanoseconds) pulses of near-infrared laser light are transmitted into the tissue and

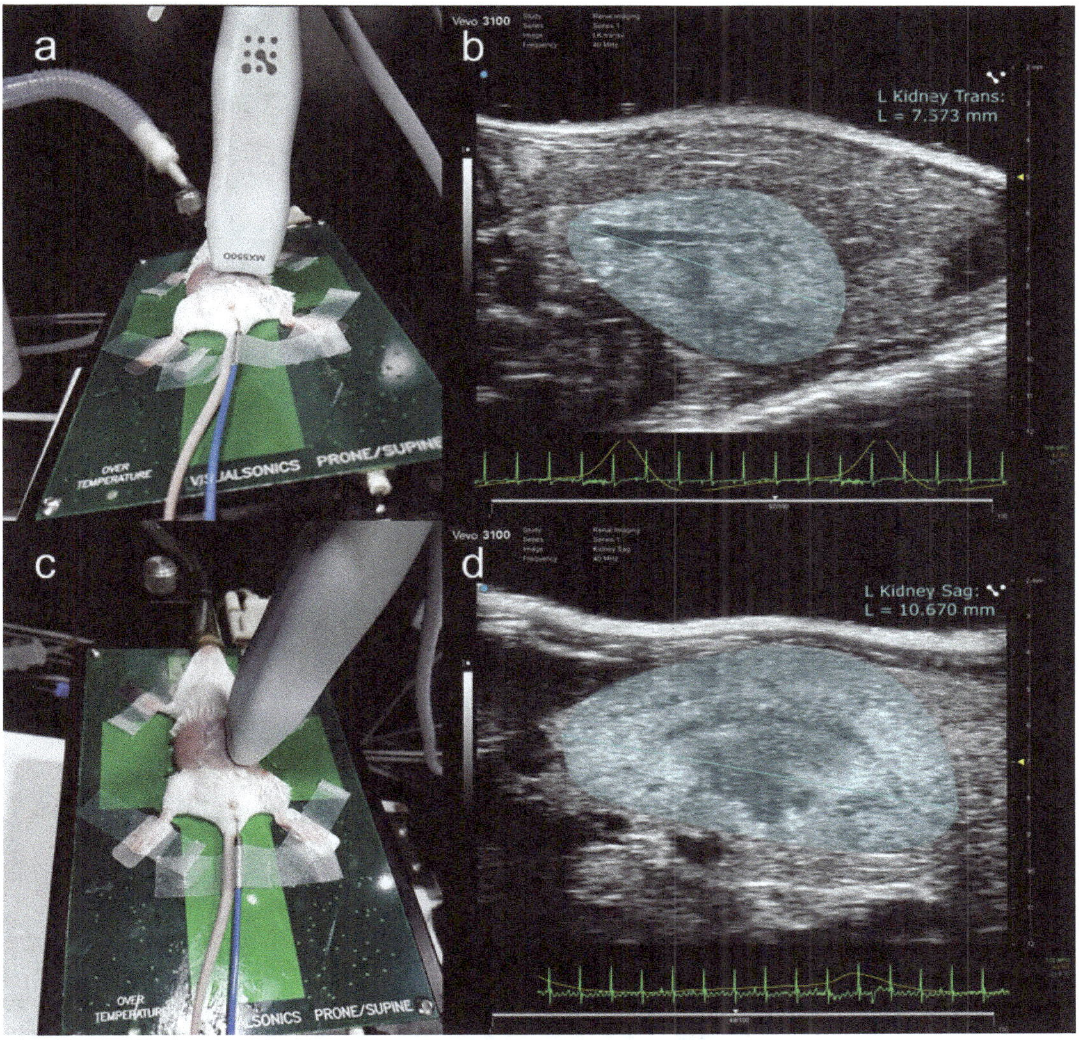

Fig. 1 Standard renal exam: animal and transducer positioning; (**a**) transverse position for left kidney imaging, (**b**) transverse US B-Mode image of the left kidney with length measurement, (**c**) sagittal position for left kidney imaging, (**d**) sagittal US B-Mode image of the left kidney with length measurement. Note the millimeter scale on the right and the physiological monitoring (ECG in green, respiration in yellow) below the US images

are selectively absorbed according to the optical properties of the tissue components. Light absorption results in a thermoelastic expansion creating a sound wave that can be localized by the ultrasound transducer and at the same resolution as the ultrasound image [4].

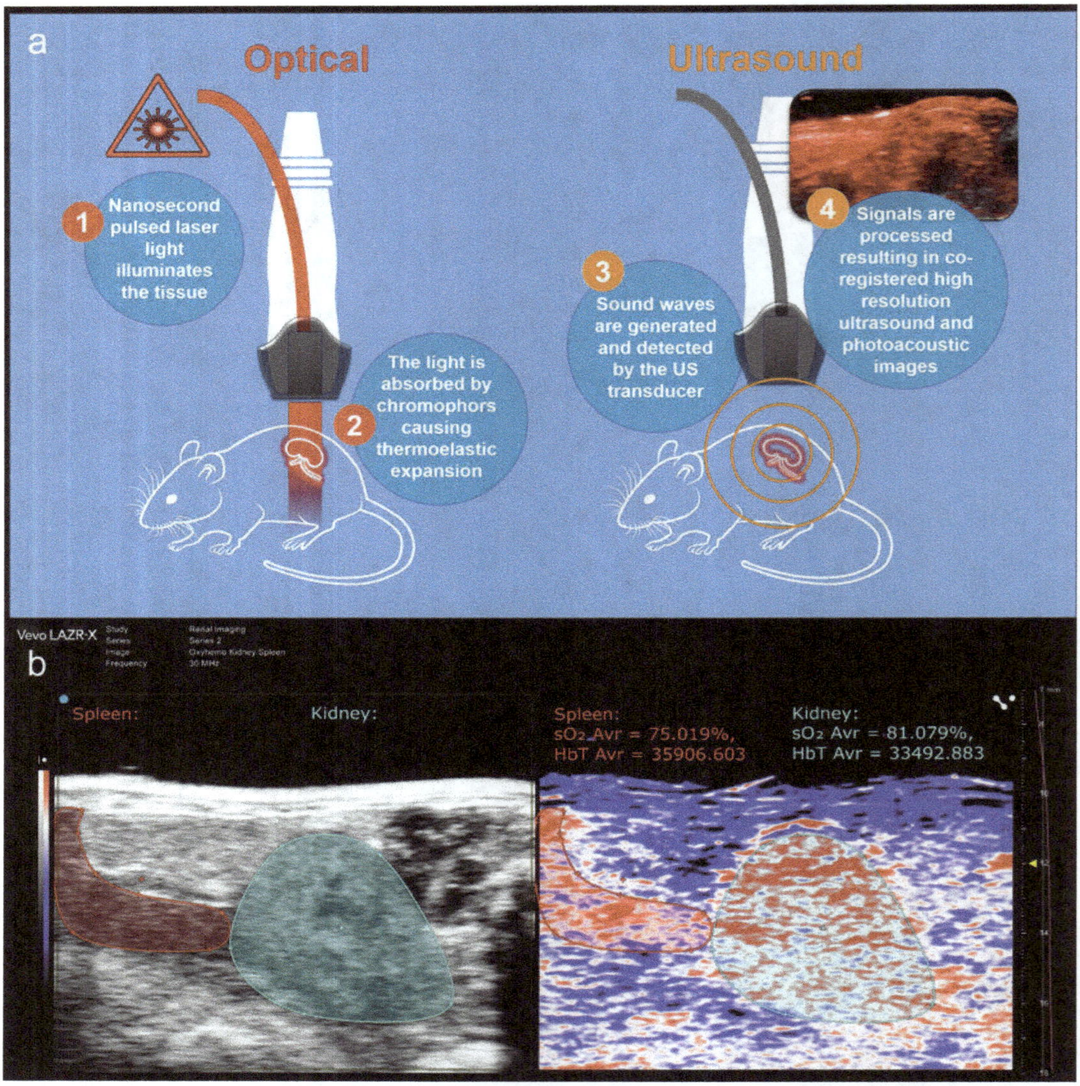

Fig. 2 Photoacoustic imaging; (**a**) the photoacoustic effect, (**b**) coregistered B-Mode image providing anatomical information (left) and photoacoustic image displaying oxygen saturation (right) in the spleen and left kidney

3 Overview of Applications

This section provides an overview of applications of high-frequency ultrasound and photoacoustic imaging in preclinical renal research. Examples of specific disease models and how multimodal imaging is applied are summarized in a brief review of selected publications in Table 1.

Table 1
Examples of specific disease models and how multimodal imaging is applied

Disease (animal model)	Usage of US and PA	Findings and Remarks	References
Polycystic kidney disease (PCK rats)	• Cyst detection • Kidney and cyst volume	Evaluation of kidneys in B-mode, power Doppler, and 3D • Quantification of kidney volume, number of cysts and cyst volume • US-based kidney volumes correlated strongly with kidney weights • US provided superior information in comparison to microscopic analysis of stained kidney sections	[12]
Type 2 diabetes (leptin-deficient (Ob/Ob) mice	• Anatomical and blood flow analysis • Renal RI and PI;	• RI and PI were higher in the ob/ob mice (RI 1.50; PI 0.81) at 21 weeks compared to lean controls (RI 0.69; PI 1.18) • Includes echocardiography and coronary flow reserve data	[13]
Orthotopic renal cell carcinoma (athymic nude mice)	• Tumor volume	• Validation of noninvasive imaging tools for monitoring of tumor growth in an orthotopic renal cell carcinoma xenograft • Tumor volumes determined by hrUS, μCT, and MRI showed a very good correlation with each other and with caliper measurements at autopsy • US examination time was very short (5 min)	[3]
Metastatic tumor xenografts Immunodeficient mice (NOD-SCID)	• Image-guided injections • Tumor localization and sizing	• To establish orthotopic xenograft models by ultrasound-guided injections into the adrenal gland and kidney (subcapsular) • Tumor location, size, and relation to the adrenal gland and kidney were monitored accurately and weekly in US • Technique is efficient, with up to 10 mice injected per 2-h session • Mice had fast recovery times of less than 15 min without procedure-related morbidity or mortality	[10]
Hydronephrosis/congenital obstructive nephropathy (megabladder (mgb) mouse)	Evaluate hydronephrosis	• Total renal length (RL) and renal pelvic anterior–posterior diameter (APD) were measured. Hydronephrosis was scored by the ratio of APD to RL • US permits easy stratification of mice into consistent pathological study groups composed of mild, moderate, and severe kidneys. This approach significantly improves the utility of this animal model	[14]

(continued)

Table 1 (continued)

Disease (animal model)	Usage of US and PA	Findings and Remarks	References
Hydronephrosis and underlying etiologies in (aging mice)	• Detection of hydronephrosis • Identification of concurrent abdominal lesions	• Underlying etiologies included pyelonephritis secondary to a preputial gland abscess and ascending urinary tract infections; cystolithiasis, infiltrative abdominal neoplasia with invasion of the renal pelvis, hilum, and parenchyma and surrounding lymph nodes; mouse urologic syndrome, and a case of spontaneous hydronephrosis with ureteritis	[6]
Acute kidney ischemia (induced by unilateral clamping in mice)	• Oxygen saturation measurements	• Longitudinal measurement of oxygen saturation shows differences between mild and severe renal injury • Kidney volume was also determined • PA provided a sensitive measure of change in sO_2 in the acute phase of AKI, with the sO_2 at 24 h after AKI being predictive of renal function in the chronic phase	[15]
Acute kidney injury (bilateral renal ischemia induced by clamping in mice)	• Renal microperfusion imaging	• Contrast-enhanced ultrasonography with high-resolution parametric perfusion maps can monitor changes in renal microvascular perfusion in space and time in mice	[16]
Acute renal ischemia induced by systemic hypoperfusion (Sprague-Dawley rats)	• Study hemorrhagic shock changes with microimaging	• After 1 h of ischemia, B-mode images documented slight changes in kidney echogenicity • Color and PW-Doppler analysis showed a reduction in renal blood flow in kidneys during the hypoperfusion with a progressive and significant change from baseline values of resistive index	[17]
Vesicoureteral reflux (C57BL6/J and C3H/HeJ inbred mice)	Monitor reflux with US contrast	• Reflux was detected in the proximal ureters and the renal pelvis bilaterally in C3H/HeJ mice • Contrast-enhanced ultrasound cystograms were established in-vivo	[18]
BALB mice	Contrast agent biodistribution in US and photoacoustic imaging	• A dual imaging contrast agent was developed to monitor kidney perfusion and organ distribution as well as whole-body biodistribution	[9]
Chronic kidney disease and cardiovascular disease (induced in C57BL/6J mice by 5/6 nephrectomy)	Assess cardiac dimensions and function	• Cardiac dysfunction and dilatation of the left ventricle was observed 8 weeks after partial nephrectomy • A treatment reversed cardiac dilatation and significantly improved cardiac dysfunction	[19]

3.1 Evaluating Kidney Size and Anatomy

B-Mode, as introduced in Measurement concepts (2.1), is used to locate the kidneys in the abdomen, observe the surrounding tissue and anatomical structure and to obtain organ size.

When viewed using ultrasound, the kidneys are located lateral of the abdominal aorta. The right kidney is positioned slightly more cranial in the thoracic cavity then the left kidney, and both can be identified by their characteristic appearance in ultrasound: the medulla in the medial portion of the kidney is darker than the cortex and surrounding the cortex, the kidney capsule appears as a bright thin line. Once the appearance of kidneys and surrounding in ultrasound are familiar, it is easy to identify any changes: Cysts are liquid-filled structures and therefore are visible as black, round structures with in the tissue. Hydronephrosis is qualitatively recognized as distension and dilatation of the renal pelvis and a method to quantify hydronephrosis based on the proportion of renal parenchyma in a longitudinal ultrasound image as been established [5] and underlying etiologies have been studied [6]. Tumor masses will appear in a different grayscale than the surrounding tissue and when becoming larger will distort the regular bean shaped form of the kidney. The observation and sizing of the kidney in 2D images can be performed in the transverse (Fig. 1a, b) and sagittal imaging (Fig. 1c, d) plane as required, based on preference. Moving through the whole organ in in both imaging planes in 2D allows to systematically screen for changes inside and also in the surroundings (e.g., ascites in the peritoneum). In addition, ultrasound imaging also may be used to study cardiovascular disease linked to chronic kidney disease [19].

Most preclinical ultrasound systems also allow to gather three-dimensional information. The principle for 3D image acquisition is similar between ultrasound and MRI where both acquire sequential 2D images with a known distance between them, determining the resolution along the *z*-axis (slice thickness). In ultrasound imaging a motor needs to be attached to move the probe across the area of interest along the *z*-axis and acquire a stack of images (Fig. 3). The consecutive 2D slices can be compiled into a 3D view, displayed in various ways, and analyzed to obtain accurate volume information of the kidneys and also cysts or tumor masses within.

3.2 Visualization of Blood Flow

When ultrasound waves are reflected by moving blood a frequency shift (Doppler shift) of the return ultrasound signal is induced that allows to display and measure blood flow. Most ultrasound systems are equipped with several imaging modes that use this Doppler effect to display blood flow in 2D images and allow for measuring blood flow velocities.

Color Doppler mode, overlaid on top of a B-Mode image for anatomical reference, displays blood flow in the area of interest in gradients of red and blue (Fig. 4b). The color gradients indicate both the direction and mean velocity of the Doppler shift: blood

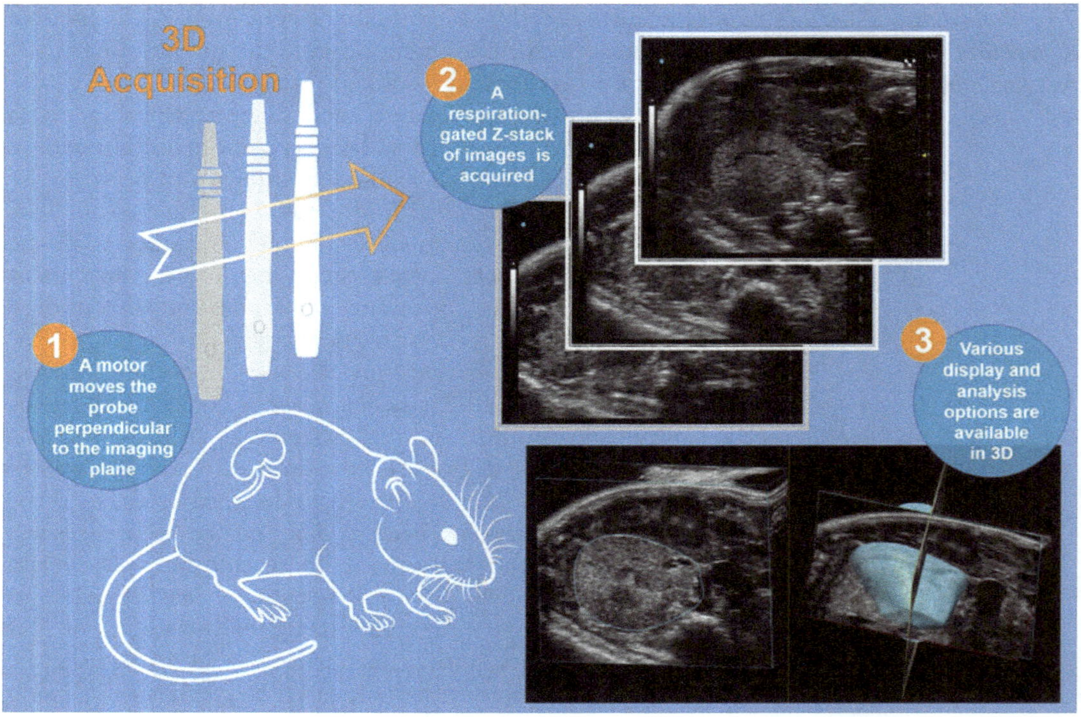

Fig. 3 Schematic workflow for 3D US image acquisition and processing

flowing toward the transducer is represented by a gradient between red (lowest velocity) and white (highest velocity) and blood flowing away from the transducer is represented by a gradient between blue (lowest velocity) and white (highest velocity). BART is an acronym commonly used to remember the colors associated with the direction of flow: Blue Away, Red Toward. Color Doppler mode is a very useful tool to identify the major and cortical vessels in the kidney and accurately guide the positioning for flow measurements, which are performed in pulsed-wave (PW) Doppler mode. To obtain a measurement, a Doppler sample volume (point where the blood flow should be measured) is placed within the vessel and the system generates a PW Doppler spectrum that displays time on the *x*-axis and flow velocity on the *y*-axis (Fig. 4d). Once PW Doppler spectrums of the renal artery and vein have been recorded, velocity measurements such as peak systolic velocity (PSV), end-diastolic velocity (EDV), and the velocity time integral (VTI) can be added. Based on these measurements, relevant parameters will be calculated as an indicator for vascular function.

- The resistive index (RI) is an example of additional analysis that may be useful. A RI of 0 is calculated for continuous flow patterns and an RI of 1 indicates a strongly pulsating flow with no flow during diastole. In the clinic an RI of the renal

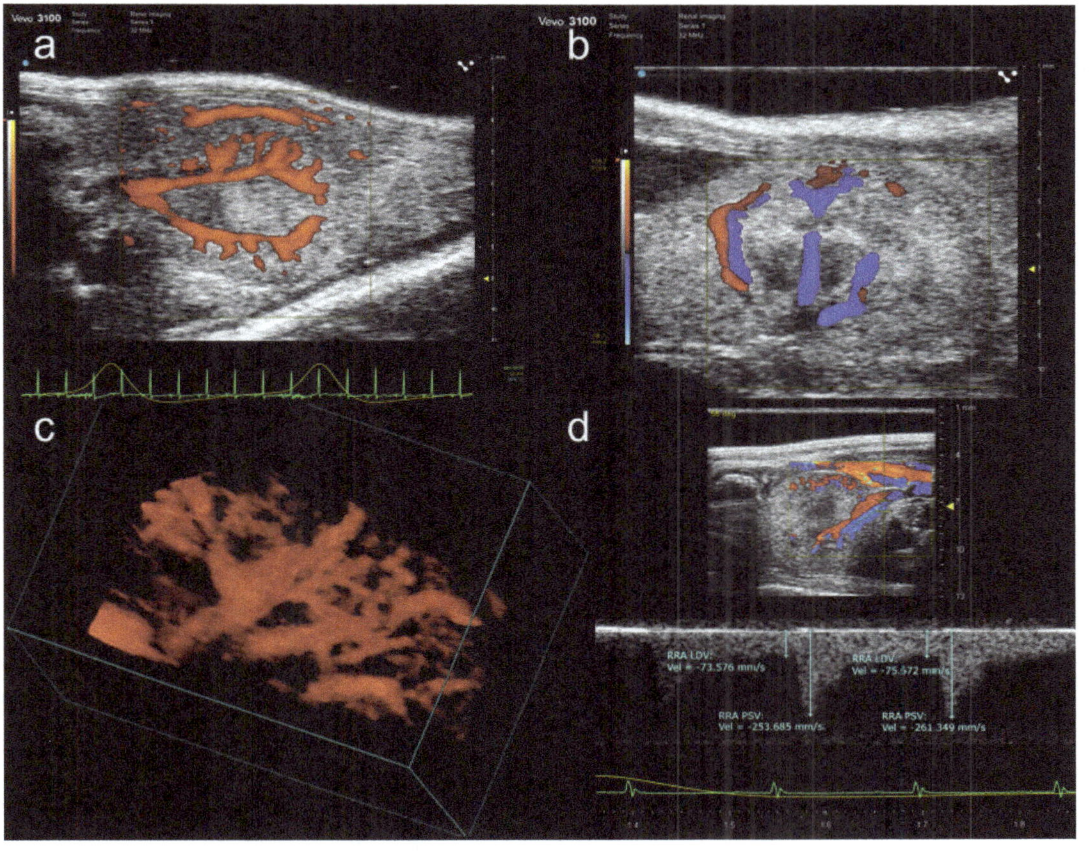

Fig. 4 Assessment of blood flow; (**a**) power Doppler signal in transverse view of the left kidney is overlaid with the B-mode image, (**b**) Blood flow in the interlobal vessels as visualized in Color Doppler Mode, in this image red and blue colors indicate arterial and venous flow, respectively; (**c**) three-dimensional rendering of Power Doppler signal of a healthy kidney, (**d**) pulse-waved Doppler profile of renal artery flow, peak systolic (PSV), and lowest diastolic velocity (LDV) measurements are shown, the sample positioning is indicated in the scout image above the flow profile

artery = 0.6 is observed in healthy adults and a rise in RI is seen as an indicator for renal disease.

$$\text{RI} = \frac{\text{PSV} - \text{EDV}}{\text{PSV}}$$

- The pulsatility index (PI) is another parameter often calculated in clinical renal diagnosis.

$$\text{PI} = \frac{\text{PSV} - \text{EDV}}{\text{VTI mean velocity}}$$

Power Doppler mode is another tool used to display and analyze blood flow within an area of interest. It is similar to color Doppler mode in detecting the occurring Doppler shift, but instead of displaying blood flow direction, it color-codes flow from orange to yellow according to signal intensity and is most useful for smaller vessels having slower blood flow (Fig. 4a).

It is crucial for PW Doppler mode and all other Doppler imaging modes, that an appropriate angle is achieved between the transmitted ultrasound beam and the blood flowing through the vessel; the imaging plane should be adjusted such that the angle between these two is less than 60 ° to provide an accurate velocity measurement.

Color and power Doppler information can also be acquired in 3D, visualizing the blood vessel structure in the entire organ (Fig. 4c). The amount of Doppler signal in a 3D volume can then be calculated. With the right animal setup, imaging both kidneys at the same time is feasible.

3.3 Perfusion Imaging

While Doppler imaging can be used to visualize blood flow in the renal artery and vein and also in the interlobar and arcuate vessels, monitoring perfusion of the kidney at capillary level requires the use of ultrasound contrast agents. Ultrasound contrast agents are very small gas bubbles (microbubbles) about 2–3 μm in diameter and encapsulated by a polymer or lipid shell (Fig. 5a). Several contrast imaging modes can be used for the detection of these microbubbles in the area of interest. Linear contrast enhanced ultrasound, the first contrast mode used at frequencies above 15 MHz, primarily relies on subtraction of background information to display the increase in echo due to the wash-in of contrast agent. Newer generation systems allow to monitor perfusion in real-time based on nonlinear fundamental detection with amplitude modulation, resulting in a higher sensitivity [7].

While ultrasound imaging to monitor perfusion requires a contrast agent and therefore intravenous access, photoacoustic imaging allows for the detection of hemoglobin and its oxygen saturation status (Fig. 2). Based on the change of hemoglobin's optical properties dependent on oxygen bound to the heme group, one can assess tissue oxygenation at a level matching BOLD (blood oxygen level–dependent) MRI [8]. It should be noted that ultrasound contrast agent and photoacoustic imaging of hemoglobin are nontoxic and harmless to the animal.

3.4 Molecular Information

Ultrasound and photoacoustic contrast agents can also be used for molecular imaging. Ultrasound contrast agents can be targeted to assess biomarker expression (Fig. 5c) but are exclusively tailored to vascular endothelium as the contrast agent does not leave the vasculature. Photoacoustic contrast agents, dyes or nanometer-sized particles, can be used for specifically targeting extravascular targets or for assessing glomeruli function and to study biodistribution [9].

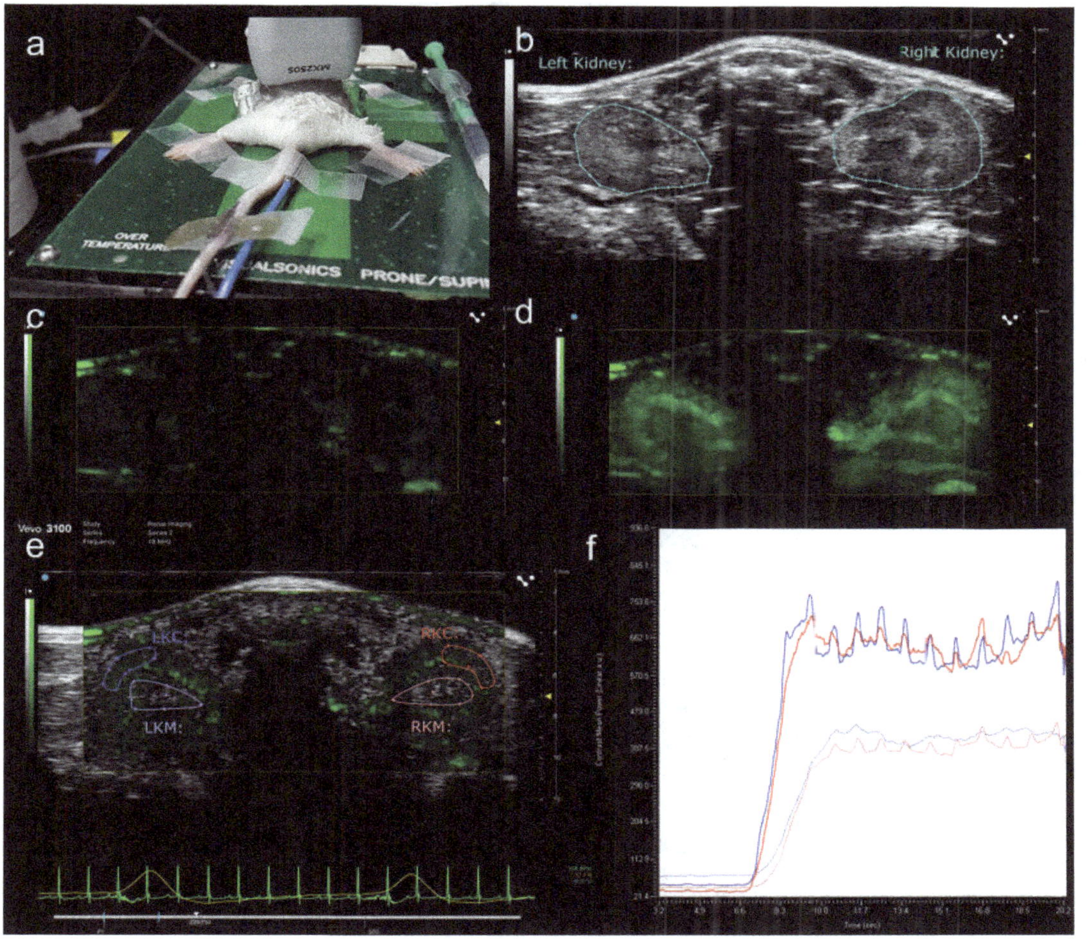

Fig. 5 Perfusion assessment of both mouse kidneys; (**a**) schematic model of a microbubble used for US contrast imaging; (**b**) animal and transducer position, (**c**) B-mode image, left and right kidney are outlined; (**d**) schematic binding of targeted contrast agent to a biomarker; Non-linear contrast image of both kidneys before (**e**) and after contrast injection (**f**). After contrast injection; for analysis, regions of interest in cortex and medulla of left (blue) and right (red) kidney are selected (**g**); a graph displays the contrast signal in these regions of interest (**h**)

3.5 Interventional Procedures

In contrast to other imaging modalities, in ultrasound and photoacoustic imaging the animal is accessible throughout the imaging session, allowing for various interventional procedures to be performed during an imaging session (Fig. 6). Using a so-called in-plane needle visualization technique, it is possible to follow the movement of a needle inside the animal in B-mode and ensure accurate placement of the needle tip for injections or aspiration. Image guided injections allow to place cells to create orthotopic tumor models or apply drug treatments precisely without the need for more invasive surgery [10]. Switching to image guided injections is an important step in the refinement of animal procedures and helps to shorten recovery time and minimize discomfort and

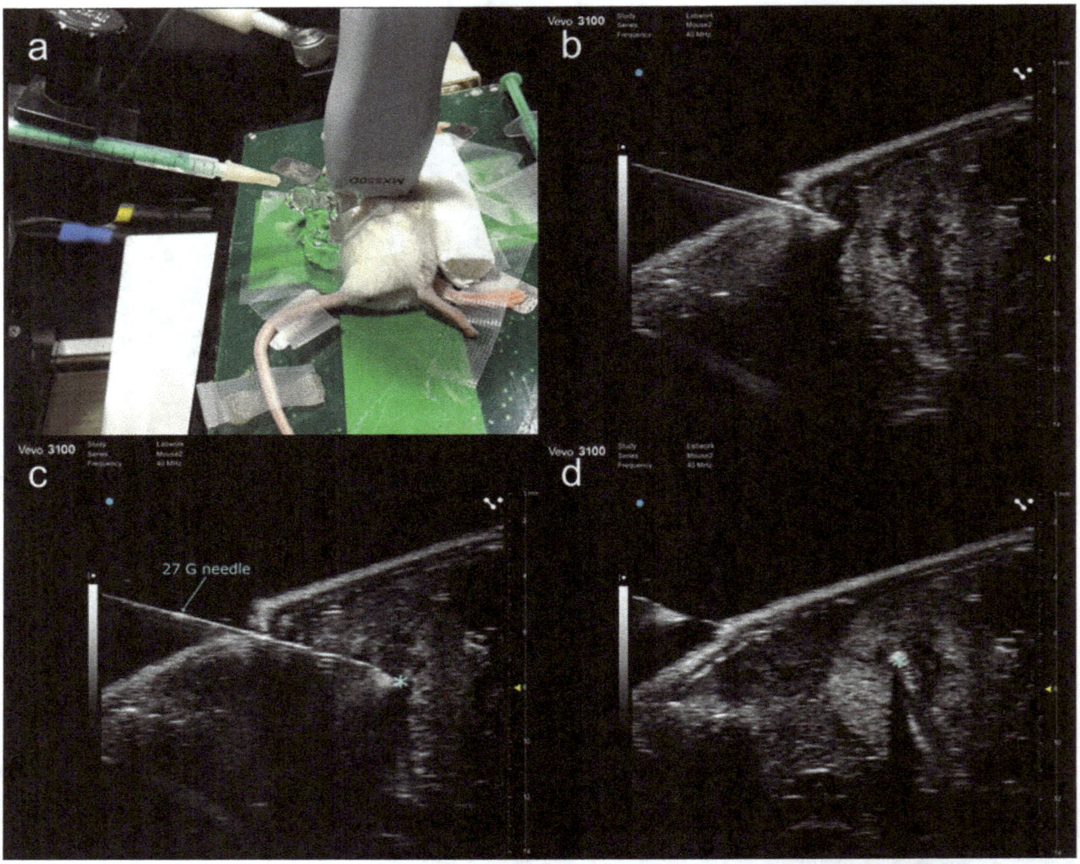

Fig. 6 Image guided injection into the left kidney of a mouse; (**a**) animal and needle positioning, (**b**) penetration of the skin, (**c**) the needle tip (marked with an asterisk) is positioned in the medulla of the kidney, (**d**) after injection of US contrast agent and needle retraction, injection site is marked with an asterisk

complications as the procedure can be performed with only light anesthesia and the procedure itself does not require postoperative analgesia. In addition the success of any given injection or aspiration can be verified in real time.

4 Protocols

4.1 Standard Renal Exam

The protocol outlined below depicts a standard renal ultrasound exam that can be performed on various ultrasound systems. If available, a system dedicated for small animal imaging using high-frequency linear transducers is be preferred due its superior resolution and sensitivity. For rats a transducer with a 50 or 75 μm resolution is appropriate and for mice a transducer with 40 μm resolution should be used. Despite the similar principle of various ultrasound systems, the availability of imaging modes, settings and analysis tools may vary. Please refer to instructions provided by the manufacturer for system-specific information and tailored work protocols.

While some brief ultrasound scans (e.g., for linear measurements, screening for pathologies or anatomical alterations) can be performed on awake animals, more comprehensive renal exams including flow measurements or volumetric analysis normally require the use of anesthesia. A brief description of isoflurane anesthesia is included below, but researchers should always carefully follow local rules and regulations.

In order to ensure reproducibility and to streamline workflow in longitudinal studies, it is recommended to store settings for all imaging modes and applications, stick to the same anesthesia type and level, as well as monitor the animal's physiologic parameters.

1. Switch on the flow of oxygen or medical air (the latter preferred for contrast enhanced ultrasound imaging) and set it to 1 L/min, place the animal in the induction box and turn on isoflurane at 4–5% until anesthesia is induced. Once a sufficient level of anesthesia is reached (loss of righting reflex), transfer the animal onto the imaging table and reduce isoflurane to 1.5–2% during imaging (depending on the animal model), or higher for interventional procedures. Make sure to switch the flow of anesthesia gas from the knock out box to the mask.
2. Place the animal in supine position if the renal exam is part of an abdominal scan; a prone position may be used to evaluate kidney structure, dimensions and volume, this position is also more suitable for image-guided injections.
3. Prepare the animal: apply eye ointment, tape the paws to the ECG leads using a small amount of ECG gel for coupling, insert a rectal probe to monitor body temperature and remove the hair in the area of interest. Animal physiology should be carefully monitored throughout the imaging session and adjustments made as necessary; for example, an additional heat lamp can be used to maintain body temperature.
4. Remove hair from the area of interest using a dedicated clipper and/or hair removal cream.
5. Apply a sufficient amount of prewarmed ultrasound gel, place the transducer in transverse position below the ribcage and start imaging in B-mode. Check the transducer orientation. In a supine position the imaging convention needs to be followed similar to MRI imaging, that is, with a transverse imaging plane the head should be behind the image, tail toward the viewer, animal's left on the right side of the screen.
6. Locate the area of interest by moving from the lower end of the ribcage toward the lower abdomen. The right kidney can be localized caudally of and adjacent to the liver. The left kidney is

located caudally of the stomach and in close proximity to spleen and the tail of the pancreas (Fig. 1a).

7. The image can be optimized by adjusting the field of view to fit the kidney, focus and gain. Localize the widest, middle part of the kidney and center the organ on the screen using the micromanipulators of the animal station. When imaging in a supine position, the animal table may be tilted sideways to bring the kidney closer to the transducer and remove shadowing caused by the intestinal tract. Save a B-Mode video clip of the transverse view for analysis (Fig. 1b).
8. Switch on color Doppler to display the blood flow in the renal artery and vein. Adjust the Doppler window to fit the position and size of the organ and fine-tune the transducer position to locate the vessels. Save a video clip, then activate pulsed-wave Doppler mode to measure blood flow in the renal artery by placing the Sample Volume gate within the artery. Align the angle of the PW Doppler with the direction of blood flow as indicated by color Doppler mode—you may need to reposition the transducer to obtain an angle smaller than 60°. Velocity, gain and baseline may be adjusted to display the flow profile and should be saved as presets in longitudinal studies. Save the blood flow profile for analysis (Fig. 4d).
9. With the transverse view centered on the screen, the sagittal view of the kidney can be displayed by rotating the transducer 90°. Confirm the longest extension of the kidney is displayed by a mid-lateral movement and save a B-Mode video clip of the sagittal view for analysis (Fig. 1d).
10. If required, intrarenal flow in the interlobar arteries can also be displayed and measured. Starting from the sagittal view, the transducer should be adjusted to the coronal plane. Fine-tune the positioning until the vessel structure (in B-Mode) and flow pattern (in color Doppler mode, Fig. 4b)) can be visualized, then switch on pulse-waved Doppler to record the flow pattern.
11. In addition a 3D data set of the area of interest can be obtained either in the transverse or sagittal view. Most commonly a 3D motor is used to move the transducer perpendicular to the imaging plane to acquire a stack of images (Fig. 3). Select a start and end position or scanning range and start 3D acquisition. Respiration gating may be applied to avoid movement artifacts due to the breathing of the animal. Once completed the data set can be processed to display a 3D view of the organ and saved for analysis.
12. A combined 3D acquisition of B-Mode and power Doppler or color Doppler may be used to also obtain blood flow information for the whole organ (Fig. 4c). In this case, power or color

Doppler should be activated before starting the 3D acquisition and the size of the window should be enlarged to cover the region of interest, the use of respiration gating and a wall filter is recommended to avoid respiration artifacts.

13. Confirm all images required for analysis have been saved. Wipe off the ultrasound gel, turn off the isoflurane and release the animal from the mouse handling table. Monitor the animal until fully recovered.

4.2 Perfusion Studies

Studying kidney perfusion in ultrasound imaging requires the intravenous injection of a contrast agent. Administration can be performed either as a continuous infusion using a pump, or as bolus injection, which can be delivered by hand but using a pump is recommended to ensure reproducibility. In addition it is possible to study reperfusion by applying a short ultrasound pulse to destroy the contrast agent within the field of view and record subsequent reperfusion. Here we would like to outline a basic perfusion study that can be included in an imaging session in combination with the standard exam. To allow for comparison, the imaging procedure should be standardized as much as possible. For a detailed review of contrast imaging in small animals and various parameters that should be considered, please refer to [11].

1. Before anesthetizing the animal, follow the instructions provided by the manufacturer to reconstitute the US contrast agent. Prepare a tail vein catheter (butterfly needle suitable for the contrast agent, fine tubing connected to syringe filled with saline).
2. Start animal anesthesia as described above. Once the animal has been moved to the animal table and eye ointment has been applied, insert the saline filled butterfly needle into the tail vein and fix the catheter with tape or tissue glue. Position and prepare the animal for imaging to obtain anatomical and blood flow information as described above using the 22–55 MHz probe (*see* Subheading 4.1).
3. Switch ultrasound transducer if required for high sensitivity detection (e.g., 15–24 MHz transducer for 2–3 μm phospholipid shell bubbles). Contrast imaging for one kidney can be performed in various positions, if perfusion of both kidneys should be observed at the same time, a prone position may be used (Fig. 5c, d). Position the animal as required and apply a small amount of gel. Avoid air bubbles as these may cause artifacts.
4. Start the nonlinear contrast (NLC) mode, adjust the imaging window, and adjust the gain so that a small amount of background signal is visible in the area of interest (Fig. 5e). Check the frame rate of the image acquisition and adjust the video clip

length to allow for sufficient acquisition time (e.g., 30 s), locate the prospective saving option on the system. If required, acquire a 3D data set before contrast injection and do not move the animal or transducer. Once the settings have been optimized it is advised to store the settings as presets.

5. Fill a new syringe with contrast agent, flush the catheter with 15 μL of saline and change to the syringe containing the contrast agent. Start the video clip with automatic storage option. After 3 s inject the bolus of 50 μL of contrast agent within 3 s using a pump for accurate injection rates. Within a few seconds a signal increase in the area of interest should be visible and the video clip will be stored automatically (Fig. 5f).
6. Change back to the syringe containing saline and flush the catheter with 15 μL and if required, record a second 3D data set using the previous settings. Circulating contrast agent will be observed for approximately 10–15 min. Once the contrast agent has been cleared a second bolus injection can be performed if required. After completing the contrast acquisition end the exam (*see* Subheading 4.1) or continue with one of the options described below.

4.3 Photoacoustic Exam to Monitor Oxygen Saturation

In addition to 2D and 3D ultrasound imaging showing renal anatomy, blood flow, and perfusion, photoacoustic (PA) imaging can add additional information by visualizing endogenous as well as exogenous contrast agents.

1. Anesthesia and animal preparation for PA imaging are identical to the procedure described above, but in order to obtain the best possible PA images the animal should be placed either in a lateral decubitus position or prone position to image both kidneys. In a prone position white gauze may be placed underneath the flanks of the animal to ensure reproducible positioning as well as optimizing light delivery.
2. Depending on the system, choose the appropriate photoacoustic transducer or the ultrasound transducer with laser fiber combination. Apply enough gel to the recess of the transducer so that it is overflowing and ensure that no bubbles are present.
3. Apply a generous amount of prewarmed, bubble-free gel to the animal. Lower the transducer into the gel just until contact is made and an image appears in B-Mode. Position the animal or transducer such that the skin line appears horizontal and at the recommended distance from the transducer. This ensures optimized and reproducible light delivery into the tissue, resulting in accurate photoacoustic data.
4. To limit the field of view to the target, adjust image depth, depth offset, and image width. If required, record ultrasound images in B-Mode or Doppler modes as described above.

5. Switch from B-mode to PA-mode, and start imaging at a single wavelength (e.g., 800 nm). First, increase the PA gain to determine if there is any signal present that may be missed with lower gain. Adjust the gain so that low-level signal can still be seen while keeping background signal (often referred to as "noise") to a minimum.
6. To compensate for light attenuation at depth, adjust the time gain compensation or fluence correction. Try to "even out" the signal throughout the depth of the image. For example, the signal at the surface of the skin can be quenched while applying a slight boost with increasing depth. All settings should be saved and reapplied in future imaging sessions.
7. Switch to oxygen detection and record a video clip for Oxygen Saturation analysis, a 3D data set may also be obtained.
8. If required, also obtain a spectral scan or a multiwavelength scans in 2D and 3D based on previously established protocols for imaging exogenous contrast agents such as dyes (e.g., Evans Blue) or nanoparticles.
9. End the exam as described above or continue to perform an interventional procedure.

4.4 Image Guided Needle Injections

Image guided interventions can be added to any imaging session as an additional step to locally administer a drug or implement cells. This procedure can be performed independently and is a fast and reliable procedure to replace a surgical intervention. Please refer to Subheading 4.1 for instructions on anesthesia, animal preparation, and imaging and follow these additional steps:

1. An analgesic treatment may be applied before the start of the procedure.
2. Prepare a syringe for injection and attach a 30G 1 in. needle. If the use of a different needle is required, please ensure the length of the shaft is sufficient for the needle to pass under the probe without the needle hub pressing against the probe casing. Fix the syringe in an injection mount to allow for precise control of the needle movement directly under the transducer, for best visualization of the needle tip the bevel should be facing upward.
3. If available, an additional micromanipulator can be placed between transducer and transducer mount, this allows to fine-tune the probe position for clear identification of the needle tip during the procedure.
4. Adjust the positioning of the needle and transducer. The needle should be aligned with and parallel to the ultrasound beam, which can be checked by placing the needle in some ultrasound gel and lowering the transducer into it (Fig. 6c). When

positioned correctly, the whole length and tip of the needle should be visible on the live image as a bright line. Once a good alignment has been achieved, movement of the needle and probe in the Y-axis should be avoided.

5. The animal may be taped to the electrodes in a prone position or in a lateral decubitus position (Fig. 6a) to inject into the contralateral kidney. In this case, taping the lower front and hind paw and tail to the electrodes will allow to monitor the animal's physiology.
6. Apply a generous amount of bubble-free gel to the area of interest. Lower transducer into the gel and bring the kidney into view. Adjust the position to have some space on the left for needle positioning.
7. If desired, set the ultrasound system up to record a long video clip by adjusting the length of the video and enable prospective saving, start recording before inserting the needle or injection as required.
8. Advance the needle forward into the gel until it is visible. By tilting and moving it up or down, the projected needle path should point to the target area within the kidney. If large blood vessels or critical organs lie within the needle pathway, reposition the animal to avoid unnecessary damage of tissue.
9. Advance the needle quickly to push through the skin, then gently move forward to place the needle tip in the target structure (Fig. 6b). If the needle slightly bends out of view during the injection, the *Y*-axis micromanipulator can be used to readjust the image. Perform the injection and wait shortly to allow for distribution then slowly retract the needle (Fig. 6d). If desired, save a video clip of the procedure.
10. End the ultrasound exam as described above and monitor the recovery of the animal. Check the animal for signs of pain or complications in regular intervals as indicated in the animal protocol (i.e., up to 24 h after injection).

4.5 Analysis

All commercially available ultrasound systems dedicated to in vivo imaging provide measurement tools for comprehensive image analysis that cover a broad range of standard applications. As data is mostly stored in proprietary file formats, analysis tools are a fundamental part of the system capabilities and convenient to use, no other third party or open source software is normally used for standard analysis. Therefore no detailed step-by-step instructions are given below. Instead the type of measurements routinely performed are outlined below and were applicable, calculations are mentioned. Depending on the ultrasound system that is used, measurements will either be added directly during the exam, afterward on the ultrasound system itself or on a dedicated offline analysis software. Please refer to the user instructions to ensure all data required for analysis is saved. Modern preclinical ultrasound and photoacoustic equipment allow for extracting the image data as DICOM or raw formats, making the data accessible in nonproprietary image analysis programs.

1. The length of the kidney in a sagittal and transverse 2D B-Mode images can be measured in mm using a line measurement.
2. In standard clinical exams, kidney volume is often calculated using the ellipsoid formula: Length × Width × Depth × 0.523. Using a 3D motor and appropriate settings a more accurate volume of the kidneys can be obtained. Depending on the software, various ways of volume reconstructions are available. Mostly the user is required to outline the organ in a few, selected frames on either the video clip or reconstructed 3D view. Based on this information an outline of the organ is created and the volume calculated. In addition to the total kidney volume, sub-volumes can be added to measure cysts, tumors or other anatomical structures. Most software packages also allow to copy volume reconstructions between imaging modes and will quantify additional parameters. In 3D Power and Color Doppler images, percent vascularity can be measured in the volume of interest. Various display options are available to visualize results.
3. In PA imaging, the PA signal intensity can be measured within an area of interest at a single wavelength and build in algorithms allow to also calculate oxygen saturation and hemoglobin content in 2D and 3D. If required, signal from endogenous or exogenous contrast agents can be separated from background using automated spectral unmixing tools.
4. Flow analysis of the renal artery or intrarenal arteries routinely include measuring peak systolic (PSV) and lowest diastolic (LDV) as well as the velocity-time-integral. If not automated in the analysis software, the Resistive Index can be calculated manually based on the first two parameters: (PSV − LDV)/PSV.
5. A basic perfusion analysis includes outlining areas of interest, for example in the kidney cortex, medulla or a tumor, to display the wash in curve of the contrast agent. Based on this curve, the time to peak, a relative measure for blood flow, and peak enhancement, a relative measure for blood volume, can be measured. If 3D data is recorded, it is also possible to observe the contrast signal before and after contrast injection and calculate the parameter percent agent.
6. For presentation purposes, ultrasound and photoacoustic imaging analysis software allows for annotations and color

coding of anatomical structures and further editing for educational purposes or publishing.

Acknowledgments

This chapter is based upon work from COST Action PARENCHIMA, supported by European Cooperation in Science and Technology (COST). COST (www.cost.eu) is a funding agency for research and innovation networks. COST Actions help connect research initiatives across Europe and enable scientists to enrich their ideas by sharing them with their peers. This boosts their research, career, and innovation.

PARENCHIMA (renalmri.org) is a community-driven Action in the COST program of the European Union, which unites more than 200 experts in renal MRI from 30 countries with the aim to improve the reproducibility and standardization of renal MRI biomarkers.

References

1. Hansen K, Nielsen M, Ewertsen C (2015) Ultrasonography of the kidney: a pictorial review. Diagnostics 6:2
2. Foster FS, Hossack J, Adamson SL (2011) Micro-ultrasound for preclinical imaging. Interface Focus 1:576–601
3. Linxweiler J, Körbel C, Müller A et al (2017) Experimental imaging in orthotopic renal cell carcinoma xenograft models: comparative evaluation of high-resolution 3D ultrasonography, in-vivo micro-CT and 9.4T MRI. Sci Rep 7:1–10
4. Needles A, Heinmiller A, Sun J et al (2013) Development and initial application of a fully integrated photoacoustic micro-ultrasound system. IEEE Trans Ultrason Ferroelectr Freq Control 60:888–897
5. Carpenter AR, Becknell B, Ingraham SE, McHugh KM (2012) Ultrasound imaging of the murine kidney. In: Michos O (ed) Kidney development. Methods in molecular biology, vol 886. Humana Press, Totowa, NJ
6. Springer DA, Allen M, Hoffman V et al (2014) Investigation and identification of etiologies involved in the development of acquired hydronephrosis in aged laboratory mice with the use of high-frequency ultrasound imaging. Pathobiol Aging Age Relat Dis 4:1–14
7. Needles A, Arditi M, Rognin NG et al (2010) Nonlinear contrast imaging with an array-based micro-ultrasound system. Ultrasound Med Biol 36:2097–2106
8. Rich LJ, Seshadri M (2015) Photoacoustic imaging of vascular hemodynamics: validation with blood oxygenation level–dependent MR imaging. Radiology 275:110–118
9. Toumia Y, Cerroni B, Trochet P et al (2018) Performances of a pristine graphene-microbubble hybrid construct as dual imaging contrast agent and assessment of its biodistribution by photoacoustic imaging. Part Part Syst Charact 35:1800066
10. Noord RAVAN, Thomas T, Krook M et al (2017) Tissue-directed implantation using ultrasound visualization for development of biologically relevant metastatic tumor xenografts. In Vivo 791:779–791
11. Hyvelin J, Tardy I, Arbogast C et al (2013) Use of ultrasound contrast agent microbubbles in preclinical research. Investig Radiol 48:1–14
12. Kapoor S, Rodriguez D, Mitchell K et al (2016) High resolution ultrasonography for assessment of renal cysts in the PCK rat model of autosomal recessive polycystic kidney disease. Kidney Blood Press Res 41:186–196
13. Westergren HU, Grönros J, Heinonen SE et al (2015) Impaired coronary and renal vascular function in spontaneously type 2 diabetic leptin-deficient mice. PLoS One 10:e0130648
14. Ingraham SE, Saha M, Carpenter AR et al (2010) Pathogenesis of renal injury in the Megabladder mouse: a genetic model of congenital obstructive nephropathy. Pediatr Res 68:500–507

15. Okumura K, Matsumoto J, Iwata Y et al (2018) Evaluation of renal oxygen saturation using photoacoustic imaging for the early prediction of chronic renal function in a model of ischemia-induced acute kidney injury. PLoS One 13:e0206461

16. Fischer K, Meral FC, Zhang Y et al (2016) High-resolution renal perfusion mapping using contrast-enhanced ultrasonography in ischemia-reperfusion injury monitors changes in renal microperfusion. Kidney Int 89:1388–1398

17. Iacobellis F, Segreto T, Berritto D et al (2018) A rat model of acute kidney injury through systemic hypoperfusion evaluated by micro-US, color and PW-Doppler. Radiol Med 124 (5):323–330

18. Paredes J, Sims-Lucas S, Wang H et al (2011) Assessing vesicoureteral reflux in live inbred mice via ultrasound with a microbubble contrast agent. AJP Ren Physiol 300: F1262–F1265

19. Yoshida A, Kanamori H, Naruse G et al (2019) (pro)renin receptor blockade ameliorates heart failure caused by chronic kidney disease. J Card Fail 25:286–300

11

MRI Mapping of the Blood Oxygenation Sensitive Parameter T_2* in the Kidney: Basic Concept

Lu-Ping Li, Bradley Hack, Erdmann Seeliger, and Pottumarthi V. Prasad

Abstract

The role of hypoxia in renal disease and injury has long been suggested but much work still remains, especially as it relates to human translation. Invasive pO_2 probes are feasible in animal models but not for human use. In addition, they only provide localized measurements. Histological methods can identify hypoxic tissue and provide a spatial distribution, but are invasive and allow only one-time point. Blood oxygenation level dependent (BOLD) MRI is a noninvasive method that can monitor relative oxygen availability across the kidney. It is based on the inherent differences in magnetic properties of oxygenated vs. deoxygenated hemoglobin. Presence of deoxyhemoglobin enhances the spin–spin relaxation rate measured using a gradient echo sequence, known as R_2^* $(= 1/T_2^*)$. While the key interest of BOLD MRI is in the application to humans, use in preclinical models is necessary primarily to validate the measurement against invasive methods, to better understand physiology and pathophysiology, and to evaluate novel interventions. Application of MRI acquisitions in preclinical settings involves several challenges both in terms of logistics and data acquisition. This section will introduce the concept of BOLD MRI and provide some illustrative applications. The following sections will discuss the technical issues associated with data acquisition and analysis.

This chapter is based upon work from the COST Action PARENCHIMA, a community-driven network funded by the European Cooperation in Science and Technology (COST) program of the European Union, which aims to improve the reproducibility and standardization of renal MRI biomarkers. This introduction chapter is complemented by two separate chapters describing the experimental procedure and data analysis.

Key words Magnetic resonance imaging (MRI), Kidney, Mice, Rats, Blood oxygenation level dependent (BOLD) MRI, Hypoxia

1 Introduction

All organs exist in a state of dynamically balanced oxygen supply as determined by blood flow and arterial oxygen content and demand as determined by metabolism. Yet renal hemodynamics and oxygenation offer a number of striking differences vs. nonrenal tissues. Most organs extract approximately 45% of available oxygen (i.e., difference between arterial and venous blood) while the kidney only

Andreas Pohlmann and Thoralf Niendorf (eds.), *Preclinical MRI of the Kidney: Methods and Protocols*, Methods in Molecular Biology, vol. 2216, https://doi.org/10.1007/978-1-0716-0978-1_10,

extracts 10–15% of available oxygen. This is in part because, on a per gram basis, whole-kidney blood flow is higher than that of most other tissues. The kidneys while receiving 20–25% of cardiac output under resting conditions, only consume about 7% of the body's total oxygen. The major determinant of renal O_2 consumption is energy-dependent tubular sodium reabsorption. Whereas O_2 consumption determines perfusion in nonrenal tissues, renal O_2 consumption is largely determined by perfusion. Increased renal blood flow is, in general, accompanied by increased glomerular filtration rate, and therefore necessitates increased energy-dependent tubular sodium reabsorption. Another particularity is the highly heterogeneous blood perfusion and oxygenation within the kidney. Virtually all of the blood flowing into the kidney perfuses the cortex. The medulla is perfused by a small fraction (about 10% of total renal blood flow) of blood that had traversed the cortex. In accordance, tissue partial pressure of oxygen (pO_2) is very low in the medulla. Three additional mechanisms substantially contribute to low renal tissue pO_2. (a) The particular architecture of the intrarenal vasculature enables shunt diffusion of O_2 from arteries to veins in the cortex as well as from descending to ascending vasa recta in the medulla. (b) The vascular architecture also promotes differential distribution of erythrocytes and plasma at certain vessel branches (plasma skimming), which results in different hematocrit and O_2 content of blood perfusing the daughter vessels. (c) The Fåhræus–Lindqvist effect lowers the hematocrit in the long and narrow vasa recta supplying the medulla, which lowers the O_2 content of blood perfusing the medulla. At the same time, a rather high metabolic rate and thus O_2 demand is required to support active reabsorption of sodium along medullary thick ascending limbs of Henle's loop (mTAL) [1]. For a comprehensive description of the causes and the degree of the heterogeneity of intrarenal perfusion and oxygenation *see* the chapter by Cantow K et al. "Quantitative Assessment of Renal Perfusion and Oxygenation by Invasive Probes: Basic Concepts."

Given these particularities in renal oxygenation, there is an interest in understanding the physiological mechanisms involved in maintaining the oxygenation status within the medulla in health and how they may be affected in disease. Acute changes to intrarenal O_2 can be caused by both changes in O_2 supply due to changes in arterial O_2 content or perfusion, changes in O_2 consumption, or a combination of the two. For example, nitric oxide (NO) regulates blood supply by relaxing smooth muscle tension of resistance vessels and inhibitors of NO formation such as L-NAME reduce renal blood flow. The resulting reduction in renal O_2 supply decreases renal tissue oxygenation as evaluated by BOLD-MRI [2]. Alternatively, loop diuretics like furosemide block the sodium–potassium–chloride transporter in the mTAL. Inhibiting this secondary active transport decreases the load of the primary active sodium–

potassium pump (Na^+/K^+ ATPase) in the mTAL. The ensuing decrease in O_2-dependent sodium reabsorption results in an increase in outer medullary pO_2. Thus, administration of furosemide is most commonly used both as a validation of the measurements [3, 4] and as a tubular functional paradigm in the clinic [5]; for detailed discussion of the pros and cons *see* the chapter by Cantow K et al. "Reversible (Patho)Physiologically Relevant Test Interventions: Rationale and Examples." Early work using atrial natriuretic peptide (ANP), which was expected to cause some increase in blood flow, caused a significant decrease in both cortical and medullary O_2 due to the net increase in O_2 consumption related to sodium transport [6]. This illustrates the distinction between monitoring oxygenation vs. perfusion or blood flow and is especially relevant in the kidney.

In the setting of kidney disease, deregulation of O_2 balance has long been studied. A recent review [7] of gene responses in six different models of acute kidney injury (gram-negative sepsis, gram-positive sepsis, ischemia reperfusion, malignant hypertension, rhabdomyolysis, and cisplatin nephrotoxicity) found that hypoxia along with oxidative stress and inflammation was the common feature of all the disease models. These acute injuries may lead to tubule cell death by apoptosis or necrosis and injured cells frequently dedifferentiated into fibroblasts. This fibrosis can lead to tubular atrophy and reduction in function, forcing the remaining tubules to use more oxygen which can cause further injury [7].

Understanding the relationship between renal oxygenation and kidney disease was predominantly based on data obtained from preclinical models with tissue pO_2 measurements using invasive microprobes [3, 6, 8]. These probes were inserted in the kidney to provide local and acute pO_2 readings. Probe position is critical and can be difficult to maintain in small animals. Alternately, pimonidazole [9] can be used to stain tissue at severe hypoxia. This histological staining method only captures hypoxia present at the moment of tissue sampling. For detailed discussion of the advantages and disadvantages of these methods *see* the chapter by Cantow K et al. "Quantitative Assessment of Renal Perfusion and Oxygenation by Invasive Probes: Basic Concepts." BOLD MRI is a noninvasive imaging technique that can be used to estimate the relative oxygen availability in tissue. It offers both spatial information (at reduced spatial resolution compared to histology) and temporal resolution (typically lower than microprobes). Figure 1 illustrates the similarity and differences between histological, microprobe, and BOLD-MRI measurements. BOLD MRI allows for longitudinal follow-up because of its noninvasive nature.

In this chapter, we will provide an overview of BOLD MRI including the basic concept involved, and a few illustrative applications of renal BOLD MRI in rodents.

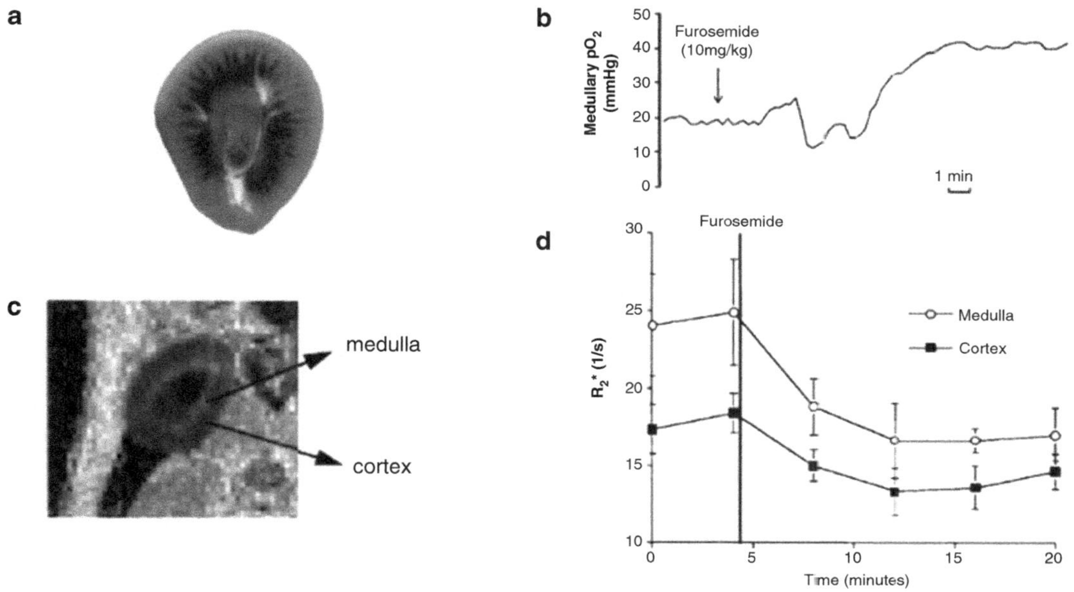

Fig. 1 (**a**) [10] A slice of rat kidney histologically stained for pimonidazole, showing the corticomedullary differences. Higher staining in the medulla is related to the increased hypoxia. This method can capture the spatial distribution of severe hypoxia within the kidney at the time of tissue sampling. (Reproduced from Zhong Z et al., *Am. J. Physiol.* 275 (*Renal Physiol.* 44): F595–F604, 1998 with permission from American Physiological Society). (**b**) [3] pO_2 microelectrode data showing the temporal changes in renal medullary pO_2 in a rat kidney and illustrates the increase in pO_2 following administration of furosemide. (Reproduced from Brezis M et al., *Am. J. Physiol.* 267 (*Renal Fluid Electrolyte Physiol.* 36): F1059–F1062, 1994 with permission from American Physiological Society). (**c**) [11] A representative slice of R_2* map in a rat kidney showing corticomedullary differences, even though the contrast is opposite compared to (**a**). The spatial resolution is also obviously lower compared to (**a**). (**d**) [11] Shows the changes in R_2* in the outer medulla and cortex after injection of furosemide. The first two points for both curves are baseline (preinjection). Both medullary and cortical R_2* drop after the injection of furosemide and stay relatively constant over the 20-min period of observation. Error bars represent standard deviation in the individual ROI measurements. This figure illustrates the merits of BOLD MRI in terms of providing both spatial and temporal information of pO_2 changes in kidneys. (Reproduced from Prasad PV et al., *J. Magn. Reson. Imaging* 1999; 9:842–846 with permission from John Wiley & Sons)

This introduction chapter is complemented by two separate chapters describing the experimental procedure and data analysis, which are part of this book.

This chapter is part of the book Pohlmann A, Niendorf T (eds) (2020) Preclinical MRI of the Kidney—Methods and Protocols. Springer, New York.

2 Measurement Concept

2.1 Basic Concept of BOLD Contrast

BOLD MRI technique uses deoxyhemoglobin (deoxyHb) as an intrinsic (or endogenous) contrast mechanism. Hemoglobin (Hb) is the primary vehicle for transporting O_2 in the blood. When O_2 is bound to Hb, it becomes oxyhemoglobin (oxyHb)

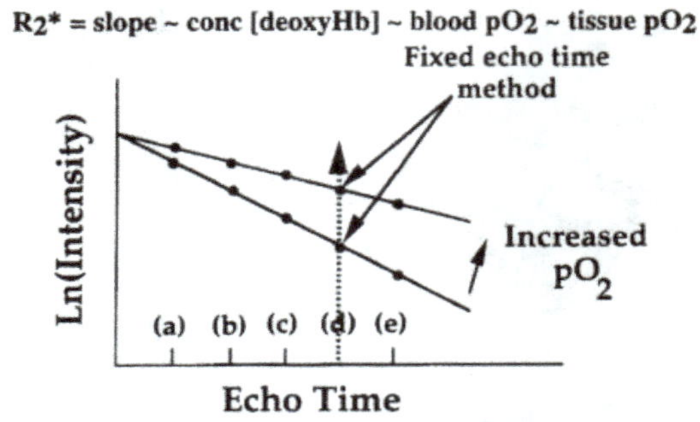

Fig. 2 [13]: Blood oxygenation level-dependent (BOLD) MRI changes qualitatively with pO_2. The deoxygenation of hemoglobin changes its magnetic characteristics, leading to changes in a parameter of magnetic resonance called R_2* (apparent spin–spin relaxation rate). R_2* can be estimated from signal intensity measurements made at several different echo times (**a–e**). The slope of Ln (intensity) vs. echo time determines R_2* and is directly related to the amount of deoxygenated blood. A decrease in the slope implies an increase in the pO_2 of blood. We can either measure the slope or obtain intensity measurements at a single echo time (e.g., **d**) to detect a difference in pO_2. Because blood pO_2 is thought to be in rapid equilibrium with tissue pO_2, changes in BOLD signal intensity or R_2* should reflect changes in the pO_2 of the tissue. (Reproduced from Prasad PV et al., Circulation. 1996 Dec 15; 94: 3271–5 with permission from American Heart Association)

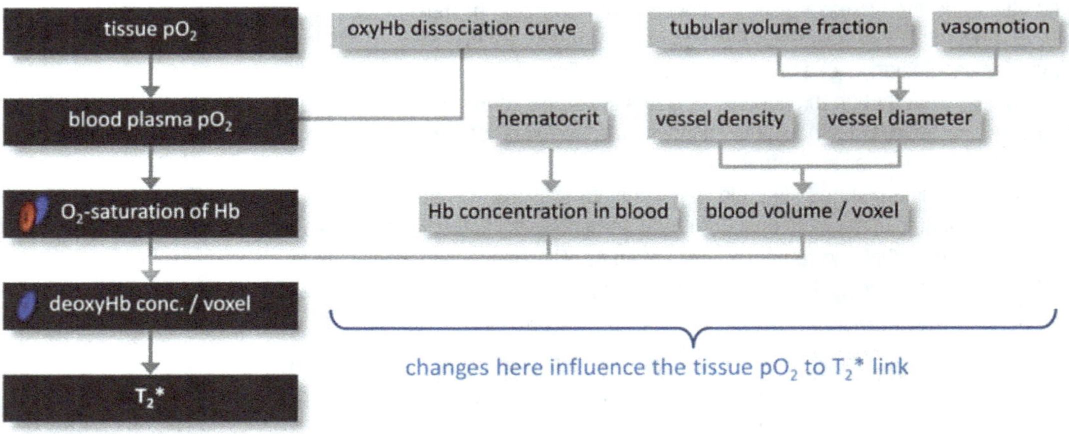

Fig. 3 [14]: Link between tissue pO_2 and T_2* (or R_2*), together with the potentially confounding factors

which is diamagnetic. When O_2 is released from Hb, it becomes deoxyhemoglobin (deoxyHb) which behaves as a paramagnet [12]. Since Hb is compartmentalized to the vascular system, the presence of deoxyHb creates local magnetic susceptibility gradients in and around blood vessels. This induces spin-dephasing so that the effective spin–spin relaxation decay of the MR signal governed by the relaxation time T_2* will be shortened when the local deoxyHb concentration is increased. This results in signal loss in T_2*-weighted imaging (e.g., gradient echo (GRE) imaging) in areas of increased deoxyHb concentration. The BOLD signal is quantitatively measured by either the effective relaxation time T_2* (s) OR relaxation rate R_2* (= $1/T_2$* and expressed in s^{-1}). T_2* and R_2* can be calculated based on GRE data acquired at different echo times (TE) and determining the slope of Ln (signal intensity) vs. TE (Fig. 2). With the assumption that hematocrit and local blood volume fraction remain unchanged (in fact, they might vary significantly), a decrease of R_2* corresponds to an increase of O_2 saturation of Hb and, assuming an unchanged oxyHb dissociation curve, in blood pO_2. Under "perfect" physiological conditions the pO_2 of capillary blood is thought to be in equilibrium with the surrounding tissue, and changes in observed R_2* could be interpreted as an indicator of changes in tissue pO_2. In many (patho)physiological scenarios however, the link between R_2* (T_2*), O_2 saturation of Hb, and tissue pO_2 is confounded by changes in various factors, which are illustrated in Fig. 3 and detailed in Subheading 2.3 [14].

The ratio of oxyHb to deoxyHb (which is the major determinant of % O_2 saturation of Hb under physiological conditions) is related to the pO_2 of blood and is governed by the oxyHb dissociation curve [15]. The renal medullary pO_2 is in the lower range of the curve. Hence a change in pO_2 will result in relatively larger change in the ratio of oxyHb to deoxyHb compared to a similar change in pO_2 of cortex. This makes BOLD MRI sensitive for following changes in pO_2 in the medulla.

2.2 BOLD MRI Acquisition Methods and Strategies for Kidney Oxygenation Measurement in Rodents

Two MR imaging techniques are used for renal BOLD MRI, namely, single shot echo planar imaging (EPI) [13] and multiple gradient echo (mGRE) sequences [4]. Functional imaging of the human brain predominantly uses single shot EPI due to the need for high temporal resolution and/or signal averaging. The ultrafast nature of EPI makes it ideal for abdominal imaging to freeze motion. It is suitable for applications with rapid changes in oxygenation and where R_2* mapping is not necessary [16]. However, it is highly sensitive to bulk magnetic susceptibility artifacts which results in image blurring, geometrical distortion, signal loss, and limited spatial resolution. The image distortion is amplified in regions with poor magnetic field homogeneity such as in the vicinity of bowels filled with gas. It is hardly used in preclinical setting, especially when using high field strength MR scanners.

mGRE sequence is currently the most widely utilized acquisition method both for human [4] and preclinical [11] applications of renal BOLD MRI. It acquires signals at multiple echo times after each excitation pulse. R_2* calculated as the slope of the straight line fitting of Ln(SI) vs. TE or by fitting the SI vs. TE data to a single decay monoexponential function. mGRE acquisitions provide improved SNR (signal-to-noise ratio), spatial resolution, and image quality compared to single shot EPI method. However, longer echo times with mGRE sequence also suffer from bulk susceptibility artifacts. In preclinical setting, motion artifacts are usually minimized using multiple averages. mGRE can suffer from phase variations between odd and even echoes when both water and fat components are present in renal tissue. Choice of echo times corresponding to in-phase or out-of-phase can minimize such artifacts. In the presence of flow, use of even echoes may be preferred.

2.3 Limitations of BOLD MRI for Absolute pO_2 Measurement

R_2* inherently depends on many parameters, primarily including R_2 the natural spin–spin relaxation rate and a susceptibility weighted component termed R_2' ($R_2^* = R_2 + R_2'$). R_2' is determined by the susceptibility component. In the context of BOLD MRI, it depends on the amount of deoxyHb present within the voxel which is determined by the combination of fractional blood volume (fraction of the voxel occupied by blood), hematocrit, and O_2 saturation of hemoglobin.

The factors confounding the relationship between R_2^*(or T_2^*) and intrarenal blood pO_2 are listed in Table 1.

BOLD MRI is inherently best suited to monitor changes in regional pO_2 which is assumed to be in a dynamic equilibrium with O_2 saturation of Hb. This inherently assumes that there are no concomitant changes in fractional blood volume, the oxyHb dissociation curve, and hematocrit. While this may be valid with certain pharmacological maneuvers, one or more of these confounders will change in various acute scenarios. Any vasodilation or vasoconstriction, either induced by pharmacologic maneuvers or by endogenous control of renal vessels, alters the blood volume fraction. Besides the vasculature, the interstitial and the tubular compartments can also experience rapid volume changes and, given the rather rigid renal capsule, can therefore modulate the blood volume fraction. The tubular volume fraction is a unique feature of the kidney; it is quite large and can rapidly change due to (a) changes in glomerular filtration, (b) alterations in tubular outflow toward the pelvis, (c) modulation of the transmural pressure gradient, and (d) changes in resorption. This is partly the motivation to establish R_2^* vs. tissue pO_2 calibration relationship. However, such calibration is strictly valid only in the model it was established in, for example, healthy animals and cannot be generalized to disease models and other species including humans. Mathematical analytical methods can be used to model the relationship between R_2' and O_2 saturation of Hb [17, 18]. However, these will require knowledge of fractional blood volume and regional hematocrit for the individual kidney. In kidneys, it is known that hematocrit is lower in the inner medulla [19]. This explains why inner medulla in rodents usually have low R_2^* values (typically lower than the cortex and erroneously indicating more availability of oxygen). Fractional blood volume is inherently an imaging specific concept and so

Table 1
Factors confounding the relationship between R_2*(or T_2*), oxygen saturation of hemoglobin, and blood pO_2

Confounding factor	Direction of effect	Examples scenarios
Blood volume fraction	Positive	Vasodilation/constriction, change in tubular volume fraction
Hematocrit	Positive	Plasma skimming, hemodilution
Oxygen–hemoglobin dissociation curve		Changes in pH, pCO_2, or temperature
Magnetic field (B_0) inhomogeneity	Positive	Bowel gas, poor shim
T_2	Positive	Edema

A "positive" direction of the effect means that an increase in the confounding factor leads to an increase in R_2* (decrease in T_2*) and hence an overestimation of the hypoxia

there is very little literature on its measurement. The ideal method to estimate fractional blood volume is by using an intravascular contrast agent such as ultrasmall paramagnetic iron oxide (USPIO) [20, 21]. Oxygen saturation of Hb is related to the pO_2 of blood by the oxyHb dissociation curve which is influenced by factors such as pH, pCO_2, and temperature. Further the inherent assumption that blood pO_2 is in a dynamic equilibrium with surrounding tissue pO_2 may not hold in disease [22]. These limitations of BOLD MRI need to be taken in to account when interpreting experimental findings as illustrated recently [14]. In order to study the detailed link between renal tissue pO_2 and T_2* in vivo, an integrated approach that combines parametric MRI and quantitative physiological measurements (MR-PHYSIOL) was proposed [23]. The MR-PHYSIOL setup was used to study the relationship between renal T_2* and tissue pO_2 and perfusion in rats. The findings indicate that changes in T_2* qualitatively reflect changes in renal tissue pO_2 induced by maneuvers including hyperoxia, suprarenal aortic occlusion, and hypoxia. Yet a closer examination of the quantitative relationships between relative changes in T_2* and in tissue pO_2 revealed discrepancies, indicating that, due to the differential changes in one or more of the confounders, simple translation of quantitative results obtained for one intervention of renal hemodynamics and oxygenation to another intervention is falling short of being appropriate. Also, taking the perfusion and oxygenation heterogeneity among the kidney layer into account, extrapolation of results obtained for one layer to others must be made with due caution [24].

2.3.1 R_2' Measurement

Given the specific interest in the susceptibility component of spin–spin relaxation rate for BOLD MRI, measurement of R_2' is desired. While there has been some effort in directly estimating R_2' using asymmetric spin-echo sequences [25], a simpler and practical method may be to perform a gradient echo and spin echo measurement to estimate R_2* and R_2 separately then calculate the difference [26]. Since R_2 can independently vary with certain pharmacological maneuvers (e.g., following L-NAME [21]), using R_2' as the BOLD MRI parameter may be more specific to the oxygenation related changes. A recent study illustrated the feasibility of using R_2' measurements to estimate blood oxygenation in rat kidneys [17]. While R_2 is not directly sensitive to BOLD effects, there is actually an indirect dependence due to diffusion effects of spins experiencing the field gradients generated by the presence of deoxyHb in the microvasculature. In this regard, R_2 has been shown to be more specific to small vessels [27], while R_2* is typically weighted by larger vessels.

2.4 Considerations Regarding Animal Preparation

- Bowel gas can create susceptibility artifacts in renal R_2* map, right lateral position helps minimize susceptibility artifacts from bowel gas.
- Respiratory motion could create artifacts and usually multiple measurements for averaging purposes can be used to minimize these. Alternately, respiratory triggering could be used but may increase the acquisition times.
- Studies indicate the choice of anesthesia has a large influence on renal R_2* [28]. This may be partly due to known effects of anesthesia on respiration, temperature, blood pressure, and hence pO_2.

3 Overview of Preclinical Applications

Noninvasive BOLD MRI is primarily attractive for the use in humans. However, there is a need for preclinical applications of the method primarily to validate the technique against invasive measures and better understand changes in different diseases.

Validation of renal BOLD MRI measurements is mostly carried out by comparing the responses to certain (patho)physiologically relevant test interventions or pharmacological maneuvers against pO_2 measurements using invasive microprobes [2, 29]. BOLD data was compared with pimonidazole staining in 10-week-old mice [30]. Interestingly, pimonidazole staining did not show differences between db/db and db/m mice, even though BOLD MRI showed significant differences (Fig. 4). This is probably related to the fact that pimonidazole detects severe hypoxia, typically $pO_2 < 10$ mmHg. There was one study in swine where the invasive probe was placed in the contralateral kidney compared to the one where BOLD MRI measurements were made [31]. This study

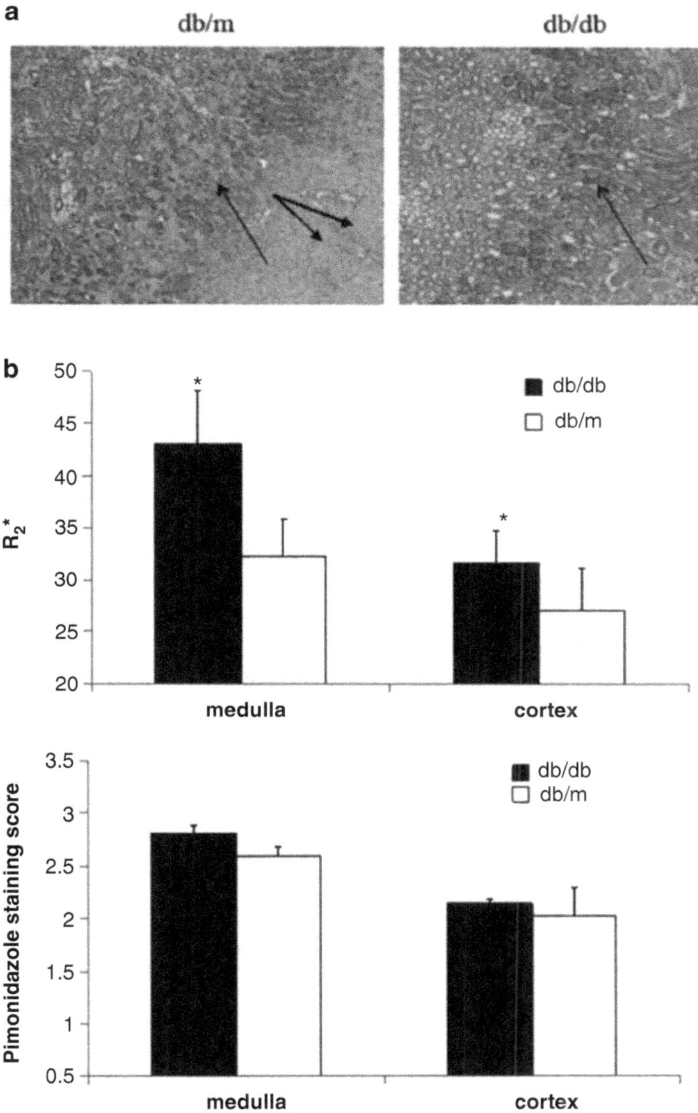

Fig. 4 [30]: (**a**) Pimonidazole immunohistochemical staining of the kidney of db/m and db/db mouse (magnification 100×). Strong pimonidazole (brown) staining of renal tubules was observed mainly in the outer medulla (single arrows) both from db/m and db/db mouse. Weaker staining was seen in the cortex of both db/db and db/m mice (double arrows). (**b**) A summary of R_2* values obtained by BOLD MRI in the medulla and cortex of 10-week-old db/db and db/m mice (upper panel). R_2* is higher in medulla than cortex in both db/db and db/m reflecting lower oxygenation in the medulla. The asterisk denotes a significant difference in R_2* between db/db and db/m in both cortex ($P < 0.04$) and medulla ($P < 0.001$). The lower panel shows the pimonidazole staining score for db/db and db/m mice of similar age (10 weeks old). The medulla had stronger staining than the cortex in both db/db and db/m reflecting increased hypoxia. No significant differences were found in the pimonidazole staining of the medulla and cortex between db/db and the db/m mice. The lack of significance with pimonidazole may be partly related to the fact that it is only sensitive to severe hypoxia, that is, $pO_2 < 10$ mmHg. (Reproduced from Prasad PV et al., Invest Radiol 2010; 45: 819–822 with permission from Wolters Kluwers Health Inc.)

proposed the use of R_2* vs. pO_2 as a calibration curve for translating BOLD MRI measurements in to pO_2 estimates. More recently, true simultaneous measurements with both BOLD MRI and invasive probes were demonstrated in rats [23]. Interventions such as hypoxia, hyperoxia, and suprarenal aortic occlusion were studied by use of this MR-PHYSIOL setup [24]. Use of high field small animal scanners is ideal for rodent applications in terms of signal-to-noise ratios. However, renal BOLD MRI can also be effectively conducted in rats using whole body scanners at both 1.5 [11] and 3 T [32] routinely used in humans which have more widespread availability. Renal BOLD MRI in mice has been shown to be feasible at 3 T using a custom surface radiofrequency loop coil for signal reception [30, 33].

Early application of renal BOLD MRI was primarily to evaluate acute effects of physiological or pharmacological maneuvers. Administration of furosemide increased medullary oxygenation predominantly due to reduction in O_2 consumption [3, 6]. Given the role of NO in essential hypertension, we have also observed differential response to administration of L-NAME in healthy rats compared to spontaneously hypertensive rats (SHR) [34]. Because the reduced NO availability in SHR is related to oxidative stress, we also observed a differential response to free radical scavenger (tempol) in SHR rats compared to controls [35].

3.1 Application to Disease Models

Acute kidney injury (AKI) is a sudden episode of kidney failure or kidney damage that happens within a few hours or a few days of an insult such as administration of nephrotoxins. AKI is common in patients who are hospitalized, patients who have underlying kidney disease, and especially in older adults. Medullary hypoxic injury plays a major role in the pathogenesis of AKI [7], as has been studied by both invasive probes and BOLD MRI in rat models of X-ray contrast induced AKI and renal ischemia/reperfusion injury [36–38].

Given the role of endothelial dysfunction in the susceptibility to contrast induced AKI, we have studied the additive effects of L-NAME, indomethacin (prostaglandin inhibitor) followed by iodinated radio-contrast medium iothalamate (Fig. 5) [32]. Using this AKI model, we compared the effects of different contrast media based on different physicochemical properties, observed large increases in R_2* in the inner-stripe of outer medulla [39]. In a similar model, we evaluated potential preventative maneuvers such as preadministration of furosemide or N-acetylcysteine (NAC, an antioxidant). We found that furosemide was effective in abolishing the increase in R_2* post-radiocontrast [40]. These observations matched with a decrease in urinary neutrophil gelatinase associated lipocalin (NGAL) measurements, a marker of tubular injury.

Unilateral ureteral obstruction (UUO) is a commonly used model of renal fibrosis [41]. However, permanent ligation of ureter

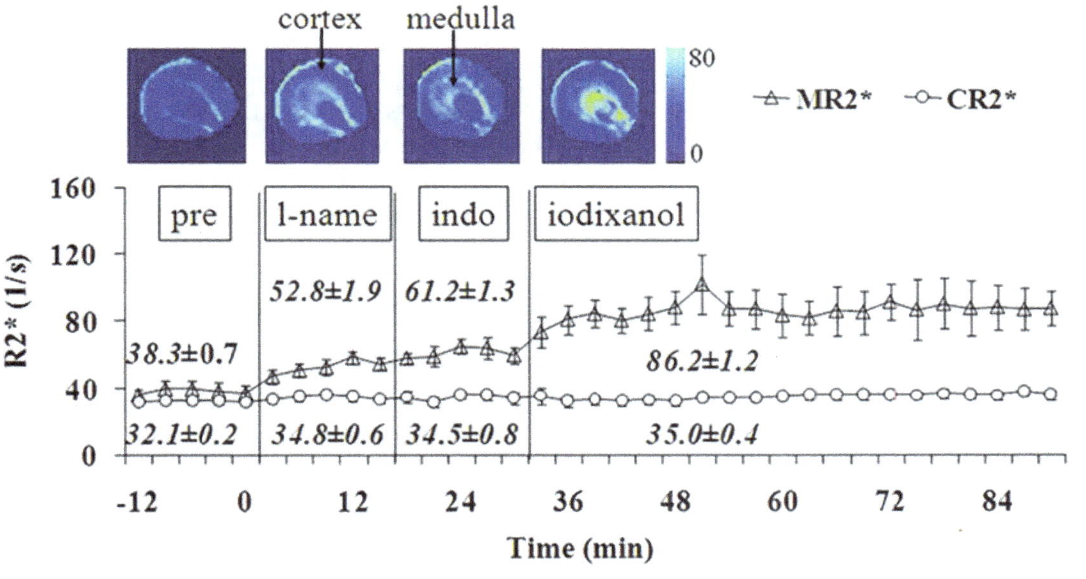

Fig. 5 [32]: Averaged (mean ± SE) renal R_2* time course from six rats in renal medulla and cortex following the administration of L-NAME, indomethacin, and radio-contrast iodixanol. The vertical lines indicate the time of administration of each of chemicals. Pre: baseline; l-name: L-NAME; indo: indomethacin. Error bars represent standard error among rats. On the top are R_2* maps generated using custom Matlab (Mathworks, Natick, MA, USA) code in one representative rat. The relative brightness in renal outer medulla suggests low oxygenation level compared to cortex. The window settings were the same in all maps. The brightness in renal outer medulla increases gradually after each chemical, suggesting the progressively decreasing of oxygenation. The R_2* maps are from baseline, following administration of L-NAME, indomethacin, and iodixanol. The arrows show the renal outer medulla and cortex where the ROIs were placed. The renal outer medulla is relatively brighter than renal cortex in baseline R_2* map, suggesting lower oxygenation level there. Each chemical contributes to the additional increased brightness in R_2* maps in the renal outer medulla, suggesting progressive hypoxia in the renal outer medulla. Bottom: shows the corresponding plot of R_2* vs. time. (Reproduced from Prasad PV et al., J. Magn. Reson. Imaging 2012; 36:1162–1167 with permission from John Wiley & Sons)

results in complete loss of renal parenchyma within couple of weeks. A reversible unilateral ureteral obstruction (rUUO) was proposed as a more representative model of chronic kidney disease (CKD) [42]. In rUUO model, the microvascular clip used to ligate the ureter is moved distally every 2 days for 6 days and then removed. BOLD MRI was used to monitor the longitudinal changes at 2 and 28 days following reversal of the UUO [43]. This application is an illustration of the advantage of a noninvasive imaging method in performing longitudinal studies within the same animal.

Acknowledgments

Work supported, in part, by grant funding from the National Institutes of Health (R01 DK093793 and R01 DK106557).

This publication is based upon work from COST Action PARENCHIMA, supported by European Cooperation in Science and Technology (COST). COST (www.cost.eu) is a funding agency for research and innovation networks. COST Actions help connect research initiatives across Europe and enable scientists to enrich their ideas by sharing them with their peers. This boosts their research, career, and innovation.

PARENCHIMA (renalmri.org) is a community-driven Action in the COST program of the European Union, which unites more than 200 experts in renal MRI from 30 countries with the aim to improve the reproducibility and standardization of renal MRI biomarkers.

References

1. Brezis M, Rosen S (1995) Hypoxia of the renal medulla--its implications for disease. N Engl J Med 332(10):647–655. https://doi.org/10.1056/NEJM199503093321006
2. Li LP, Ji L, Santos EA, Dunkle E, Pierchala L, Prasad P (2009) Effect of nitric oxide synthase inhibition on intrarenal oxygenation as evaluated by blood oxygenation level-dependent magnetic resonance imaging. Investig Radiol 44(2):67–73. https://doi.org/10.1097/RLI.0b013e3181900975
3. Brezis M, Agmon Y, Epstein FH (1994) Determinants of intrarenal oxygenation. I. Effects of diuretics. Am J Physiol 267(6 Pt 2): F1059–F1062
4. Prasad PV, Chen Q, Goldfarb JW, Epstein FH, Edelman RR (1997) Breath-hold R2* mapping with a multiple gradient-recalled echo sequence: application to the evaluation of intrarenal oxygenation. J Magn Reson Imaging 7(6):1163–1165
5. Prasad PV, Li LP, Thacker JM, Li W, Hack B, Kohn O, Sprague SM (2019) Cortical perfusion and tubular function as evaluated by magnetic resonance imaging correlates with annual loss in renal function in moderate chronic kidney disease. Am J Nephrol 49(2):114–124. https://doi.org/10.1159/000496161
6. Brezis M, Heyman SN, Epstein FH (1994) Determinants of intrarenal oxygenation. II. Hemodynamic effects. Am J Physiol 267 (6 Pt 2):F1063–F1068
7. Hultstrom M, Becirovic-Agic M, Jonsson S (2018) Comparison of acute kidney injury of different etiology reveals in-common mechanisms of tissue damage. Physiol Genomics 50 (3):127–141. https://doi.org/10.1152/physiolgenomics.00037.2017
8. Aukland K, Krog J (1960) Renal oxygen tension. Nature 188:671. https://doi.org/10.1038/188671a0
9. Rosenberger C, Rosen S, Paliege A, Heyman SN (2009) Pimonidazole adduct immunohistochemistry in the rat kidney: detection of tissue hypoxia. Methods Mol Biol 466:161–174. https://doi.org/10.1007/978-1-59745-352-3_12
10. Zhong Z, Arteel GE, Connor HD, Yin M, Frankenberg MV, Stachlewitz RF, Raleigh JA, Mason RP, Thurman RG (1998) Cyclosporin A increases hypoxia and free radical production in rat kidneys: prevention by dietary glycine. Am J Phys 275(4):F595–F604. https://doi.org/10.1152/ajprenal.1998.275.4.F595
11. Priatna A, Epstein FH, Spokes K, Prasad PV (1999) Evaluation of changes in intrarenal oxygenation in rats using multiple gradient-recalled echo (mGRE) sequence. J Magn Reson Imaging 9(6):842–846
12. Buxton RB (2013) The physics of functional magnetic resonance imaging (fMRI). Rep Prog Phys 76(9):096601. https://doi.org/10.1088/0034-4885/76/9/096601
13. Prasad PV, Edelman RR, Epstein FH (1996) Noninvasive evaluation of intrarenal oxygenation with BOLD MRI. Circulation 94 (12):3271–3275. https://doi.org/10.1161/01.cir.94.12.3271

14. Niendorf T, Pohlmann A, Arakelyan K, Flemming B, Cantow K, Hentschel J, Grosenick D, Ladwig M, Reimann H, Klix S, Waiczies S, Seeliger E (2015) How bold is blood oxygenation level-dependent (BOLD) magnetic resonance imaging of the kidney? Opportunities, challenges and future directions. Acta Physiol 213(1):19–38. https://doi.org/10.1111/apha.12393

15. Severinghaus JW (1979) Simple, accurate equations for human blood O2 dissociation computations. J Appl Physiol Respir Environ Exerc Physiol 46(3):599–602. https://doi.org/10.1152/jappl.1979.46.3.599

16. Schachinger H, Klarhofer M, Linder L, Drewe J, Scheffler K (2006) Angiotensin II decreases the renal MRI blood oxygenation level-dependent signal. Hypertension 47 (6):1062–1066. https://doi.org/10.1161/01.HYP.0000220109.98142.a3

17. Thacker J, Zhang JL, Franklin T, Prasad P (2017) BOLD quantified renal pO2 is sensitive to pharmacological challenges in rats. Magn Reson Med 78(1):297–302. https://doi.org/10.1002/mrm.26367

18. Zhang JL, Morrell G, Rusinek H, Warner L, Vivier PH, Cheung AK, Lerman LO, Lee VS (2014) Measurement of renal tissue oxygenation with blood oxygen level-dependent MRI and oxygen transit modeling. Am J Physiol Renal Physiol 306(6):F579–F587. https://doi.org/10.1152/ajprenal.00575.2013

19. Zimmerhackl B, Robertson CR, Jamison RL (1985) The microcirculation of the renal medulla. Circ Res 57(5):657–667

20. Pohlmann A, Cantow K, Huelnhagen T, Grosenick D, Dos Santos PJ, Boehmert L, Gladytz T, Waiczies S, Flemming B, Seeliger E, Niendorf T (2017) Experimental MRI monitoring of renal blood volume fraction variations en route to renal magnetic resonance oximetry. Tomography 3(4):188–200. https://doi.org/10.18383/j.tom.2017.00012

21. Storey P, Ji L, Li LP, Prasad PV (2011) Sensitivity of USPIO-enhanced R2 imaging to dynamic blood volume changes in the rat kidney. J Magn Reson Imaging 33(5):1091–1099. https://doi.org/10.1002/jmri.22526

22. Evans RG, Leong CL, Anderson WP, O'Connor PM (2007) Don't be so BOLD: potential limitations in the use of BOLD MRI for studies of renal oxygenation. Kidney Int 71 (12):1327–1328; author reply 1328. https://doi.org/10.1038/sj.ki.5002321

23. Cantow K, Arakelyan K, Seeliger E, Niendorf T, Pohlmann A (2016) Assessment of renal hemodynamics and oxygenation by simultaneous magnetic resonance imaging (MRI) and quantitative invasive physiological measurements. Methods Mol Biol 1397:129–154. https://doi.org/10.1007/978-1-4939-3353-2_11

24. Pohlmann A, Arakelyan K, Hentschel J, Cantow K, Flemming B, Ladwig M, Waiczies S, Seeliger E, Niendorf T (2014) Detailing the relation between renal T2* and renal tissue pO2 using an integrated approach of parametric magnetic resonance imaging and invasive physiological measurements. Investig Radiol 49(8):547–560. https://doi.org/10.1097/RLI.0000000000000054

25. Zhang X, Zhang Y, Yang X, Wang X, An H, Zhang J, Fang J (2013) Feasibility of noninvasive quantitative measurements of intrarenal R (2)' in humans using an asymmetric spin echo echo planar imaging sequence. NMR Biomed 26(1):91–97. https://doi.org/10.1002/nbm.2823

26. Yang X, Cao J, Wang X, Li X, Xu Y, Jiang X (2008) Evaluation of renal oxygenation in rat by using R2' at 3-T magnetic resonance: initial observation. Acad Radiol 15(7):912–918. https://doi.org/10.1016/j.acra.2008.01.015

27. Boxerman JL, Hamberg LM, Rosen BR, Weisskoff RM (1995) MR contrast due to intravascular magnetic susceptibility perturbations. Magn Reson Med 34(4):555–566

28. Niles DJ, Gordon JW, Fain SB (2015) Effect of anesthesia on renal R2 * measured by blood oxygen level-dependent MRI. NMR Biomed 28(7):811–817. https://doi org/10.1002/nbm.3314

29. dos Santos EA, Li LP, Ji L, Prasad PV (2007) Early changes with diabetes in renal medullary hemodynamics as evaluated by fiberoptic probes and BOLD magnetic resonance imaging. Investig Radiol 42(3):157–162. https://doi.org/10.1097/01.rli.0000252492.96709.36

30. Prasad P, Li LP, Halter S, Cabray J, Ye M, Batlle D (2010) Evaluation of renal hypoxia in diabetic mice by BOLD MRI. Invest Radiol 45 (12):819–822. https://doi.org/10.1097/RLI.0b013e3181ec9b02

31. Pedersen M, Dissing TH, Morkenborg J, Stodkilde-Jorgensen H, Hansen LH, Pedersen LB, Grenier N, Frokiaer J (2005) Validation of quantitative BOLD MRI measurements in kidney: application to unilateral ureteral obstruction. Kidney Int 67(6):2305–2312. https://doi.org/10.1111/j.1523-1755.2005.00334.x

32. Li LP, Franklin T, Du H, Papadopoulou-Rosenzweig M, Carbray J, Solomon R, Prasad PV (2012) Intrarenal oxygenation by blood

oxygenation level-dependent MRI in contrast nephropathy model: effect of the viscosity and dose. J Magn Reson Imaging 36 (5):1162–1167. https://doi.org/10.1002/jmri.23747

33. Li LP, Ji L, Lindsay S, Prasad PV (2007) Evaluation of intrarenal oxygenation in mice by BOLD MRI on a 3.0T human whole-body scanner. J Magn Reson Imaging 25 (3):635–638. https://doi.org/10.1002/jmri.20841

34. Li L, Storey P, Kim D, Li W, Prasad P (2003) Kidneys in hypertensive rats show reduced response to nitric oxide synthase inhibition as evaluated by BOLD MRI. J Magn Reson Imaging 17(6):671–675. https://doi.org/10.1002/jmri.10301

35. Li LP, Li BS, Storey P, Fogelson L, Li W, Prasad P (2005) Effect of free radical scavenger (tempol) on intrarenal oxygenation in hypertensive rats as evaluated by BOLD MRI. J Magn Reson Imaging 21(3):245–248. https://doi.org/10.1002/jmri.20260

36. Hoff U, Lukitsch I, Chaykovska L, Ladwig M, Arnold C, Manthati VL, Fuller TF, Schneider W, Gollasch M, Muller DN, Flemming B, Seeliger E, Luft FC, Falck JR, Dragun D, Schunck WH (2011) Inhibition of 20-HETE synthesis and action protects the kidney from ischemia/reperfusion injury. Kidney Int 79(1):57–65. https://doi.org/10.1038/ki.2010.377

37. Arakelyan K, Cantow K, Hentschel J, Flemming B, Pohlmann A, Ladwig M, Niendorf T, Seeliger E (2013) Early effects of an x-ray contrast medium on renal T2 */T2 MRI as compared to short-term hyperoxia, hypoxia and aortic occlusion in rats. Acta Physiol 208(2):202–213. https://doi.org/10.1111/apha.12094

38. Seeliger E, Flemming B, Wronski T, Ladwig M, Arakelyan K, Godes M, Mockel M, Persson PB (2007) Viscosity of contrast media perturbs renal hemodynamics. J Am Soc Nephrol 18 (11):2912–2920. https://doi.org/10.1681/ASN.2006111216

39. Li LP, Lu J, Zhou Y, Papadopoulou MV, Franklin T, Bokhary U, Solomon R, Sen A, Prasad PV (2014) Evaluation of intrarenal oxygenation in iodinated contrast-induced acute kidney injury-susceptible rats by blood oxygen level-dependent magnetic resonance imaging. Invest Radiol 49:403–410. https://doi.org/10.1097/RLI.0000000000000031

40. Li LP, Thacker J, Lu J, Franklin T, Zhou Y, Papadopoulou MV, Solomon R, Prasad PV (2014) Efficacy of preventive interventions for iodinated contrast-induced acute kidney injury evaluated by intrarenal oxygenation as an early marker. Invest Radiol 49(10):647–652. https://doi.org/10.1097/RLI.0000000000000065

41. Togao O, Doi S, Kuro-o M, Masaki T, Yorioka N, Takahashi M (2010) Assessment of renal fibrosis with diffusion-weighted MR imaging: study with murine model of unilateral ureteral obstruction. Radiology 255 (3):772–780. https://doi.org/10.1148/radiol.10091735

42. Puri TS, Shakaib MI, Chang A, Mathew L, Olayinka O, Minto AW, Sarav M, Hack BK, Quigg RJ (2010) Chronic kidney disease induced in mice by reversible unilateral ureteral obstruction is dependent on genetic background. Am J Physiol Renal Physiol 298(4): F1024–F1032. https://doi.org/10.1152/ajprenal.00384.2009

43. Haque ME, Franklin T, Bokhary U, Mathew L, Hack BK, Chang A, Puri TS, Prasad PV (2014) Longitudinal changes in MRI markers in a reversible unilateral ureteral obstruction mouse model: preliminary experience. J Magn Reson Imaging 39(4):835–841. https://doi.org/10.1002/jmri.24235

12

Reversible (Patho)Physiologically Relevant Test Interventions: Rationale and Examples

Kathleen Cantow, Mechthild Ladwig-Wiegard, Bert Flemming, Andrea Fekete, Adam Hosszu, and Erdmann Seeliger

Abstract

Renal tissue hypoperfusion and hypoxia are early key elements in the pathophysiology of acute kidney injury of various origins, and may also promote progression from acute injury to chronic kidney disease. Here we describe test interventions that are used to study the control of renal hemodynamics and oxygenation in experimental animals in the context of kidney-specific control of hemodynamics and oxygenation. The rationale behind the use of the individual tests, the physiological responses of renal hemodynamics and oxygenation, the use in preclinical studies, and the possible application in humans are discussed.

This chapter is based upon work from the COST Action PARENCHIMA, a community-driven network funded by the European Cooperation in Science and Technology (COST) program of the European Union, which aims to improve the reproducibility and standardization of renal MRI biomarkers.

Key words Renal hemodynamics and oxygenation, In vivo methods, Rats, Test interventions

1 Introduction

Kidney diseases are a global health burden with steadily increasing incidence and prevalence [1–5]. Animal studies indicate that acute kidney injuries (AKI) of various origins share one common link in the pathophysiological chain of events, ultimately leading to AKI, as well as to progression from AKI to chronic kidney diseases (CKD): imbalance between renal oxygen delivery and oxygen demand [6–14]. Renal tissue hypoperfusion and hypoxia have also been suggested to play a pivotal role in the pathophysiology of other kidney diseases including diabetic kidney disease [15–19]. These pathophysiological concepts have largely been generated by preclinical studies that used either invasive quantitative probes or noninvasive functional magnetic resonance imaging (MRI) techniques to gain insight into renal hemodynamics and oxygenation. Thus, making ultimate statements on the role of renal hypoperfusion and hypoxia for these renal disorders is elusive

Andreas Pohlmann and Thoralf Niendorf (eds.), *Preclinical MRI of the Kidney: Methods and Protocols*, Methods in Molecular Biology, vol. 2216, https://doi.org/10.1007/978-1-0716-0978-1_4,

because in vivo assessment of renal hemodynamics and oxygenation constitutes a challenge.

All modalities available in today's experimental and translational research practice have inherent shortcomings and methodological constraints. Invasiveness is the major disadvantage of the gold standard physiological probes such as perivascular flow probes for measurement of total renal blood flow, laser-Doppler-optodes for assessment of local tissue perfusion, and Clark-type electrodes or fluorescence-quenching optodes for measurements of local tissue partial pressure of oxygen (pO_2), which precludes their use in humans. While functional MRI including blood oxygenation-sensitized T_2* (aka blood oxygenation level-dependent MRI; BOLD-MRI) offers noninvasive techniques to obtain insight into renal perfusion and oxygenation, its major weakness is its qualitative nature. Before it can be used for quantitative characterization of renal tissue perfusion and oxygenation, it needs to be calibrated with the gold standard invasive techniques in various (patho)-physiological scenarios [20–24].

The control of renal hemodynamics and oxygenation under physiological as well as under pathophysiological conditions is complex and differs considerably from nonrenal tissue [8, 21, 23, 25–27]. Due to the considerable capacity of the organism's homeostatic control systems to—at least partially—compensate for disturbances of, or injury to, certain control elements, these alterations are often not easily detectable when studied by measuring baseline data only. In order to disentangle these complexities, dedicated reversible test interventions are conceptually appealing. In fact, such interventions can serve three main purposes. First, they are used to gain more insight into the control of renal hemodynamics and oxygenation in healthy animals and in animal models of various kidney diseases [8, 12, 25, 28–37]. Second, the tests are used to assess whether a given drug or contrast agent has beneficial or unwarranted effects on the control of renal hemodynamics and oxygenation [38–40]. Finally, dedicated reversible tests are used to achieve calibration of functional MRI data [22, 23].

In this chapter, specifics of the control of renal hemodynamics and oxygenation are outlined first. Then, the individual test procedures are described, and the rationale behind their use, the physiological response of renal hemodynamics and oxygenation, the use in preclinical studies and the possible application in humans are discussed.

This chapter is part of the book Pohlmann A, Niendorf T (eds) (2020) Preclinical MRI of the Kidney—Methods and Protocols. Springer, New York.

2 Specifics of Renal Hemodynamics and Oxygenation

Renal hemodynamics and oxygenation offer a number of striking differences when compared to nonrenal tissue. First, total renal blood flow (RBF) is huge when compared to virtually all other organs on a per gram basis: the kidneys receive about 20% of the cardiac output under resting conditions. Yet the distribution of blood perfusion differs substantially between the layers: while 100% of blood flowing into the kidney reaches the cortex, only 15% of blood that previously passes through the cortex, will reach the medulla. Even intralayer (cortex, outer medulla, and inner medulla) perfusion is quite heterogeneous [8, 41, 42]. In accordance with the high total RBF, the kidneys' oxygen extraction (the difference between the O_2 content in the renal arterial and the renal venous blood) is low as compared to the majority of nonrenal tissues. Yet the partial pressure of oxygen (pO_2) is low in the medulla and also varies considerably within the respective layers, in accordance with the different blood flow distribution [21, 23, 26, 43–47].

Second, the kidney differs from all other organs with regard to the relationship between metabolism and perfusion. More than 26 thousand millimoles of sodium (Na^+) are filtered in the human glomeruli every day, equivalent to more than 1.5 kg of table salt. To achieve sodium balance, the amount of salt excreted by the kidneys must exactly match the amount of ingested salt minus the amount of extrarenal loss. Thus, more than 99% of the filtered sodium must usually be reabsorbed from the tubules. Tubular resorption relies on active transport processes, which account for about 85% of the kidney's energy expenditure and therefore its O_2 consumption. The more sodium is filtered in the glomeruli, the more must be reabsorbed. As glomerular filtration rate (GFR), under the majority of circumstances, increases with increasing RBF, renal O_2 consumption also usually increases with increasing renal perfusion. This is in contradistinction to all other organs, where metabolism determines perfusion [8, 48].

Third, hormones such as angiotensin II and epinephrine, sympathetic vasomotor nerves, and paracrine mediators such as nitric oxide or adenosine, that control resistance vessels in nonrenal tissues, impinge on intrarenal resistance vessels too, thereby altering renal O_2 delivery. However, in the kidney, they additionally affect tubular sodium resorption and thus O_2 consumption. Furthermore, their effect on postglomerular vessels can result in divergent responses of RBF and GFR. Finally, adenosine exerts vasodilation in virtually all nonrenal vascular beds, but vasoconstriction in the renal cortex [8, 25, 48, 49].

Fourth, the kidney is equipped with efficient mechanisms of autoregulation, that is, the ability to dampen or even to abolish the effects that changes in renal arterial pressure would otherwise inevitably have on RBF and GFR. The almost perfect autoregulation of RBF and GFR probably relies on the fact that not just one, but three mechanisms are involved. The first one, the myogenic response (aka Bayliss effect) acts not only on renal resistance vessels but also on brain and gut vessels. The second mechanism, the tubuloglomerular feedback (TGF), and the third one, hitherto just named "third mechanism", are kidney-specific. Renal autoregulatory mechanisms, in particular the TGF and the third mechanism, have been suggested to serve the purpose of balancing O_2 delivery, that is, RBF with metabolic and O_2 demands arising from tubular reabsorption. The outer medulla is particularly prone to imbalance between O_2 delivery and demand since this layer exhibits a high O_2 demand but low pO_2 [21, 34, 35, 50–52].

Fifth, intrarenal perfusion is also affected by changes in tubular volume. The tubular volume fraction is quite large and can rapidly change due to alterations in GFR, in tubular outflow toward the pelvis, in tubular fluid resorption, and modulation of the transmural pressure gradient. Since the renal capsule is rather tough, changes in tubular volume will result in circular distension or compression of intrarenal vessels [23, 36].

Finally, in addition to the heterogeneous intrarenal blood perfusion, three other factors substantially contribute to the low tissue pO_2 and, in particular, to the "physiological hypoxia" in the medulla. First, there is a considerable shunt diffusion of O_2 from arteries to veins in the cortex and from descending to ascending vasa recta in the medulla [53–55]. Second, the Fåhræus–Lindqvist effect lowers the hematocrit in the vasa recta supplying the medulla, which lowers the O_2 content of blood perfusing parts of the medulla [41, 42]. Third, plasma skimming at intrarenal vessel branches results in different hematocrit and therefore O_2 content of blood perfusing the daughter vessels [41, 56].

3 Dedicated Reversible Test Interventions

3.1 Short Periods of Occlusion of the Renal Artery or Renal Vein

Occlusions of the renal artery (alternatively: the suprarenal aorta) or of the renal vein emulate clinical conditions in which deficient renal perfusion results in deterioration of intrarenal oxygenation. If maintained for longer periods of time these conditions can cause AKI [57–59]. The rationale for performing both of these tests is that renal arterial occlusion and renal venous occlusion have similar effects with regard to renal perfusion and oxygenation, yet opposing effects with regard to intrarenal blood volume. With the onset of aortic occlusion, the inflow of blood into the kidney is abruptly stopped while outflow via the renal vein continues until pressures in intrarenal vessels and in the vena cava are equalized. With the onset of renal venous occlusion, outflow of blood is abruptly stopped while inflow via the artery does not cease until the arterial pressure-induced distension of intrarenal vessels is counterbalanced by the resistance of the renal tissue including the rather tough capsule [22, 39, 60].

In both cases, renal tissue perfusion rapidly decreases and eventually approaches zero flow. As renal O_2 consumption remains unaltered at the early stage of occlusions, a rapid and massive decline in renal tissue pO_2 results, which, in turn, also reduces blood pO_2 and the O_2 saturation of hemoglobin (StO_2) in the intrarenal (micro)vasculature. This intrarenal deoxygenation of hemoglobin (Hb) is aggravated by a progressive rightward shift of the oxyHb dissociation curve during the occlusion due to the intrarenal accumulation of carbon dioxide (CO_2) [22, 39, 60].

Yet the opposing changes of renal blood volume have an impact on renal tissue oxygenation. The decrease in tissue pO_2 at the onset of the venous occlusion is much slower than at the onset of the arterial occlusion. While renal O_2 consumption is similar during both kinds of occlusions, the transiently maintained inflow of oxygenated blood at the onset of venous occlusion increases the intrarenal reservoir of O_2 [22, 39, 60].

The opposing changes in renal blood volume have a massive impact on the changes in blood oxygenation-sensitized T_2^* (and its reciprocal value, R_2^*), because T_2^* reflects the amount of deoxygenated Hb (deoxyHb) per tissue volume (voxel) [23]. In case of the venous occlusion with its increase in the vascular volume fraction and thus the increasing amount of deoxyHb per volume, tissue T_2^* massively decreases [60]. With the arterial occlusion's decrease of deoxyHb per volume, the decrease in T_2^* is small. In fact, it was found significantly smaller than the decrease in T_2^* measured during hypoxemia (8% inspiratory oxygen fraction), which is diametrically opposed to the effects of arterial occlusion versus hypoxemia on tissue pO_2 (*see* Fig. 1) [22, 23, 36].

Short-time (1–3 min) occlusions of the renal artery (or of the suprarenal aorta) have been used in several studies for different scientific purposes. In order to gauge the effects on T_2^* and T_2 of bolus injections of an X-ray contrast medium into the thoracic aorta of healthy rats, the effect of arterial occlusion (and that of hypoxemia) was quantified in the same rats [36]. En route to calibration of T_2^* with quantitative physiological measurements by means of a dedicated hybrid MR-PHYSIOL setup (*see* the chapter by Cantow K et al. "Monitoring Renal Hemodynamics and Oxygenation by Invasive Probes: Experimental Protocol"), suprarenal aortic occlusion was used [22]. In order to ascertain that the superparamagnetic iron oxide nanoparticle (USPIO) preparation, ferumoxytol is suitable as a contrast medium for MR-based assessment of the renal blood volume fraction; its possible unwarranted effects on control of renal hemodynamics and oxygenation were tested by interventions including suprarenal aortic occlusion in rats (*see* Fig. 2)

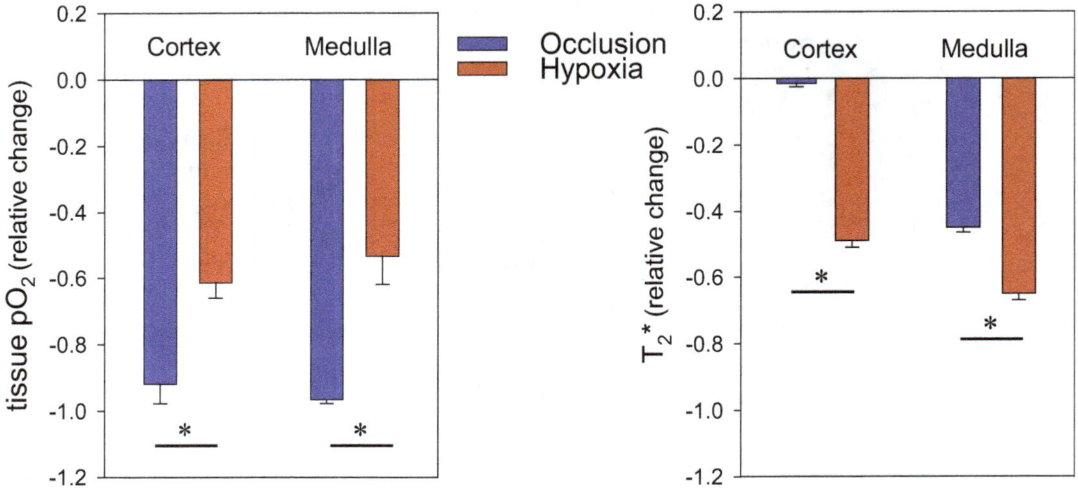

Fig. 1 Comparison of relative changes in renal cortical and medullary tissue pO_2 quantified by invasive gold standard fluorescence quenching optodes (left panel) versus relative changes in renal cortical and medullary T_2^* (so-called BOLD-MRI, right panel), during short-term occlusion of the suprarenal aorta and short-term hypoxia (8% inspiratory O_2 fraction), respectively, in anesthetized rats. Data are mean ± SEM, redrawn from Refs. 22, 36

[38]. Implementing a setup that combines classical invasive probes for RBF, tissue perfusion, and pO_2 with newly developed near infrared spectroscopy (NIRS) techniques that enable monitoring of the amount of Hb per tissue volume and the O_2 saturation of Hb (StO_2) of intrarenal blood (termed PHYSIOL-NIRS), aortic occlusion was used as one of the test interventions [39]. By means of a dedicated deconvolution procedure developed by our group, the time course of RBF upon the release of the occlusion can be analyzed. This "step-response" analysis allows us to determine the strength of each of the three mechanisms of RBF autoregulation in the whole kidney in vivo, in both healthy rats and rat models of AKI [30, 34, 35].

Short-time (1–3 min) occlusions of the renal vein were also used for different purposes. In order to establish an optimum dose of the USPIO ferumoxytol in rats for the purpose of T_2*-based quantification of the renal blood volume fraction in a 9.4T small animal scanner, renal venous occlusion was chosen as the combined effects of the decrease in O_2 delivery and the increase in the blood volume fraction; thus, deoxyHb per volume was expected to result in a most prominent decrease in T_2* (*see* Fig. 3) [60].

Both renal arterial occlusion and renal venous occlusion was performed in the same healthy rats in the PHYSIOL-NIRS setup in order to directly compare their effects [39].

As the implementation of vascular occluders necessitates invasive techniques, these tests can be performed in preclinical studies only.

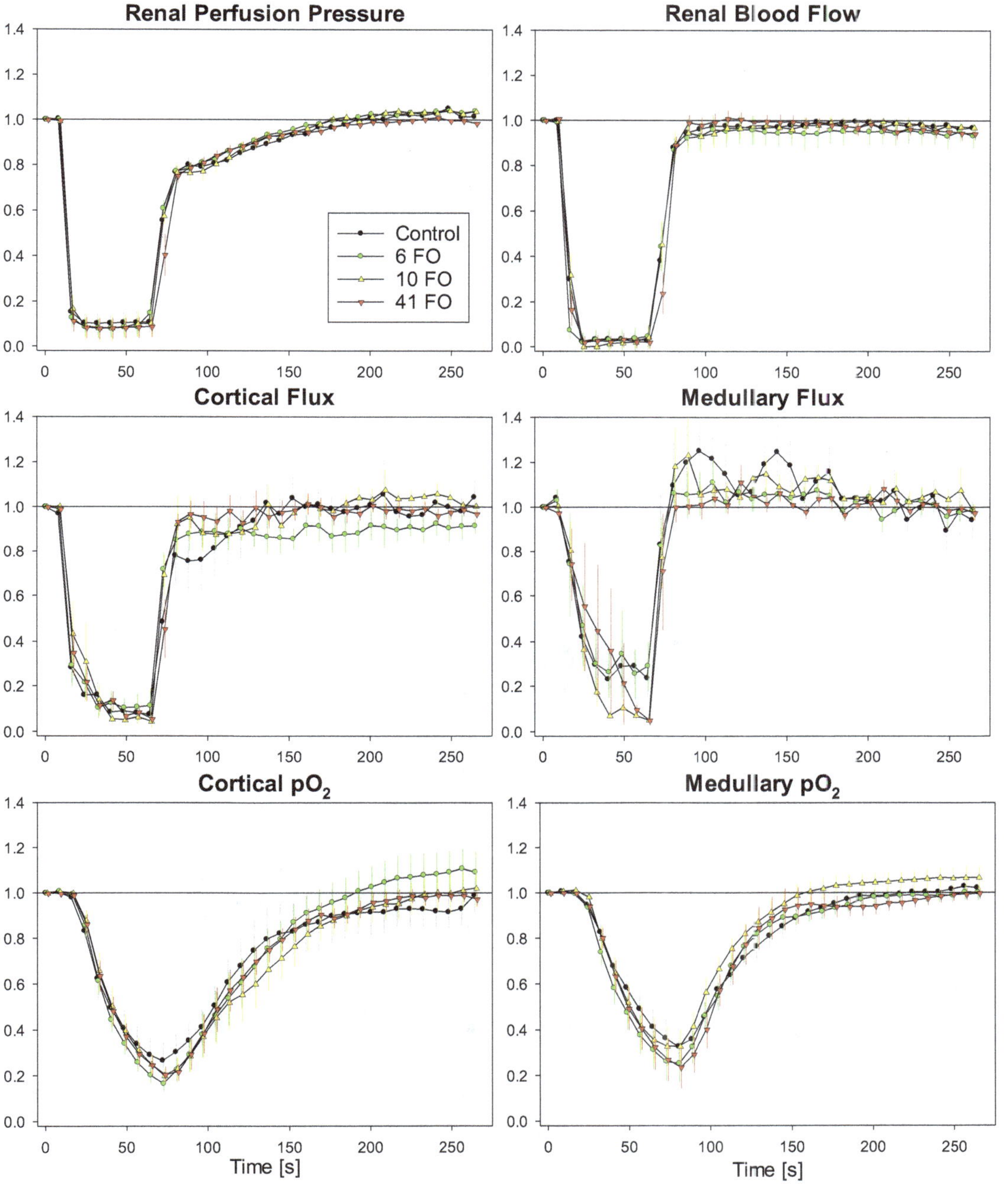

Fig. 2 In order to study whether the USPIO preparation, ferumoxytol (FO), exerts unwarranted effects on regulation of renal hemodynamics and oxygenation, a short-term suprarenal aortic occlusion was employed as test intervention in anesthetized rats [38]. Here, the relative changes (mean ± SEM) in hemodynamics and tissue oxygenation are depicted with FO dosages of 6, 10, and 41 mg Fe/kg body mass, or vehicle (Control)

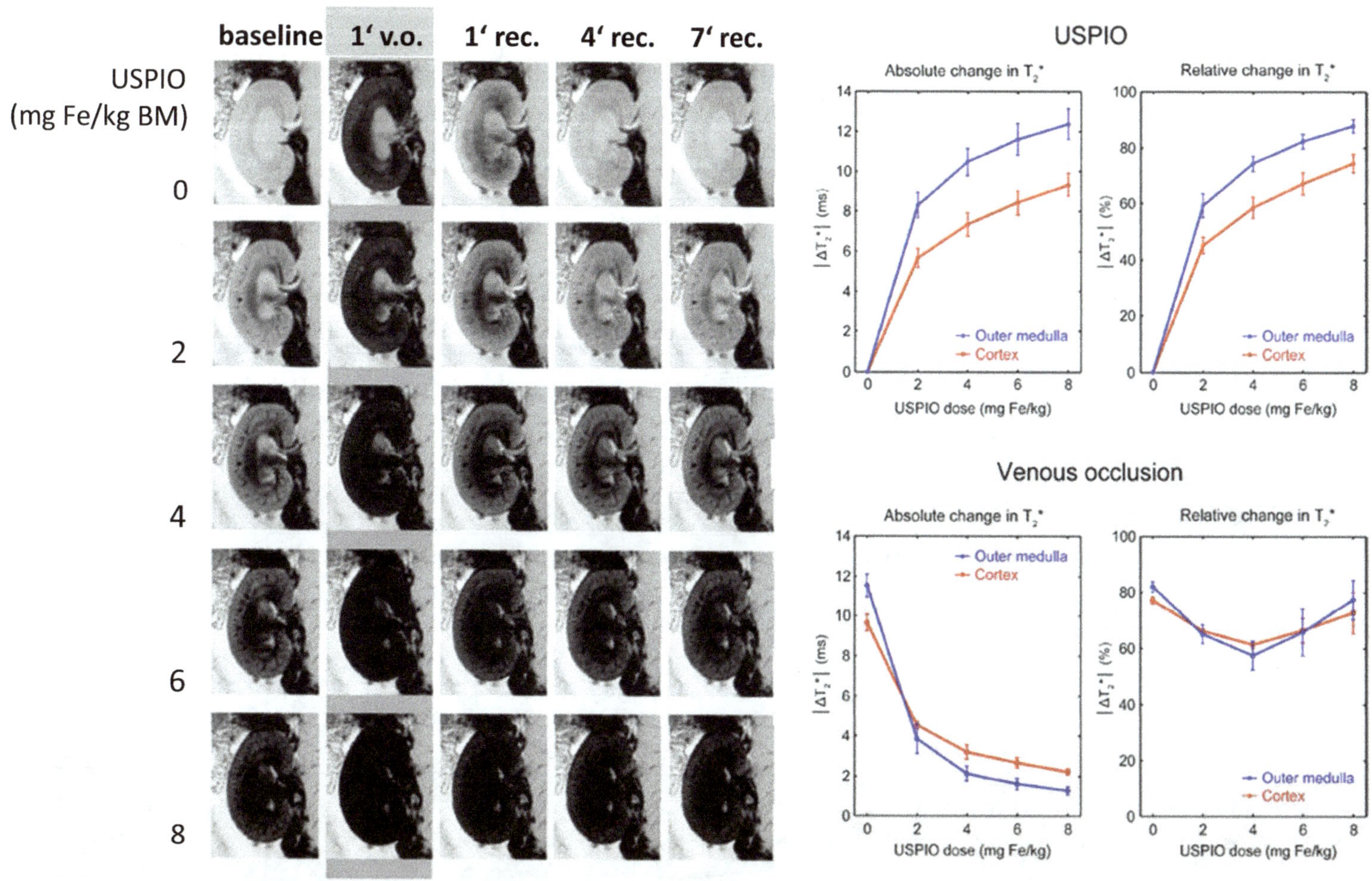

Fig. 3 Left panel: T_2*-weighted images (echo time = 3.6 ms, spatial resolution = 226 × 422 μm) obtained by a 9.4 T small animal MR scanner (Bruker Biospin, Biospec 94/20) of a rat kidney in vivo at baseline, during occlusion of the renal vein (v.o.), and at the beginning of the recovery phase (rec.) without the USPIO ferumoxytol (top row), and with four increasing doses of ferumoxytol [60]. Right panels: Comparison of the renal cortical and medullary T_2* sensitivity to USPIO injection and the T_2* sensitivity to the venous occlusion at different USPIO doses. Data are mean ± SEM ($n = 4$ rats) of cortical and medullary ROIs [60]

3.2 Servocontrolled Changes in Renal Arterial Pressure

Dynamic changes in renal arterial pressure according to different time courses of pressure reduction followed by pressure restoration—be it staircasewise or rampwise changes—enable insights into control of renal hemodynamics and oxygenation including the degree of autoregulation's efficiency and the contributions of the three autoregulatory mechanisms in vivo. This is achieved by a servocontrol system developed by our group, that was utilized to help disentangle the complexities of renal physiology and pathophysiology [30, 31, 33, 34]. Moreover, a study that employed such an intervention in a rat model that emulates an early stage of diabetic kidney disease (a type 1 diabetes mellitus–like model induced by administration of streptozotocin 4 weeks before obtaining the data on renal perfusion and oxygenation) unmasked alterations in the control of renal perfusion and oxygenation that would have gone undetected when only baseline data had been obtained [32]. Data on medullary tissue pO_2 obtained by invasive probes in this model have been inconsistent, which, among other reasons, may be caused by the spatial heterogeneity of pO_2 within the renal medulla [15–17]. A recent study did not find any significant differences in baseline data on RBF and cortical and medullary tissue pO_2 among healthy control rats, diabetic rats, and diabetic rats treated with the antidiabetic liraglutide (a glucagon-like peptide 1 agonist approved for patients suffering from type 2 diabetes). However, as depicted by Fig. 4, the response to ramp-wise reduction and restoration of renal arterial pressure differed considerably among these groups [32].

Again, as the implementation of a vascular occluder necessitates invasive techniques, such studies can be performed in preclinical studies only.

3.3 Short Periods of Changes in the Inspiratory Gas Mixture

Hyperoxia, hypoxia, and hypercapnia primarily alter blood oxygenation. Renal O_2 delivery is determined by renal perfusion and by the arterial O_2 content. The latter is determined, among other factors, by the inspiratory fraction of oxygen (FiO_2), and, due to the effect of CO_2 on the oxyHb dissociation curve, also by the inspiratory fraction of CO_2 ($FiCO_2$).

Increasing the FiO_2 from 21% (normoxia) to 100% (hyperoxia) results in a substantial increase in arterial pO_2 (usually four- to fivefold), whereas the increase in arterial O_2 content is very small, because most of the Hb in arterial blood is already O_2 saturated under normoxic conditions. Yet the increase in arterial pO_2 enhances the driving force for diffusion of O_2 from intrarenal vessels to tissue as well as from intrarenal arteries to veins. As a consequence, the increase in renal tissue pO_2 is substantial, whereby medullary pO_2 increases less than cortical pO_2, due to arteriovenous diffusive O_2 shunting, which reduces the O_2 content of arterial blood that perfuses the medulla [22, 26, 39, 53–55]. Renal T_2^* changes exerted by hyperoxia are small

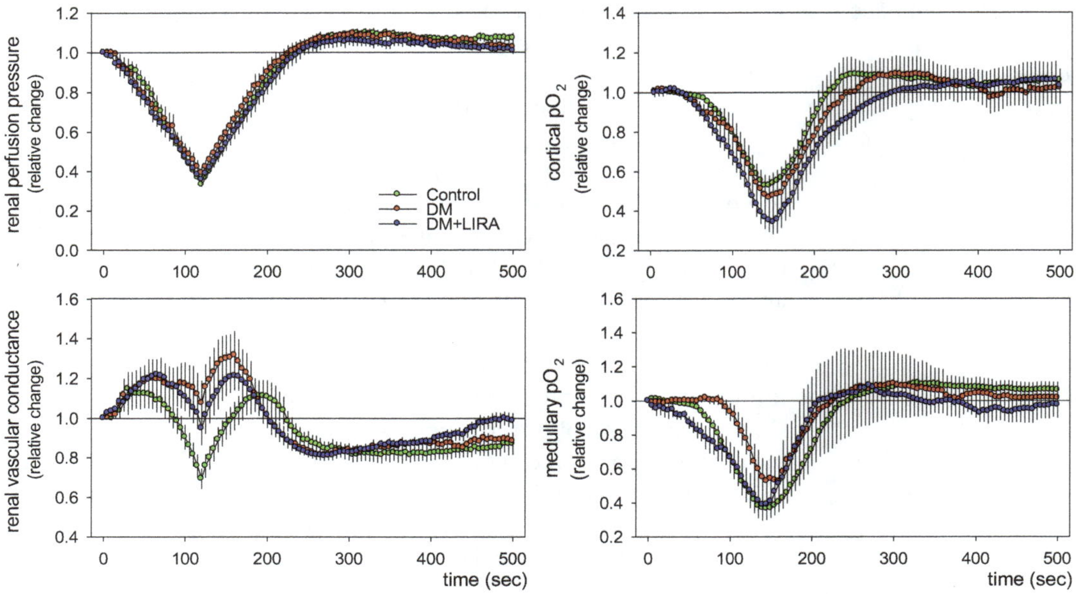

Fig. 4 Changes of invasively measured parameters of renal hemodynamics and oxygenation during ramp-wise reduction in renal perfusion pressure followed by ramp-wise pressure restoration in anesthetized rats. Conductance values (the reciprocal of vascular resistance) were calculated by dividing the respective perfusion values by renal perfusion pressure, in order to distinguish flow changes that result from passive circular distension/compression of vessels from those actively exerted by vascular smooth muscles. Three groups were studied: a healthy control group, a group in which a diabetes mellitus type 1-like disorder (DM) was induced by streptozotocin 4 weeks before obtaining the data, and a third group in which DM was induced and the antidiabetic liraglutide administered for 3 weeks (DM + LIRA). Values (mean $\pm$ SEM) are given as relative changes from baseline [32]

[22]. While the amount of deoxyHb in arterial blood is barely changed, the increase in blood pO_2 in intrarenal veins that results from the higher arteriovenous pO_2 difference decreases venous deoxyHb. While primarily altering blood oxygenation, the hyperoxic stimulus has also secondary effects: it results in vasoconstriction, preferentially in nonrenal vascular beds, which leads to an increase in arterial pressure [22, 31, 39].

The primary effect of reducing the FiO_2 (typically to either 8% or 10%, with durations of 3–12 min, in rat studies) is a decrease in oxygenation of arterial blood (hypoxemia) with the consequent reduction in renal O_2 supply. With ongoing O_2 consumption, this does per se result in a decrease in renal tissue pO_2. Yet renal O_2 supply is further diminished by hypoxia-induced extrarenal vasodilation that results in a drop in arterial pressure with ensuing decrease in RBF [22, 31, 39, 59]. Whether this is aggravated of alleviated by constriction or dilation, respectively, of the renal vasculature depends on the degree of hypoxia: in anesthetized rats, FiO_2 of 8% results in renal vasoconstriction while 10% results in vasodilation [22, 31, 39]. The combined effect of hypoxemia and reduced RBF on renal O_2 supply leads to a major mismatch with O_2 consumption, that massively reduces tissue pO_2 as well as T_2* (*see* Fig. 1) [22, 39]. A further secondary effect of arterial hypoxemia is increased ventilation triggered by arterial chemoreceptors. The ensuing decrease in arterial pCO_2 shifts the oxyHb dissociation curve to the left, that is, O_2 is hindered from being released by Hb, which further aggravates the tissue hypoxia [61, 62].

With the hypercapnic stimulus (increasing $FiCO_2$ to 5%) the opposite effect is achieved, namely a rightward shift of the oxyHb dissociation curve. This would per se result in a decrease in StO_2 and an increase in blood and tissue pO_2. However, while the increase in tissue pO_2 is substantial, the StO_2 decrease is meagre [39]. The major reason that StO_2 does not decrease much is that increased pCO_2 of arterial blood is a very strong stimulus for ventilation, again mediated by arterial chemoreceptors [61, 62].

Hyperoxic, hypoxic, and hypercapnic tests have been used in a multitude of preclinical in vivo studies. With regard to the kidney this includes but is not limited to studies on the control of renal hemodynamics and oxygenation in healthy animals and models of kidney diseases [26, 27, 31, 53–55, 59], experiments that aimed at calibration of T_2* by means of the MR-PHYSIOL setup (*see* Fig. 5), [22] studies on the T_2* effect of an X-ray contrast medium, [36] assessment of possible unwarranted effects of the USPIO ferumoxytol, [38] and experiments en route to the PHYSIOL-NIRS setup [39].

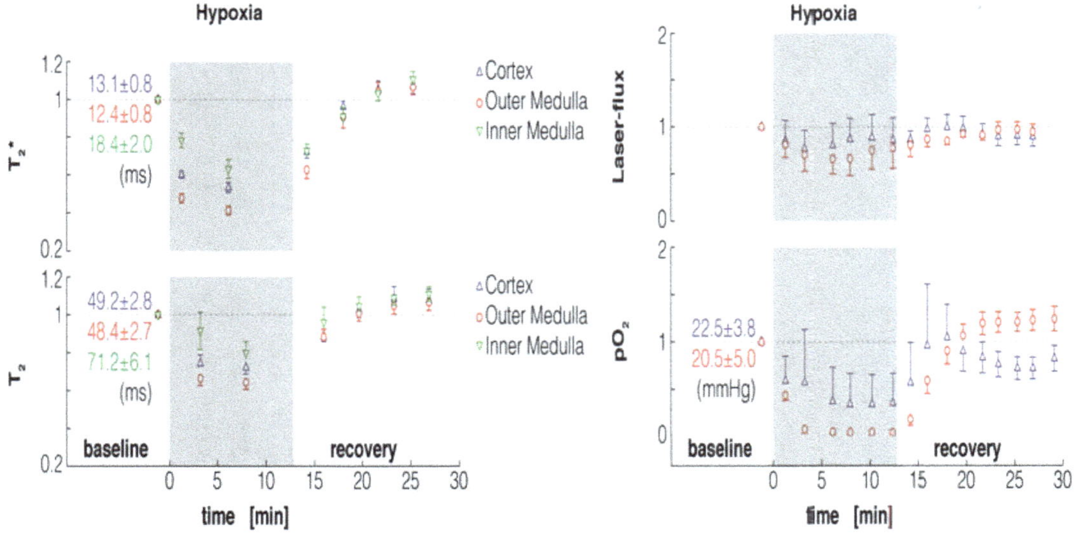

Fig. 5 Time courses of selected invasively measured data and MR parameters acquired simultaneously throughout baseline, a period of hypoxia (FiO_2 = 8%), and recovery in anesthetized rats by means of a dedicated MR-PHYSIOL hybrid setup (for details see text). Data (mean ± SEM) are relative changes from baseline, redrawn from Ref. 22

Given the broad therapeutic use of pure oxygen, short-term tests with 100% FiO_2 should pose no problem for studies in humans, whereas hypoxic challenges are precluded in humans, for obvious ethical reasons. Hypercapnia has been used for decades in humans, in particular, for the study of cerebrovascular reactivity, and should thus be employed in preclinical and clinical studies on renal hemodynamics and oxygenation as well [63, 64].

3.4 Administration of Drugs and Endogenous Vasoactive Substances

Furosemide is the "classic" loop diuretic: its major action is the inhibition of the sodium–potassium–two-chloride cotransporter in the apical membrane of tubular epithelial cells of the thick ascending limb of Henle's loop. The primary effect is an increase in urine flow rate and in urinary sodium and potassium excretion. As less tubular resorption necessitates less renal O_2 consumption, administration of furosemide leads to an increase in renal tissue pO_2 [65, 66]. In accordance, increases in renal T_2* (or decreases in its reciprocal value R_2*) have been observed in a multitude of preclinical as well as clinical studies (*see* Fig. 6) [37, 66–69]. It must be noted, however, that the increase in T_2* upon furosemide does not solely rely on improved oxygenation. First, the increase in tubular fluid downstream of the thick ascending limb will increase the transmural pressure gradient, thereby compressing intrarenal

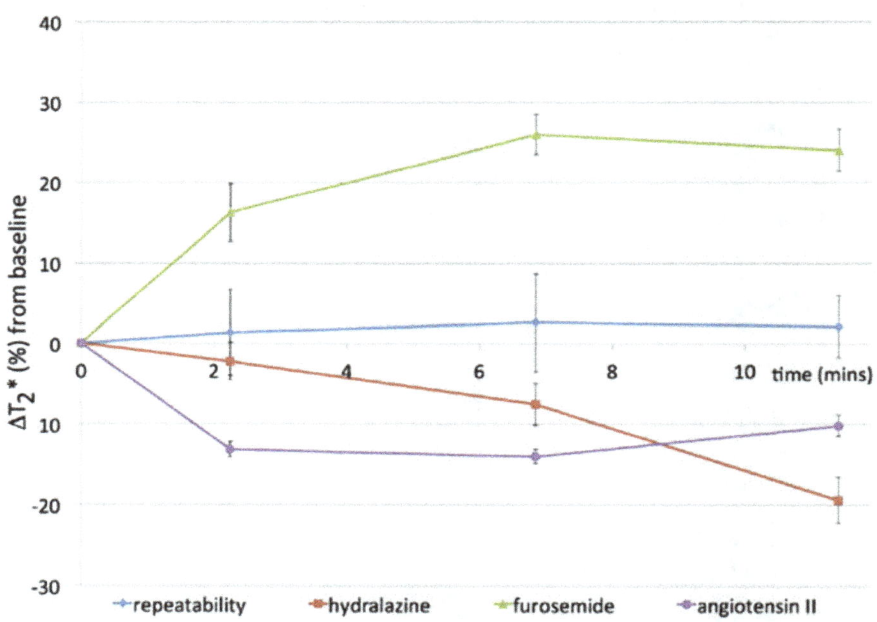

Fig. 6 Effect of injections of furosemide (5 mg/kg body mass), hydralazine (5 mg/kg), angiotensin II (0.5 μg/min/kg), and saline (repeatability) on renal BOLD as recorded by means of a 1.5 T clinical MR scanner (Magnetom Avanto, Siemens Healthcare), using a multiple gradient echo sequence (TR = 300 ms, TE = 5, 10, 20, 30, and 40 ms, voxel size 0.6 × 0.6 mm in-plane and 5 mm slice thickness) in rats in vivo. Data are mean ± SEM of median ROI values [37]

vessels with the ensuing decrease in the amount of deoxyHb per tissue volume. Second, furosemide inhibits the TGF, thereby compromising renal autoregulation with the possible consequence of an increase in RBF [34, 35, 50].

The use of the furosemide test in both preclinical and clinical MR studies is nowadays as widespread that it is almost regarded as a gold standard. However, whether it fulfils all expectations regarding its use as a diagnostic tool in patients suffering from various kidney diseases, remains to be seen [68].

Administration of furosemide is a reversible intervention insofar as its direct effects vanish with the excretion of the drug. However, it leaves the organism with deficits in water, sodium, and potassium. These should ideally be replenished—be it per os or by means of infusions of a balanced electrolyte solution.

Bolus injections of adenosine cause a rapid drop in arterial pressure due to its vasodilatory effect on nonrenal resistance vessels. In the renal cortical vascular bed, it exerts vasoconstriction [39, 49]. The consequence of these two effects is a substantial decrease in RBF followed by a smaller decrease in cortical tissue pO_2. All these effects vanish rapidly, lasting less than a minute for the hemodynamics and less than 2 min for the cortical pO_2 in rats [39].

Whereas the role of adenosine in various renal control mechanisms including the TGF as well as the potentially beneficial effect of adenosine receptor antagonists for prevention of X-ray contrast media-induced AKI have been intensively studied, [49, 70] the adenosine test has seldom been used to study renal hemodynamics and oxygenation. This may appear surprising, as injections of adenosine—be it intravenously or into coronary arteries—in patients suffering from coronary disease is quite established [71, 72]. While the risk for a decrease in renal cortical pO_2 in patients must not be ignored—even if it is lasting less than 2 min, the test should at least find wider use in preclinical studies.

Acknowledgments

This work was funded, in part (Kathleen Cantow and Erdmann Seeliger) by the German Research Foundation (Gefoerdert durch die Deutsche Forschungsgemeinschaft (DFG), Project number/ Projektnummer 394046635, SFB 1365, RENOPROTECTION). The authors wish to thank Ariane Anger and Andrea Gerhardt for expert technical assistance.

This chapter is based upon work from COST Action PAR ENCHIMA, supported by European Cooperation in Science and Technology (COST). COST (www.cost.eu) is a funding agency for research and innovation networks. COST Actions help connect research initiatives across Europe and enable scientists to enrich their ideas by sharing them with their peers. This boosts their research, career, and innovation.

PARENCHIMA (renalmri.org) is a community-driven Action in the COST program of the European Union, which unites more than 200 experts in renal MRI from 30 countries with the aim to improve the reproducibility and standardization of renal MRI biomarkers.

References

1. Fortrie G, de Geus HRH, Betjes MGH (2019) The aftermath of acute kidney injury: a narrative review of long-term mortality and renal function. Crit Care 23(1):24. https://doi.org/10.1186/s13054-019-2314-z
2. Selby NM, Taal MW (2019) Long-term outcomes after AKI-a major unmet clinical need. Kidney Int 95(1):21–23. https://doi.org/10.1016/j.kint.2018.09.005
3. Zuk A, Bonventre JV (2019) Recent advances in acute kidney injury and its consequences and impact on chronic kidney disease. Curr Opin Nephrol Hypertens 28(4):397–405. https://doi.org/10.1097/mnh.0000000000000504
4. Levin A, Tonelli M, Bonventre J, Coresh J, Donner JA, Fogo AB, Fox CS, Gansevoort RT, Heerspink HJL, Jardine M, Kasiske B, Kottgen A, Kretzler M, Levey AS, Luyckx VA, Mehta R, Moe O, Obrador G, Pannu N, Parikh CR, Perkovic V, Pollock C, Stenvinkel P, Tuttle KR, Wheeler DC, Eckardt KU (2017) Global kidney health 2017 and beyond: a roadmap for closing gaps in care, research, and policy. Lancet 390(10105):1888–1917. https://doi.org/10.1016/s0140-6736(17)30788-2
5. Bello AK, Levin A, Tonelli M, Okpechi IG, Feehally J, Harris D, Jindal K, Salako BL, Rateb A, Osman MA, Qarni B, Saad S, Lunney M, Wiebe N, Ye F, Johnson DW (2017) Assessment of global kidney health care status. JAMA 317(18):1864–1881. https://doi.org/10.1001/jama.2017.4046
6. Brezis M, Rosen S (1995) Hypoxia of the renal medulla--its implications for disease. N Engl J Med 332:647–655
7. Seeliger E, Sendeski M, Rihal CS, Persson PB (2012) Contrast-induced kidney injury: mechanisms, risk factors, and prevention. Eur Heart J 33(16):2007–2015
8. Evans RG, Ince C, Joles JA, Smith DW, May CN, O'Connor PM, Gardiner BS (2013) Haemodynamic influences on kidney oxygenation: the clinical implications of integrative physiology. Clin Exp Pharmacol Physiol 40:106–122
9. Evans RG, Ow CP, Bie P (2015) The chronic hypoxia hypothesis: the search for the smoking gun goes on. Am J Physiol Renal Physiol 308(2):F101–F102
10. Shu S, Wang Y, Zheng M, Liu Z, Cai J, Tang C, Dong Z (2019) Hypoxia and hypoxia-inducible factors in kidney injury and repair. Cell 8(3):207. https://doi.org/10.3390/cells8030207
11. Hultstrom M, Becirovic-Agic M, Jonsson S (2018) Comparison of acute kidney injury of different etiology reveals in-common mechanisms of tissue damage. Physiol Genomics 50(3):127–141. https://doi.org/10.1152/physiolgenomics.00037.2017
12. Calzavacca P, Evans RG, Bailey M, Bellomo R, May CN (2015) Cortical and medullary tissue perfusion and oxygenation in experimental septic acute kidney injury. Crit Care Med 43(10):e431–e439
13. Fähling M, Seeliger E, Patzak A, Persson PB (2017) Understanding and preventing contrast-induced acute kidney injury. Nat Rev Nephrol 13(3):169–180
14. Ma S, Evans RG, Iguchi N, Tare M, Parkington HC, Bellomo R, May CN, Lankadeva YR (2019) Sepsis-induced acute kidney injury: a disease of the microcirculation. Microcirculation 26(2):e12483. https://doi.org/10.1111/micc.12483
15. Palm F, Carlsson PO, Hansell P, Hellberg O, Nygren A, Liss P (2003) Altered response in renal blood flow and oxygen tension to contrast media in diabetic rats. Acta Radiol 44(3):347–353
16. Palm F, Cederberg J, Hansell P, Liss P, Carlsson PO (2003) Reactive oxygen species cause diabetes-induced decrease in renal oxygen tension. Diabetologia 46(8):1153–1160
17. dos Santos EA, Li LP, Ji L, Prasad PV (2007) Early changes with diabetes in renal medullary hemodynamics as evaluated by fiberoptic probes and BOLD magnetic resonance imaging. Investig Radiol 42(3):157–162. https://

doi.org/10.1097/01.rli.0000252492.96709.36

18. Calvin AD, Misra S, Pflueger A (2010) Contrast-induced acute kidney injury and diabetic nephropathy. Nat Rev Nephrol 6(11):679–688
19. Hansell P, Welch WJ, Blantz RC, Palm F (2013) Determinants of kidney oxygen consumption and their relationship to tissue oxygen tension in diabetes and hypertension. Clin Exp Pharmacol Physiol 40(2):123–137
20. Evans RG, Gardiner BS, Smith DW, O'Connor PM (2008) Methods for studying the physiology of kidney oxygenation. Clin Exp Pharmacol Physiol 35(12):1405–1412
21. Pohlmann A, Cantow K, Hentschel J, Arakelyan K, Ladwig M, Flemming B, Hoff U, Persson PB, Seeliger E, Niendorf T (2013) Linking non-invasive parametric MRI with invasive physiological measurements (MR-PHYSIOL): towards a hybrid and integrated approach for investigation of acute kidney injury in rats. Acta Physiol (Oxf) 207(4):673–689
22. Pohlmann A, Arakelyan K, Hentschel J, Cantow K, Flemming B, Ladwig M, Waiczies S, Seeliger E, Niendorf T (2014) Detailing the relation between renal T2* and renal tissue pO2 using an integrated approach of parametric magnetic resonance imaging and invasive physiological measurements. Investig Radiol 49(8):547–560
23. Niendorf T, Pohlmann A, Arakelyan K, Flemming B, Cantow K, Hentschel J, Grosenick D, Ladwig M, Reimann H, Klix S, Waiczies S, Seeliger E (2015) How BOLD is blood oxygenation-dependent (BOLD) magnetic resonance imaging of the kidney? Opportunities, challenges and future directions. Acta Physiol (Oxf) 213(1):19–38
24. Hirakawa Y, Tanaka T, Nangaku M (2017) Renal hypoxia in CKD; pathophysiology and detecting methods. Front Physiol 8:99. https://doi.org/10.3389/fphys.2017.00099
25. Calzavacca P, Evans RG, Bailey M, Bellomo R, May CN (2015) Variable responses of regional renal oxygenation and perfusion to vasoactive agents in awake sheep. Am J Physiol Regul Integr Comp Physiol 309(10):R1226–R1233
26. Evans RG, Gardiner BS, Smith DW, O'Connor PM (2008) Intrarenal oxygenation: unique challenges and the biophysical basis of homeostasis. Am J Physiol Renal Physiol 295(5):1259–1270
27. Evans RG, Goddard D, Eppel GA, O'Connor PM (2011) Factors that render the kidney susceptible to tissue hypoxia in hypoxemia. Am J Physiol Regul Integr Comp Physiol 300(4):R931–R940
28. Emans TW, Janssen BJ, Pinkham MI, Ow CP, Evans RG, Joles JA, Malpas SC, Krediet CT, Koeners MP (2016) Exogenous and endogenous angiotensin-II decrease renal cortical oxygen tension in conscious rats by limiting renal blood flow. J Physiol 594(21):6287–6300. https://doi.org/10.1113/jp270731
29. Evans RG, Madden AC, Denton KM (2000) Diversity of responses of renal cortical and medullary blood flow to vasoconstrictors in conscious rabbits. Acta Physiol Scand 169(4):297–308
30. Seeliger E, Flemming B, Wronski T, Ladwig M, Arakelyan K, Godes M, Mockel M, Persson PB (2007) Viscosity of contrast media perturbs renal hemodynamics. J Am Soc Nephrol 18(11):2912–2920
31. Flemming B, Seeliger E, Wronski T, Steer K, Arenz N, Persson PB (2000) Oxygen and renal hemodynamics in the conscious rat. J Am Soc Nephrol 11(1):18–24
32. Ferrara F, Cantow K, Flemming B, Skalweit A, Ladwig M, Fähling M, Seeliger E (2017) Effects of liraglutide on control of renal hemodynamics and oxygenation in diabetic rats. Acta Physiol (Oxf) 219(Suppl. 711):38
33. Flemming B, Arenz N, Seeliger E, Wronski T, Steer K, Persson PB (2001) Time-dependent autoregulation of renal blood flow in conscious rats. J Am Soc Nephrol 12(11):2253–2262
34. Seeliger E, Wronski T, Ladwig M, Dobrowolski L, Vogel T, Godes M, Persson PB, Flemming B (2009) The renin-angiotensin system and the third mechanism of renal blood flow autoregulation. Am J Physiol Renal Physiol 296(6):F1334–F1345
35. Wronski T, Seeliger E, Persson PB, Forner C, Fichtner C, Scheller J, Flemming B (2003) The step response: a method to characterize mechanisms of renal blood flow autoregulation. Am J Physiol Renal Physiol 285(4):F758–F764
36. Arakelyan K, Cantow K, Hentschel J, Flemming B, Pohlmann A, Ladwig M, Niendorf T, Seeliger E (2013) Early effects of an x-ray contrast medium on renal T_2*/T_2 MRI as compared to short-term hyperoxia, hypoxia and aortic occlusion in rats. Acta Physiol 208(2):202–213
37. Jerome NP, Boult JK, Orton MR, d'Arcy J, Collins DJ, Leach MO, Koh DM, Robinson SP (2016) Modulation of renal oxygenation and perfusion in rat kidney monitored by quantitative diffusion and blood oxygen level dependent magnetic resonance imaging on a

clinical 1.5T platform. BMC Nephrol 17 (1):142. https://doi.org/10.1186/s12882-016-0356-x

38. Cantow K, Pohlmann A, Flemming B, Ferrara F, Waiczies S, Grosenick D, Niendorf T, Seeliger E (2016) Acute effects of ferumoxytol on regulation of renal hemodynamics and oxygenation. Sci Rep 6:29965. https://doi.org/10.1038/srep29965
39. Grosenick D, Cantow K, Arakelyan K, Wabnitz H, Flemming B, Skalweit A, Ladwig M, Macdonald R, Niendorf T, Seeliger E (2015) Detailing renal hemodynamics and oxygenation in rats by a combined near-infrared spectroscopy and invasive probe approach. Biomed Opt Express 6(2):309–323
40. Seeliger E, Cantow K, Arakelyan K, Ladwig M, Persson PB, Flemming B (2014) Low-dose nitrite alleviates early effects of an X-ray contrast medium on renal hemodynamics and oxygenation in rats. Investig Radiol 49(2):70–77
41. Edwards A, Silldforff EP, Pallone TL (2000) The renal medullary microcirculation. Front Biosci 5:E36–E52
42. Zimmerhackl BL, Robertson CR, Jamison RL (1987) The medullary microcirculation. Kidney Int 31(2):641–647
43. Schurek HJ (1988) Kidney medullary hypoxia: a key to understanding acute renal failure? die Nierenmarkhypoxie: ein Schlussel zum Verstandnis des akuten Nierenversagens? Klin Wochenschr 66(18):828–835
44. Baumgartl H, Leichtweiss HP, Lubbers DW, Weiss C, Huland H (1972) The oxygen supply of the dog kidney: measurements of intrarenal pO_2. Microvasc Res 4(3):247–257
45. Lubbers DW, Baumgartl H (1997) Heterogeneities and profiles of oxygen pressure in brain and kidney as examples of the pO_2 distribution in the living tissue. Kidney Int 51(2):372–380
46. Evans RG, Ow CPC (2018) Heterogeneity of renal cortical oxygenation: seeing is believing. Kidney Int 93(6):1278–1280. https://doi.org/10.1016/j.kint.2018.01.039
47. Hirakawa Y, Mizukami K, Yoshihara T, Takahashi I, Khulan P, Honda T, Mimura I, Tanaka T, Tobita S, Nangaku M (2018) Intravital phosphorescence lifetime imaging of the renal cortex accurately measures renal hypoxia. Kidney Int 93(6):1483–1489. https://doi.org/10.1016/j.kint.2018.01.015
48. Evans RG, Harrop GK, Ngo JP, Ow CP, O'Connor PM (2014) Basal renal O_2 consumption and the efficiency of O_2 utilization for Na^+ reabsorption. Am J Physiol Renal Physiol 306(5):F551–F560
49. Vallon V, Muhlbauer B, Osswald H (2006) Adenosine and kidney function. Physiol Rev 86(3):901–940
50. Just A (2007) Mechanisms of renal blood flow autoregulation: dynamics and contributions. Am J Physiol Regul Integr Comp Physiol 292 (1):R1–R17
51. O'Connor PM (2006) Renal oxygen delivery: matching delivery to metabolic demand. Clin Exp Pharmacol Physiol 33(10):961–967
52. Blantz RC, Weir MR (2004) Are the oxygen costs of kidney function highly regulated? Curr Opin Nephrol Hypertens 13(1):67–71
53. Schurek HJ, Jost U, Baumgartl H, Bertram H, Heckmann U (1990) Evidence for a preglomerular oxygen diffusion shunt in rat renal cortex. Am J Physiol 259(6 Pt 2):F910–F915
54. Ngo JP, Ow CP, Gardiner BS, Kar S, Pearson JT, Smith DW, Evans RG (2016) Diffusive shunting of gases and other molecules in the renal vasculature: physiological and evolutionary significance. Am J Physiol Regul Integr Comp Physiol 311(5):R797–r810. https://doi.org/10.1152/ajpregu.00246.2016
55. Leong CL, Anderson WP, O'Connor PM, Evans RG (2007) Evidence that renal arterial-venous oxygen shunting contributes to dynamic regulation of renal oxygenation. Am J Physiol Renal Physiol 292:F1726–F1733
56. Pappenheimer JR, Kinter WB (1956) Hematocrit ratio of blood within mammalian kidney and its significance for renal hemodynamics. Am J Physiol 185:377
57. Hoff U, Lukitsch I, Chaykovska L, Ladwig M, Arnold C, Manthati VL, Fuller TF, Schneider W, Gollasch M, Muller DN, Flemming B, Seeliger E, Luft FC, Falck JR, Dragun D, Schunck WH (2011) Inhibition of 20-HETE synthesis and action protects the kidney from ischemia/reperfusion injury. Kidney Int 79(1):57–65
58. Hosszu A, Antal Z, Lenart L, Hodrea J, Koszegi S, Balogh DB, Banki NF, Wagner L, Denes A, Hamar P, Degrell P, Vannay A, Szabo AJ, Fekete A (2017) sigma1-receptor Agonism protects against renal ischemia-reperfusion injury. J Am Soc Nephrol 28(1):152–165. https://doi.org/10.1681/asn.2015070772
59. Cantow K, Flemming B, Ladwig-Wiegard M, Persson PB, Seeliger E (2017) Low dose nitrite improves reoxygenation following renal ischemia in rats. Sci Rep 7(1):14597–15058
60. Pohlmann A, Cantow K, Huelnhagen T, Grosenick D, Dos Santos PJ, Boehmert L, Gladytz T, Waiczies S, Flemming B, Seeliger E, Niendorf T (2017) Experimental MRI monitoring of renal blood volume

fraction variations En route to renal magnetic resonance oximetry. Tomography 3 (4):188–200. https://doi.org/10.18383/j.tom.2017.00012

61. Kumar P (2009) Systemic effects resulting from carotid body stimulation-invited article. Adv Exp Med Biol 648:223–233. https://doi.org/10.1007/978-90-481-2259-2_26
62. Lahiri S, Forster RE 2nd (2003) CO_2/H(+) sensing: peripheral and central chemoreception. Int J Biochem Cell Biol 35 (10):1413–1435
63. Catchlove SJ, Pipingas A, Hughes ME, Macpherson H (2018) Magnetic resonance imaging for assessment of cerebrovascular reactivity and its relationship to cognition: a systematic review. BMC Neurosci 19(1):21. https://doi.org/10.1186/s12868-018-0421-4
64. Corfield DR, McKay LC (2016) Regional cerebrovascular responses to hypercapnia and hypoxia. Adv Exp Med Biol 903:157–167. https://doi.org/10.1007/978-1-4899-7678-9_11
65. Brezis M, Agmon Y, Epstein FH (1994) Determinants of intrarenal oxygenation. I. Effects of diuretics. Am J Physiol 267(6 Pt 2): F1059–F1062. https://doi.org/10.1152/ajprenal.1994.267.6.F1059
66. Warner L, Glockner JF, Woollard J, Textor SC, Romero JC, Lerman LO (2011) Determinations of renal cortical and medullary oxygenation using blood oxygen level-dependent magnetic resonance imaging and selective diuretics. Investig Radiol 46(1):41–47. https://doi.org/10.1097/RLI.0b013e3181f0213f
67. Prasad PV, Edelman RR, Epstein FH (1996) Noninvasive evaluation of intrarenal oxygenation with BOLD MRI. Circulation 94 (12):3271–3275. https://doi.org/10.1161/01.cir.94.12.3271
68. Palmucci S, Mammino L, Caltabiano DC, Costanzo V, Foti PV, Mauro LA, Farina R, Profitta ME, Sinagra N, Ettorre GC, Veroux M, Basile A (2019) Diffusion-MR in kidney transplant recipients: is diuretic stimulation a useful diagnostic tool for improving differentiation between functioning and non-functioning kidneys? Clin Imaging 53:97–104. https://doi.org/10.1016/j.clinimag.2018.10.003
69. Haddock B, Larsson HBW, Francis S, Andersen UB (2019) Human renal response to furosemide: simultaneous oxygenation and perfusion measurements in cortex and medulla. Acta Physiol (Oxf) 227:e13292. https://doi.org/10.1111/apha.13292
70. Welch WJ (2002) Adenosine A1 receptor antagonists in the kidney: effects in fluid-retaining disorders. Curr Opin Pharmacol 2 (2):165–170
71. Gili S, Barbero U, Errigo D, De Luca G, Biondi-Zoccai G, Leone AM, Iannaccone M, Montefusco A, Omede P, Moretti C, D'Amico M, Gaita F, D'Ascenzo F (2018) Intracoronary versus intravenous adenosine to assess fractional flow reserve: a systematic review and meta-analysis. J Cardiovasc Med (Hagerstown) 19(6):274–283. https://doi.org/10.2459/jcm.0000000000000652
72. Solerno R, Pedroni P, Mariani J, Sarmiento R (2018) Comparison of sodium nitroprusside and adenosine for fractional flow reserve assessment: a systematic review and meta-analysis. Expert Rev Cardiovasc Ther 16(10):765–770. https://doi.org/10.1080/14779072.2018.1513789

13

Renal Diffusion-Weighted Imaging (DWI) for Apparent Diffusion Coefficient (ADC), Intravoxel Incoherent Motion (IVIM), and Diffusion Tensor Imaging (DTI): Basic Concepts

Neil Peter Jerome, Anna Caroli, and Alexandra Ljimani

Abstract

The specialized function of the kidney is reflected in its unique structure, characterized by juxtaposition of disorganized and ordered elements, including renal glomerula, capillaries, and tubules. The key role of the kidney in blood filtration, and changes in filtration rate and blood flow associated with pathological conditions, make it possible to investigate kidney function using the motion of water molecules in renal tissue. Diffusion-weighted imaging (DWI) is a versatile modality that sensitizes observable signal to water motion, and can inform on the complexity of the tissue microstructure. Several DWI acquisition strategies are available, as are different analysis strategies, and models that attempt to capture not only simple diffusion effects, but also perfusion, compartmentalization, and anisotropy. This chapter introduces the basic concepts of DWI alongside common acquisition schemes and models, and gives an overview of specific DWI applications for animal models of renal disease.

This chapter is based upon work from the COST Action PARENCHIMA, a community-driven network funded by the European Cooperation in Science and Technology (COST) program of the European Union, which aims to improve the reproducibility and standardization of renal MRI biomarkers. This introduction chapter is complemented by two separate chapters describing the experimental procedure and data analysis.

Key words MRI, Kidney, Diffusion, Diffusion-weighted imaging (DWI), Apparent diffusion coefficient (ADC), Intravoxel incoherent motion (IVIM), Mouse, Rat

1 Introduction

The dominant role of magnetic resonance imaging (MRI), and in particular diffusion-weighted imaging (DWI), in the diagnosis and monitoring of renal disease is driven by the ability to provide simultaneous assessment of kidney anatomy and function. In addition to the potential to avoid or reduce the need for biopsy, which is invasive and subject to sampling bias, the use of functional imaging techniques such as DWI allow examination of tissue microstructure in vivo as well as the potential for challenge protocols using administered agents. In particular, in view of the controversial study on

Andreas Pohlmann and Thoralf Niendorf (eds.), *Preclinical MRI of the Kidney: Methods and Protocols*, Methods in Molecular Biology, vol. 2216, https://doi.org/10.1007/978-1-0716-0978-1_11, © The Author(s) 2021

gadolinium-containing MR contrast agents with regard to nephrogenic systemic fibrosis (NSF) [1] or possible gadolinium deposits in the central nervous system (CNS) [2], contrast-free examination techniques are to be preferred, especially in patients with impaired renal function.

Diffusion-weighted imaging comes in many variants, from simple to complex schemes, all based on indirect observation of water molecular motion, that are sensitive to changes in renal perfusion and tubular flow, alterations of cellularity arising from inflammation, edema, or hyperplasia, and from fibrosis. A recent review of the application of renal DWI in humans [3] gives an overview of research performed so far and illustrates renal DWI potential in the clinic. The authors in particular conclude that DWI is well-placed to investigate decline of renal function as well as to monitor disease progression in both acute and chronic kidney diseases, while noting that complexity of the diffusion signal makes biological validation difficult.

The strengths of DWI are not without accompanying drawbacks, however, which include the relatively long acquisition times required for advanced DWI protocols, an increased susceptibility to image artifacts, and an overall decreased spatial resolution due to the imaging sequences used. Careful consideration of both the research question to be addressed and the optimal acquisition parameters to be used, together with acquisition of complementary MRI modalities, can ameliorate some of these issues.

This chapter discusses the underlying phenomena and contrast mechanisms of diffusion-weighted imaging. It is complemented by two separate chapters describing experimental procedure and data analysis, which are part of this book.

This chapter is part of the book Pohlmann A, Niendorf T (eds) (2020) Preclinical MRI of the Kidney—Methods and Protocols. Springer, New York.

2 Diffusion Weighted Imaging Concepts

2.1 Fundamental Concept

MRI signal arising from water protons in vivo is sensitive to the exact nature of the tissue, including not only how the spins interact with the tissue lattice and other spins through T_1 and T_2 relaxation mechanisms, but also the tendency of water molecules to physically move around, or diffuse, over time. The use of the term diffusion-weighted imaging is a general catch-all term for any imaging using pulsed field gradients for motion sensitization. DWI is sensitive to the nature and degree of proton movement, which depends on tissue microstructure, therefore representing an informative component of research and clinical MRI protocols.

The use of pulsed gradient fields added to a MRI readout sequence, in a dephase-rephase cycle commonly implemented as a polarity-reversed pair or as equal pulses placed either side of a spin-echo pulse, causes a loss of the MRI signal proportional to the

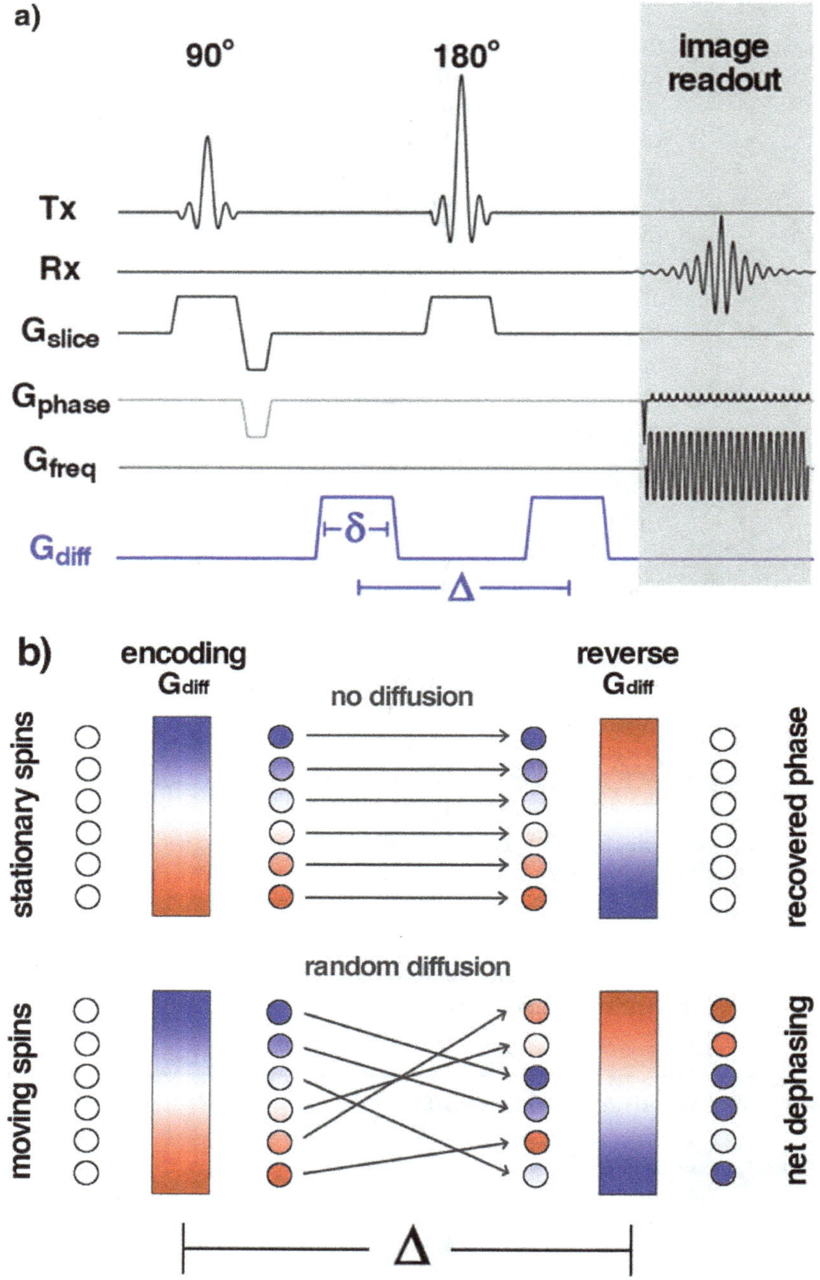

Fig. 1 Illustration of (**a**) DWI pulse sequence, showing the diffusion gradients (lower line, in blue) for a spin-echo echo-planar readout sequence. (**b**) Schematic one-dimensional illustration of the net dephasing of spins dependent on their motion. The initial gradient pulse adds an additional phase (red and blue being +/− additions to the static magnetic field) by transiently modulating the Larmor frequency of the spins. The amount of additional phase is defined by the spin location along the gradient pulse direction (here up/down for simplicity). During the diffusion time Δ, spins have an opportunity to diffuse according to their tissue environment. The reverse pulse (in practice the same polarity, but acting as reversed in combination with the 180° spin-echo pulse) restores the phase offset for spins that have not moved (upper section), whereas moving spins do not receive equal dephase and rephase shifts, leading to a net phase shift (indicated by remaining color) and an overall signal loss

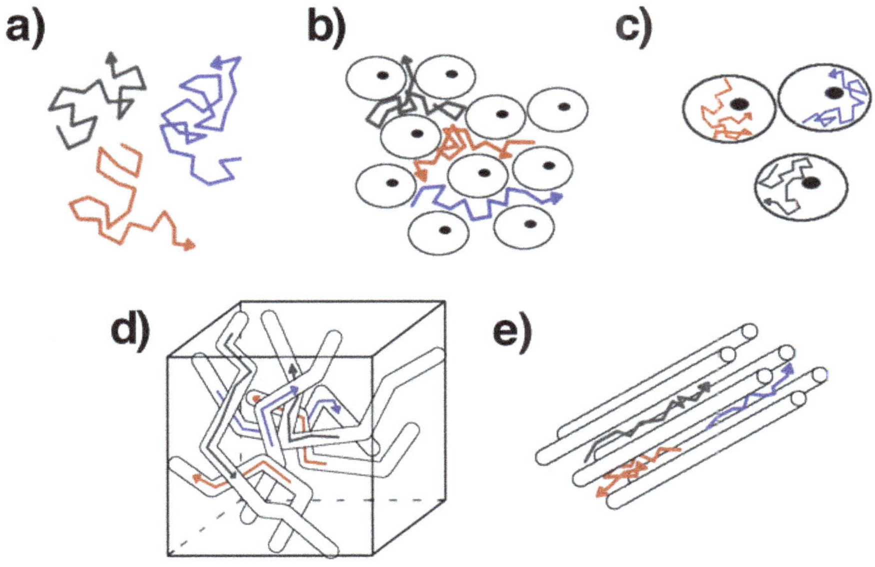

Fig. 2 Schematic summary of motion types that can be investigated by diffusion imaging. Illustrative paths for water molecules are shown for: (**a**) free diffusion, also called Gaussian or true diffusion, that is a random motion; (**b**) apparent hindered diffusion in the tissue, where the microstructure alter true diffusion by introducing barriers; (**c**) apparent diffusion restriction, for example within cells (**d**) pseudodiffusion, denoting motion due to flow in vessels or tubules; and (**e**) diffusion directionality caused by structural elements

overall mis-match of the pulses experienced by spins that have changed location (Fig. 1). The larger the distance covered by water molecules (and the proton spins therein) between the gradient pulses, the greater the mismatch of pulses experienced by the spins, and the greater the overall signal destruction from the net spin dephasing. Over time, this basic DWI concept has been implemented into a raft of specialized sequences, targeted and optimized for different applications.

2.2 Water Motion and Relation to Microstructure

In a large, single-compartment system, free diffusion of water molecules is a truly chaotic, random phenomenon known as Brownian motion, and might go on indefinitely (Fig. 2a). Here, the average displacement of molecules over time is described by an increasingly wide distribution, Gaussian (or normal) in nature, centered on the starting position and characterized by a *diffusion coefficient*. In biological tissues, water molecules interact with surrounding structures (cell walls, extracellular matrix, and so forth), which act as barriers causing an alteration and possible restriction in diffusion (Fig. 2b, c). Tissue microstructure may also contain flow elements, or structure with directional preference (Fig. 2d, e). The observed diffusion coefficient from an imaging voxel, which may contain a complex mix of diffusion environments, is thus an empirical parameter, the *apparent diffusion coefficient (ADC)* measured in mm^2/s. Since tissue microstructure is a major determinant of apparent diffusion, pathological conditions affecting microstructure cause an alteration in ADC.

The length scale of diffusion imaging, that is the average distance covered by water molecules during the DWI experiment, is determined as a balance of the average speed of the water molecules in their environment and the diffusion time allowed in the acquisition. Moreover, it is possible to see signal characteristic of molecules whose motion is restricted to certain structures if the length scale exceeds the structure dimensions. This, for example, allows for the inference of intracellular water motion and thus cell size in appropriately designed DWI protocols [4].

In the kidney, nonrandom perfusion and tubular flow, which manifest as pseudodiffusion processes, as well as the high degree of directional order in the renal structure, add complexity to the investigation of water molecule motion. Specific signal interpretation models have been developed to account for an additional (or sometimes more than one) pseudodiffusion compartment, generally possessing a pseudodiffusion coefficient of a higher magnitude than that of true diffusion. Similarly, additional models assessing diffusion along multiple explicit directions have been developed to provide information on directional motion as well as on the relative anisotropy of the tissue.

Since the complexity of diffusion signal interpretation models is intrinsically tied to the complexity of image acquisition protocols, DWI acquisition and analysis cannot be considered and discussed independently (*see* **Note 1**). The choice of acquisition parameters will determine and/or limit the possible signal interpretation models, and therefore acquisition must be carefully designed, with the expected analysis in mind. In particular, DWI acquisitions are often lengthy, and there is always pressure to limit their duration when transferred to clinical practice to minimize patient discomfort. When planning renal DWI studies in the preclinical setting, it is thus important to consider also their translational potential, and the additional value that more complex acquisitions offer in relation to the extra scan time required.

3 Diffusion Modeling

The degree of diffusion weighting applied to an image is conventionally reported as its *b*-value, where *b* is a compound parameter, expressed in s/mm^2, arising from the specifics of the pulsed gradients used to sensitize the signal to spin motion. The *b*-value is limited by the gradient hardware, but values of several thousand are commonly achievable. Given that the incomplete rephasing of displaced water molecules explicitly leads to a loss of signal, increased diffusion weighting is ultimately limited by signal-to-noise and in general is performed with a lower spatial resolution than images acquired using other MRI modalities. Sufficiently high *b*-values may reduce the signal to the level of background noise, and in these cases either these data can be excluded, or an explicit noise term added to the analysis.

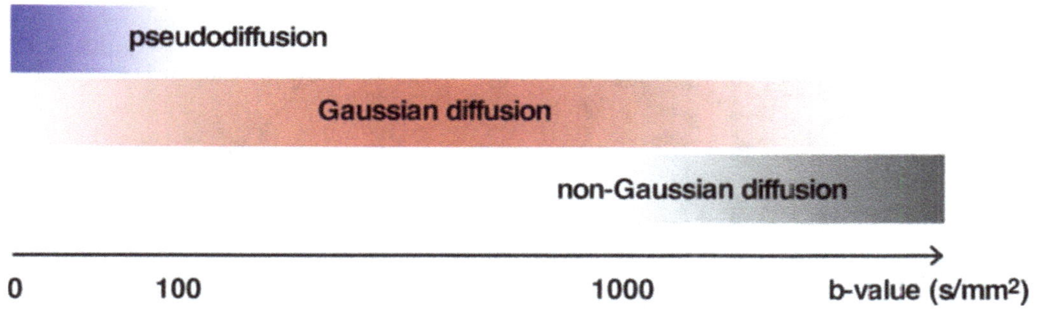

Fig. 3 Different diffusion weightings, summarized by the compound parameter *b*-value, give rise to diffusion signal that is influenced by different diffusion regimes. Intuitive, though necessarily simplified, interpretations of these diffusion phenomena include (1) pseudodiffusion, observed at low *b*-values and reflecting vessel and tubular flow; (2) Gaussian (or random) diffusion, reflecting diffusion of water molecules in the renal tissue and thus informing on renal microstructure and cellularity; and (3) non-Gaussian diffusion, observed at high *b*-values and providing additional information on tissue microstructure. In addition to *b*-value, diffusion time, delay, and direction parameters influence the observed DWI signal

The range of *b*-values used in a diffusion imaging protocol defines which diffusion components will be present and/or dominate the signal, and thus will influence the analysis. The simplified illustration in Fig. 3 gives a rough guideline to the *b*-value ranges where different diffusion phenomena can be detected, though it is important to appreciate the simplifications made when attempting to model diffusion processes in tissue, and that *b*-value magnitude alone is not sufficient to describe the experiment.

In some circumstances, such as the spatial localization of tumors, it may be sufficient to simply observe the hyperintense signal of highly cellular regions on a single diffusion-weighted image of sufficient *b*-value to provide increased contrast (although at lower overall signal). Diffusion-weighted images have an underlying T_2 weighting arising from the longer TE required to allow for inclusion of the diffusion-sensitizing pulses, which can be confounding where long-T_2 regions (e.g., free water) can be mistaken for low diffusion areas—this is known as the T_2 *shine-through* effect [5]. In most applications, however, modeling of the DWI signal behavior, across a set of matched images varying only in the applied *b*-values, removes the T_2 influence and gives quantitative parameters that are, in theory, comparable across studies (*see* **Note 2**).

In the following sections, several diffusion signal interpretation models relevant to renal studies are described, though this is far from an exhaustive list of models or mathematical representations available. Choice of DWI protocols are often selected in terms of the additional value that they may offer in relation to their additional complexity and duration, and with a particular diffusion model and analysis scheme in mind (*see* **Note 3**).

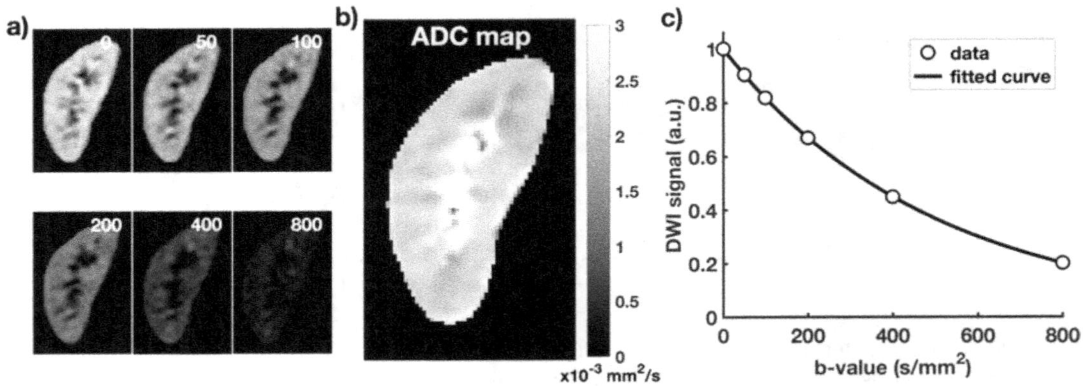

Fig. 4 Monoexponential ADC model. (**a**) Example DWI images acquired with different *b*-values (given in s/mm^2) from a healthy kidney, and (**b**) the ADC map resulting from fitting a monoexponential model. Signal-to-noise ratio, depending on T_2, spatial resolution, and the underlying diffusion itself, decreases with the increase in *b*-value. (**c**) Schematic illustration of an ideal ADC curve fit to noiseless data. Analysis methods are discussed in detail in the chapter by Jerome NP et al. "Analysis of Renal Diffusion-Weighted Imaging (DWI) Using Apparent Diffusion Coefficient (ADC) and Intravoxel Incoherent Motion (IVIM) Models"

3.1 Monoexponential Apparent Diffusion Coefficient (ADC)

The simplest and most widely used model to interpret the DWI signal is a single compartment model, summarizing all motion components (from diffusion, flow, etc.) in a single coefficient (ADC, *see* **Note 4**). The resulting ADC maps (*see* Fig. 4) are derived from the fitting of the DWI signal, across all *b*-values on a voxel-wise basis, of a single-exponential model according to the following formula:

$$S_{(\mathrm{b})} = S_{(\mathrm{total})} \cdot \exp\left(-\frac{\mathrm{TE}}{T_2}\right) \cdot \exp\left(-b.\mathrm{ADC}\right) \tag{1}$$

where $S_{(\mathrm{b})}$ and $S_{(\mathrm{total})}$ represent the signal observed at a particular *b*-value, and the overall equilibrium signal (at $b = 0$ s/mm^2 and TE $= 0$ ms) respectively. Since the echo time TE is usually not varied across images with different diffusion weightings, the first two terms are often summarized as S_0, the signal at a *b*-value of zero, and the formula simplifies as follows:

$$S_{(\mathrm{b})} = S_0 \cdot \exp\left(-b.\mathrm{ADC}\right) \tag{2}$$

Despite the DWI signal not being truly monoexponential, and ADC being a purely empirical parameter summarizing different factors contributing to the diffusion signal, ADC can still be considered as a sensitive and useful biomarker [6, 7].

The monoexponential model requires acquisition of a minimum of 2 *b*-values. The lower value is commonly set as zero by default, although this leads to what is known as a perfusion-sensitive ADC; choosing a minimum *b*-value of approximately

100–200 s/mm^2 removes this influence to give a perfusion-insensitive ADC. The highest b-value is normally chosen as the maximum value while retaining sufficient signal, commonly in the range 700–1000 s/mm^2 [8], although non-Gaussian processes may become relevant at this upper limit (Fig. 3). The coefficient derived from the analysis is always referred to as ADC, although it is important to note that if the underlying signal curve is not mono-exponential the measured ADC strongly depends on the b-values chosen [9], and so is not necessarily comparable across studies. Main advantages of the simple monoexponential equation is the short acquisition time required, and the general robustness of ADC as a marker of diffusion [10]. The monoexponential model is also suited to DWI studies with multiple b-values, with additional data points allowing for estimation of ADC uncertainties.

3.2 Intravoxel Incoherent Motion (IVIM)

One advanced model to interpret the diffusion imaging signal is the intravoxel incoherent motion (IVIM) model. Originally proposed by Le Bihan for the assessment of microcapillary perfusion in the brain [11], the model is generally applicable if a number of assumptions are fulfilled, and represents a popular choice for attempting to separate diffusion from flowing components [12].

In this model, a second compartment is included in the signal interpretation to describe the flow-based motion of water molecules in blood capillaries and tubules that, if assumed to randomly occur in all directions, appears as an accelerated diffusion process (Fig. 5).

The pseudodiffusion component associated with flow is described by the pseudodiffusion coefficient D^* that, since flow is faster than diffusion, is approximately an order of magnitude larger

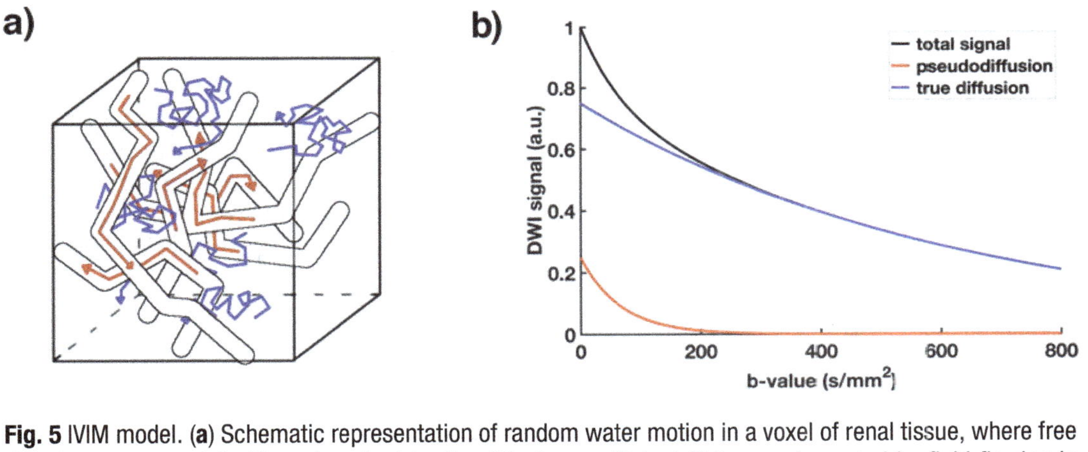

Fig. 5 IVIM model. (**a**) Schematic representation of random water motion in a voxel of renal tissue, where free diffusion component (in blue, described by the diffusion coefficient D) is complemented by fluid flowing in capillaries and tubules (in red, described by the pseudodiffusion coefficient D^*). (**b**) Contributions of true diffusion and pseudodiffusion to the observed diffusion signal decay—pseudodiffusion is substantially faster than true diffusion, and so is only observed at low b-values

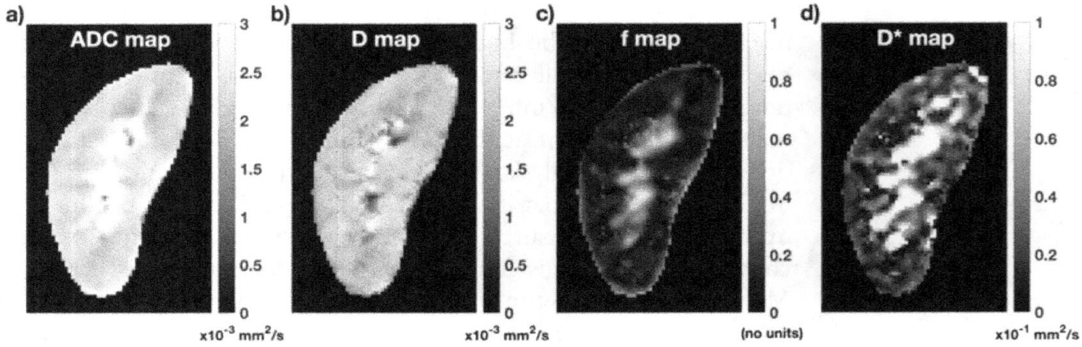

Fig. 6 Representative parametric maps resulting from DWI model fitting. (**a**) ADC map, resulting from monoexponential model fitting. (**b**) Pure diffusion *D*, (**c**) pseudodiffusion fraction *f*, and (**d**) pseudodiffusion *D** maps, resulting from IVIM model fitting over several *b*-values. DWI-based parameters show contrast between the cortex, medulla, and renal hilum. Some extreme values are seen as a consequence of respiratory motion at the lower boundary of the kidney. Parameters associated with pseudodiffusion, *f* and *D**, commonly give maps with higher noise

than the true diffusion coefficient D. The components have relative signal contributions given by the pseudodiffusion fraction (f), and the overall IVIM model is described by the following equation:

$$S_{(\mathrm{b})} = S_0.((1-f).\exp(-b.D) + f.\exp(-b.D^*)) \qquad (3)$$

implicitly assuming that there is no exchange between the compartments, and that the associated compartmental T_2 values are the same. Since this is known not to be true in certain circumstances [13, 14], it is important to note that the derived pseudodiffusion coefficient D^* and pseudodiffusion fraction f are nevertheless empirical and should strictly be considered reflective of and not, as often stated, a direct measure of perfusion or flow.

The use of the IVIM model requires substantially more complex analyses than the monoexponential model (analyses are discussed in the chapter by Jerome NP et al. "Analysis of Renal Diffusion-Weighted Imaging (DWI) Using Apparent Diffusion Coefficient (ADC) and Intravoxel Incoherent Motion (IVIM) Models"), and more care to reliably separate pure diffusion from pseudodiffusion components. IVIM analysis tools are increasingly being offered by MRI manufacturers, although the choice of model fitting methods may significantly influence the derived parameters from the more complex model [15, 16]. Parametric maps resulting from IVIM analysis show the similarity of D coefficient with ADC, and the increased noise that is characteristic of the pseudodiffusion parameters f and D^* (Fig. 6).

The main feature of any DWI acquisition intended for IVIM analysis is the increased number of *b*-values required, especially low *b*-values that sample the signal curve before the pseudodiffusion component has decayed (Fig. 5). Simplified versions of the IVIM approach usually attempt to limit the acquisition time by using fewer *b*-values, the minimum being three for a segmented fitting that does not attempt to measure D^* [15, 17–19]. Additional complications of multiple *b*-value acquisitions are the increased sensitivity to movement, and the known difficulty of providing repeatable pseudodiffusion parameters compared to diffusion [20–22].

3.3 Diffusion Tensor Imaging (DTI)

If the directionality (or loss thereof) of diffusion arising from tissue structure is of interest, for example as an indication of loss of function or invasion of relevant tissue, consideration of the diffusion signal decay along specified direction, expressed as a tensor, allows calculation of an ellipsoid that represents the diffusion propagator in three dimensions. In the simplified case of isotropic diffusion, diffusion is equal in all directions and the ellipsoid is a sphere. Diffusion isotropy is assumed, though often unstated, in both the monoexponential and IVIM models described above. Conversely, in diffusion tensor imaging (DTI), diffusion-sensitizing gradients are applied along a number of prespecified directions, which are included in the model used to interpret the diffusion imaging signal. In DTI, the diffusion is assumed to be Gaussian and to follow a monoexponential signal decay.

The degree of direction-dependency of the diffusion signal is captured by the fractional anisotropy (*FA*) parameter, ranging from 0 (complete isotropy) to 1 (complete anisotropy) and derived from the relative dimensions of the diffusion ellipsoid according to the following equation:

$$\mathrm{FA} = \sqrt{\frac{3\left[(\lambda_1 - \mathrm{MD})^2 + (\lambda_2 - \mathrm{MD})^2 + (\lambda_3 - \mathrm{MD})^2\right]}{2\left({\lambda_1}^2 + {\lambda_2}^2 + {\lambda_3}^2\right)}} \tag{4}$$

where λ_i represent the eigenvalues of the corresponding diffusion eigenvectors, meaning diffusion coefficients along each of the principal ellipsoid axes, and MD represents mean diffusivity, given by the following:

$$\mathrm{MD} = (\lambda_1 + \lambda_2 + \lambda_3)/3 \tag{5}$$

Directional diffusion coefficients can be reported for each individual direction (λ_i) or along the major and minor axes of the ellipsoid (λ_1 and λ_{trans}, the latter computed as average of the transverse axes coefficients). Given their complexity and alternative formulations, DTI equations used in any study should be clearly stated [23, 24].

Similar to IVIM, DTI requires the acquisition of substantially more images than the basic DWI scheme, although for DTI the number of directions of the applied diffusion-sensitizing gradients is increased rather than the number of *b*-values. In order to define

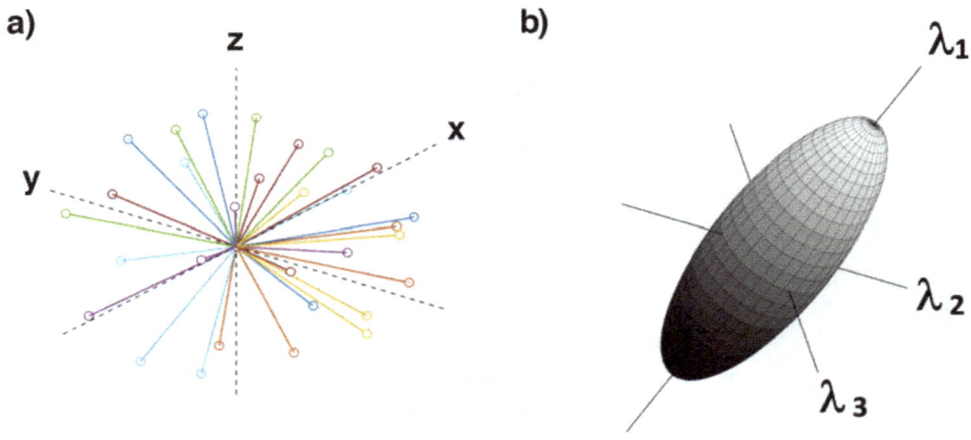

Fig. 7 Illustration of diffusion tensor imaging principles. (**a**) Diffusion vectors in q-space, representing diffusion gradients of equal magnitude applied along different directions (in this case $n = 30$) to investigate tissue anisotropy. (**b**) Corresponding diffusion propagator ellipsoid, where λ_i represent diffusion magnitude along each of the principal ellipsoid axes (i.e., eigenvalues of the principal eigenvectors). Measures of anisotropy, derived from these eigenvalues, are able to describe diffusion with directional preference

the tensor, a minimum of six different directions must be acquired alongside the $b = 0$ image (which, not being diffusion-weighted, has no directionality), but to reduce noise sensitivity it is common to acquire more, up to 30 or even 60 directions. Diffusion directions are usually equally distributed over the surface of a sphere, forming a "shell" in diffusion space (also called q-space), although user-defined vector sets are acceptable as long as there is sufficient sampling of the diffusion directions (Fig. 7).

The DTI technique was developed for application in the brain, but can provide relevant information in the kidney as well. Color and brightness of fractional anisotropy maps indicate orientation and degree of anisotropic diffusion, and can be portrayed as small ellipsoids, which are oriented and color-coded according to the direction of strongest diffusion, to illustrate tissue structure (similar to tractography in brain white matter). Maps of mean diffusivity resemble conventional diffusion coefficient maps (Fig. 8).

Given the large number of images required for DTI analysis, it is common to acquire only one shell in q-space, corresponding to a single non-zero b-value chosen based on the target tissue and expected signal-to-noise ratio. For body applications, this is much lower than for the brain, and is commonly within the range 500–1000 s/mm^2. More complex acquisition strategies are available, including multiple shells, as well as the option to retroactively ignore the directional information and calculate ADC.

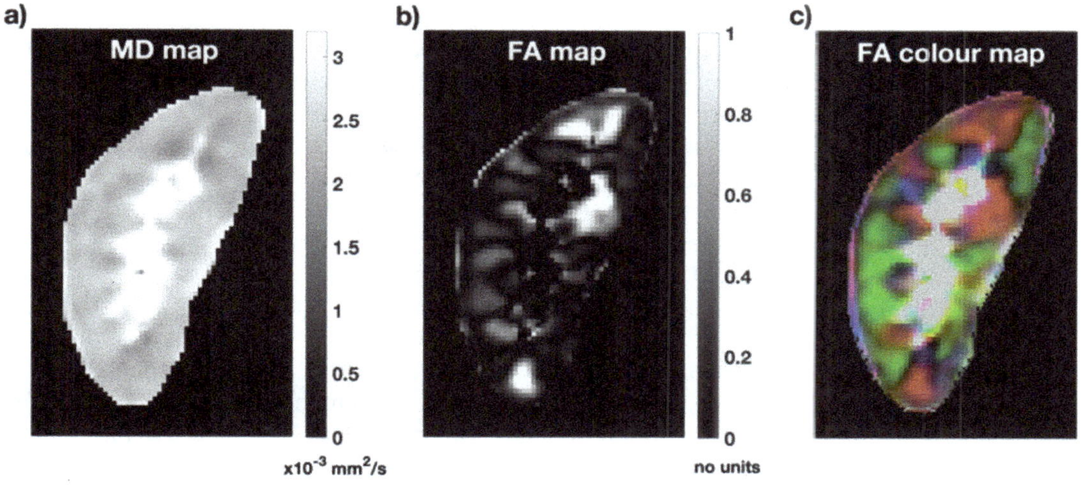

Fig. 8 Representative parametric maps resulting from diffusion tensor imaging analysis of a healthy kidney. (**a**) Mean diffusion (MD) map. (**b**) Fractional anisotropy (FA) map in gray scale. (**c**) FA map in color scale, illustrating the direction of the λ_1 eigenvector

4 Diffusion Imaging in the Kidney

A more detailed review of the applications of renal diffusion imaging in humans was recently conducted by the international COST Action PARENCHIMA [3]. Much of the literature summarized therein, predominantly using the most established ADC but also including IVIM and DTI measures, reports a correlation between diffusion metrics and eGFR decline [25–29] or fibrosis [30–32], in patients with diabetes and other chronic kidney disease (CKD) [33–38], as well as in kidney allograft recipients [30, 39, 40].

Preclinical studies also demonstrate the broad connection of ADC with renal disease, with both ADC and DTI studies having links to renal fibrosis from acute ureteral obstruction [41–45] and diabetes [46, 47]. Preclinical studies also allow for study of the effects of potential contrast agents [48–50]. The development of novel DWI-based biomarkers may yet rely on biological validation and an improvement in specificity [51].

5 Diffusion Acquisition Considerations

In diffusion imaging, most trade-offs are about keeping the acquisition time reasonable and, similar to other MRI modalities, acquiring signal-to-noise ratio sufficient to provide reliable results. Preclinical imaging protocols are less constrained by time than clinical protocols, and so allow for longer scanning that may take advantage of increased averaging or alternate acquisition schemes.

Since increasing the number of acquired averages to give sufficient signal-to-noise quickly becomes prohibitive, DWI is normally acquired with lower spatial resolution than anatomical T_1- or T_2-weighted images. Number and repeats of each *b*-value depend on time available and intended analysis strategy, and are thus specific to each study and/or scanner. By default, most MR scanners will acquire three orthogonal directions (which may or may not be available as separate images [52]) for all nonzero *b*-values in order to calculate the ***trace image***, implicitly assuming isotropic diffusion. Such schemes ultimately determine the exact sampling and thus the format of the resulting data. Furthermore, most diffusion imaging sequences allow for specification of several diffusion schemes (often with vendor-specific names and implementations), which trade-off between image quality and diffusion direction specifics. Such schemes may involve multiple "shots" to acquire k-space [31, 53], smaller field-of-view excitation through combination pulses [54], as well as variations on the gradient scheme such as bipolar encoding, designed to reduce distortion from eddy currents [55, 56]. In general, diffusion-weighted images may require an explicit postprocessing protocol as part of the analysis (*see* **Note 5**).

Since the acquisition of high *b*-values requires a larger TE in order to accommodate the pulses, the choice of the maximum *b*-value is a compromise between precision of diffusion estimates over a suitably chosen *b*-value range, and the available signal (*see* **Note 6**). DWI sequence variants that explicitly probe the effects of the diffusion time Δ as well as TE illustrate the importance of not neglecting potential influences of the acquisition parameters on the diffusion signal [13, 57].

Other significant factors in diffusion imaging arise directly from the use of echo-planar imaging (EPI) readout sequences, which although suitably fast gives images which are susceptible to distortion artifacts arising from high use of gradients (finite slew rates, eddy currents, nonlinearity, and so forth) and local susceptibility differences at tissue boundaries (and especially at tissue–air boundaries). Distortion correction can thus be necessary in diffusion imaging, and may involve prospective planning (e.g., phase-reversal images) [58] as well as retrospective processing (e.g., registration) [59].

Additional DWI protocols, such as those including flow compensation [60], alternate strategies to EPI readout [53, 61], and steady-state free precession sequences [62–64] and the influence of physiological factors on the DWI [65], have been reported in literature and may provide tools for ameliorating specific physiological and instrumental factors.

6 Notes

1. The specifics of diffusion imaging data acquisition and intended analysis strongly influence each other, and thus both should be borne in mind while planning a new study. Whenever possible, overly specific acquisition protocols should be avoided to allow for data reuse through additional retrospective analysis, and cross-study comparisons.
2. Many acquisition parameters influence the resulting diffusion-related parameters, making comparison across studies challenging. In the absence of widely accepted standardized protocols, it may be advantageous to consider the extent to which comparison with other studies will be possible.
3. As with all MRI studies, but of particular importance in diffusion imaging, care should be taken to report the adopted protocol as completely as possible. This necessarily includes the acquisition scheme and parameters, but also extends to the analysis algorithms.
4. The majority of diffusion models contain a parameter that attempts to capture the underlying tissue diffusion—ADC, (IVIM) *D*, (DTI) MD, and so on. While superficially similar and reflective of tissue structure, they are not precisely equivalent given the different assumptions implicit in the models they derive from.
5. The most common readout for diffusion imaging is the echo planar imaging (EPI) sequence, which is susceptible to artifacts and distortion; an adequate post-processing scheme is required. Analysis of DWI is discussed in more detail in the chapter by Jerome NP et al. "Analysis of Renal Diffusion-Weighted Imaging (DWI) Using Apparent Diffusion Coefficient (ADC) and Intravoxel Incoherent Motion (IVIM) Models."
6. Since diffusion contrast is created by deliberate dephasing and thus loss of the MR signal, sufficient signal-to-noise ratio is critical to ensure good quality data and successful analysis. Failure to assess the signal-to-noise ratio or account for the noise floor may introduce bias in the estimate of diffusion parameters.

Acknowledgments

NPJ wishes to acknowledge support from the liaison Committee between the Central Norway Regional Health Authority and the Norwegian University of Science and Technology (Project nr. 90065000).

This chapter is based upon work from COST Action PARENCH IMA, supported by European Cooperation in Science and Technology (COST). COST (www.cost.eu) is a funding agency for research and innovation networks. COST Actions help connect research initiatives across Europe and enable scientists to enrich their ideas by sharing them with their peers. This boosts their research, career, and innovation.
PARENCHIMA (renalmri.org) is a community-driven Action in the COST program of the European Union, which unites more than 200 experts in renal MRI from 30 countries with the aim to improve the reproducibility and standardization of renal MRI biomarkers.

References

1. Roditi G, Maki JH, Oliveira G, Michaely HJ (2009) Renovascular imaging in the NSF era. J Magn Reson Imaging 30:1323–1334
2. Olchowy C, Cebulski K, Łasecki M et al (2017) The presence of the gadolinium-based contrast agent depositions in the brain and symptoms of gadolinium neurotoxicity-a systematic review. PLoS One 12:1–14
3. Caroli A, Schneider M, Friedli I et al (2018) Diffusion-weighted magnetic resonance imaging to assess diffuse renal pathology: a systematic review and statement paper. Nephrol Dial Transplant 33:ii29–ii40
4. Panagiotaki E, Chan RW, Dikaios N et al (2015) Microstructural characterization of normal and malignant human prostate tissue with vascular, extracellular, and restricted diffusion for cytometry in tumours magnetic resonance imaging. Investig Radiol 50:218–227
5. Cheng L, Blackledge MD, Collins DJ et al (2016) T2-adjusted computed diffusion-weighted imaging: a novel method to enhance tumour visualisation. Comput Biol Med 79:92–98
6. Eisenberger U, Theony HC, Boesch C et al (2014) Living renal allograft transplantation : diffusion-weighted MR imaging in longitudinal follow-up of the donated and the remaining kidney. Radiology 270:800–808
7. Thoeny HC, De Keyzer F (2011) Diffusion-weighted MR imaging of native and transplanted kidneys. Radiology 259:25–38
8. Saritas EU, Lee JH, Nishimura DG (2011) SNR dependence of optimal parameters for apparent diffusion coefficient measurements. IEEE Trans Med Imaging 30:424–437
9. Zhang JL, Sigmund EE, Rusinek H et al (2012) Optimization of b-value sampling for diffusion-weighted imaging of the kidney. Magn Reson Med 67:89–97
10. Winfield JM, Tunariu N, Rata M et al (2017) Extracranial soft-tissue tumors: repeatability of apparent diffusion coefficient estimates from diffusion-weighted MR imaging. Radiology 284:88–99
11. Le Bihan D, Breton E, Lallemand D et al (1988) Separation of diffusion and perfusion in intravoxel incoherent motion MR imaging. Radiology 168:497–505
12. Ljimani A, Lanzman RS, Müller-Lutz A et al (2018) Non-gaussian diffusion evaluation of the human kidney by Padé exponent model. J Magn Reson Imaging 47:160–167
13. Jerome NP, D'Arcy JA, Feiweier T et al (2016) Extended T2-IVIM model for correction of TE dependence of pseudo-diffusion volume fraction in clinical diffusion-weighted magnetic resonance imaging. Phys Med Biol 61: N667–N680
14. Lemke A, Laun FB, Simon D et al (2010) An in vivo verification of the intravoxel incoherent motion effect in diffusion-weighted imaging of the abdomen. Magn Reson Med 64:1580–1585
15. Meeus EM, Novak J, Withey SB et al (2017) Evaluation of intravoxel incoherent motion fitting methods in low-perfused tissue. J Magn Reson Imaging 45:1325–1334
16. Vidić I, Jerome NP, Bathen TF et al (2019) Accuracy of breast cancer lesion classification using intravoxel incoherent motion diffusion-weighted imaging is improved by the inclusion of global or local prior knowledge with bayesian methods. J Magn Reson Imaging 50:1478–1488
17. Cho GY, Moy L, Zhang JL et al (2015) Comparison of fitting methods and b-value

sampling strategies for intravoxel incoherent motion in breast cancer. Magn Reson Med 74:1077–1085

18. Gurney-Champion OJ, Klaassen R, Froeling M et al (2018) Comparison of six fit algorithms for the intravoxel incoherent motion model of diffusionweighted magnetic resonance imaging data of pancreatic cancer patients. PLoS One 13:1–18
19. Jalnefjord O, Andersson M, Montelius M et al (2018) Comparison of methods for estimation of the intravoxel incoherent motion (IVIM) diffusion coefficient (D) and perfusion fraction (f). MAGMA 31(6):715–723. https://doi.org/10.1007/s10334-018-0697-5
20. Jerome NP, Boult JKR, Orton MR et al (2016) Modulation of renal oxygenation and perfusion in rat kidney monitored by quantitative diffusion and blood oxygen level dependent magnetic resonance imaging on a clinical 1.5T platform. BMC Nephrol 17:142
21. Jerome NP, Miyazaki K, Collins DJ et al (2016) Repeatability of derived parameters from histograms following non-Gaussian diffusion modelling of diffusion-weighted imaging in a paediatric oncological cohort. Eur Radiol 27:345–353
22. Orton MR, Jerome NP, Rata M, Koh D-M (2018) IVIM in the body: a general overview. In: Le Bihan D, Iima M, Federau C, Sigmund EE (eds) Intravoxel incoherent motion MRI Princ. Appl. Pan Stanford Publishing Pte. Ltd., pp 145–174
23. Kingsley PB (2006) Introduction to diffusion tensor imaging mathematics : part II. Anisotropy, diffusion- weighting factors, and gradient encoding schemes. Concepts Magn Reson Part A 28A:123–154
24. Kingsley PB (2006) Introduction to diffusion tensor imaging mathematics: part I. tensors, rotations, and eigenvectors. Concepts Magn Reson Part A 28A:101–122
25. Ding J, Chen J, Jiang Z et al (2016) Is low b-factors-based apparent diffusion coefficient helpful in assessing renal dysfunction? Radiol Med 121:6–11
26. Ding J, Chen J, Jiang Z et al (2016) Assessment of renal dysfunction with diffusion-weighted imaging: comparing intra-voxel incoherent motion (IVIM) with a mono-exponential model. Acta Radiol 57:507–512
27. Li Q, Wu X, Qiu L et al (2013) Diffusion-weighted MRI in the assessment of split renal function: comparison of navigator-triggered prospective acquisition correction and breath-hold acquisition. Am J Roentgenol 200:113–119
28. Prasad PV, Thacker J, Li LP et al (2015) Multi-parametric evaluation of chronic kidney disease by MRI: a preliminary cross-sectional study. PLoS One 10:1–14
29. Özçelik Ü, Çevik H et al (2017) Evaluation of transplanted kidneys and comparison with healthy volunteers and kidney donors with diffusion-weighted magnetic resonance imaging: initial experience. Exp Clin Transplant. https://doi.org/10.6002/ect.2016.0341
30. Friedli I, Crowe LA, Berchtold L et al (2016) New magnetic resonance imaging index for renal fibrosis assessment: a comparison between diffusion-weighted imaging and T1 mapping with histological validation. Sci Rep 6:1–15
31. Friedli I, Crowe LA, de Perrot T et al (2017) Comparison of readout-segmented and conventional single-shot for echo-planar diffusion-weighted imaging in the assessment of kidney interstitial fibrosis. J Magn Reson Imaging 46:1631–1640
32. Zhao J, Wang ZJ, Liu M et al (2014) Assessment of renal fibrosis in chronic kidney disease using diffusion-weighted MRI. Clin Radiol 69:1117–1122
33. Inoue T, Kozawa E, Okada H et al (2011) Noninvasive evaluation of kidney hypoxia and fibrosis using magnetic resonance imaging. J Am Soc Nephrol 22:1429–1434
34. Liu Z, Xu Y, Zhang J et al (2015) Chronic kidney disease: pathological and functional assessment with diffusion tensor imaging at 3T MR. Eur Radiol 25:652–660
35. Rona G, Pasaoglu L, Ozkayar N et al (2016) Functional evaluation of secondary renal amyloidosis with diffusion-weighted MR imaging. Ren Fail 38:249–255
36. Wang WJ, Pui MH, Guo Y et al (2014) 3T magnetic resonance diffusion tensor imaging in chronic kidney disease. Abdom Imaging 39:770–775
37. Emre T, Kiliçkesmez Ö, Büker A et al (2016) Renal function and diffusion-weighted imaging: a new method to diagnose kidney failure before losing half function. Radiol Med 121:163–172
38. Çakmak P, Yağci AB, Dursun B et al (2014) Renal diffusion-weighted imaging in diabetic nephropathy: correlation with clinical stages of disease. Diagnostic Interv Radiol 20:374–378
39. Palmucci S, Cappello G, Attinà G et al (2015) Diffusion weighted imaging and diffusion tensor imaging in the evaluation of transplanted kidneys. Eur J Radiol Open 2:71–80

40. Hueper K, Khalifa AA, Bräsen JH et al (2016) Diffusion-weighted imaging and diffusion tensor imaging detect delayed graft function and correlate with allograft fibrosis in patients early after kidney transplantation. J Magn Reson Imaging 44:112–121
41. Haque ME, Franklin T, Bokhary U et al (2014) Longitudinal changes in MRI markers in a reversible unilateral ureteral obstruction mouse model: preliminary experience. J Magn Reson Imaging 39:835–841
42. Hu G, Yang Z, Liang W et al (2019) Intravoxel incoherent motion and arterial spin labeling MRI analysis of reversible unilateral ureteral obstruction in rats. J Magn Reson Imaging 50:288–296
43. Togao O, Doi S, Kuro-o M et al (2010) Assessment of renal fibrosis with diffusion-weighted MR Imaging: study with murine model purpose: methods: results: conclusion. Radiology 255:772–780
44. Wang F, Takahashi KK, Li H et al (2018) Assessment of unilateral ureter obstruction with multi-parametric MRI. Magn Reson Med 79:2216–2227
45. Pons M, Leporq B, Ali L et al (2018) Renal parenchyma impairment characterization in partial unilateral ureteral obstruction in mice with intravoxel incoherent motion-MRI. NMR Biomed 31:1–9
46. Kaimori JY, Isaka Y, Hatanaka M et al (2017) Visualization of kidney fibrosis in diabetic nephropathy by long diffusion tensor imaging MRI with spin-echo sequence. Sci Rep 7:2–9
47. Yan YY, Hartono S, Hennedige T et al (2017) Intravoxel incoherent motion and diffusion tensor imaging of early renal fibrosis induced in a murine model of streptozotocin induced diabetes. Magn Reson Imaging 38:71–76
48. Jost G, Lenhard DC, Sieber MA et al (2011) Changes of renal water diffusion coefficient after application of iodinated contrast agents: effect of viscosity. Investig Radiol 46:796–800
49. Wang Y, Ren K, Liu Y et al (2017) Application of BOLD MRI and DTI for the evaluation of renal effect related to viscosity of iodinated contrast agent in a rat model. J Magn Reson Imaging 46:1320–1331
50. Liang L, Chen WB, KWY C et al (2016) Using intravoxel incoherent motion MR imaging to study the renal pathophysiological process of contrast-induced acute kidney injury in rats: comparison with conventional DWI and arterial spin labelling. Eur Radiol 26:1597–1605
51. Thoeny HC, Grenier N (2010) Science to practice: can diffusion-weighted MR imaging findings be used as biomarkers to monitor the progression of renal fibrosis? Radiology 255:667–668
52. Jerome NP, Orton MR, D'Arcy JA et al (2015) Use of the temporal median and trimmed mean mitigates effects of respiratory motion in multiple-acquisition abdominal diffusion imaging. Phys Med Biol 60:N9–N20
53. Wu CJ, Wang Q, Zhang J et al (2016) Readout-segmented echo-planar imaging in diffusion-weighted imaging of the kidney: comparison with single-shot echo-planar imaging in image quality. Abdom Radiol 41:100–108
54. He YL, Hausmann D, Morelli JN et al (2016) Renal zoomed EPI-DWI with spatially-selective radiofrequency excitation pulses in two dimensions. Eur J Radiol 85:1773–1777
55. Furuta A, Isoda H, Yamashita R et al (2014) Comparison of monopolar and bipolar diffusion weighted imaging sequences for detection of small hepatic metastases. Eur J Radiol 83:1626–1630
56. Kyriazi S, Blackledge M, Collins DJ, Desouza NM (2010) Optimising diffusion-weighted imaging in the abdomen and pelvis: comparison of image quality between monopolar and bipolar single-shot spin-echo echo-planar sequences. Eur Radiol 20:2422–2431
57. Clark CA, Hedehus M, Moseley ME (2001) Diffusion time dependence of the apparent diffusion tensor in healthy human brain and white matter disease. Magn Reson Med 45:1126–1129
58. Holland D, Kuperman JM, Dale AM (2010) Efficient correction of inhomogeneous static magnetic field-induced distortion in echo planar imaging. NeuroImage 50:175–183
59. Guyader J-M, Bernardin L, Douglas NHM et al (2015) Influence of image registration on apparent diffusion coefficient images computed from free-breathing diffusion MR images of the abdomen. J Magn Reson Imaging 42:315–330
60. Wetscherek A, Stieltjes B, Laun FB (2015) Flow-compensated intravoxel incoherent motion diffusion imaging. Magn Reson Med 74:410–419
61. Friedli I, Crowe LA, Viallon M et al (2015) Improvement of renal diffusion-weighted magnetic resonance imaging with readout-segmented echo-planar imaging at 3T. Magn Reson Imaging 33:701–708

62. Delalande C, De Zwart JA, Trillaud H et al (1999) An echo-shifted gradient-echo MRI method for efficient diffusion weighting. Magn Reson Med 41:1000–1008
63. Ding S, Trillaud H, Yongbi M et al (1995) High resolution renal diffusion imaging using a modified steady-state free precession sequence. Magn Reson Med 34:586–595
64. Lu L, Erokwu B, Lee G et al (2012) Diffusion-prepared fast imaging with steady-state free precession (DP-FISP): a rapid diffusion MRI technique at 7 T. Magn Reson Med 68:868–873
65. Lanzman RS, Ljimani A, Müller-Lutz A et al (2019) Assessment of time-resolved renal diffusion parameters over the entire cardiac cycle. Magn Reson Imaging 55:1–6

14

Quantitative Assessment of Renal Perfusion and Oxygenation by Invasive Probes: Basic Concepts

Kathleen Cantow, Roger G. Evans, Dirk Grosenick, Thomas Gladytz, Thoralf Niendorf, Bert Flemming, and Erdmann Seeliger

Abstract

Renal tissue hypoperfusion and hypoxia are early key elements in the pathophysiology of acute kidney injury of various origins, and may also promote progression from acute injury to chronic kidney disease. Here we describe basic principles of methodology to quantify renal hemodynamics and tissue oxygenation by means of invasive probes in experimental animals. Advantages and disadvantages of the various methods are discussed in the context of the heterogeneity of renal tissue perfusion and oxygenation.

This chapter is based upon work from the COST Action PARENCHIMA, a community-driven network funded by the European Cooperation in Science and Technology (COST) program of the European Union, which aims to improve the reproducibility and standardization of renal MRI biomarkers. This introduction chapter is complemented by a separate chapter describing the experimental procedure and data analysis.

Key words Renal hemodynamics and oxygenation, In vivo methods, Quantitative invasive probes

1 Introduction

Kidney diseases are a global health burden with steadily increasing prevalence and incidence [1–5]. Animal studies have provided evidence that acute kidney injury (AKI) of various origins shares a common link in the pathophysiological chain of events, ultimately leading to AKI, as well as to progression from AKI to chronic kidney disease (CKD): imbalance between renal oxygen delivery and oxygen demand [3, 6–13]. Renal tissue hypoperfusion and hypoxia have also been suggested to play a pivotal role in the pathophysiology of other kidney diseases including diabetic kidney disease [14–16].

The majority of the preclinical studies that generated this concept utilized a set of invasive probes to measure renal hemodynamics and oxygenation in anesthetized animals [12, 14, 17–20]. These methods have also been used (1) to study mechanisms of

Andreas Pohlmann and Thoralf Niendorf (eds.), *Preclinical MRI of the Kidney: Methods and Protocols*, Methods in Molecular Biology, vol. 2216, https://doi.org/10.1007/978-1-0716-0978-1_6, © The Author(s) 2021

physiological control of renal hemodynamics and oxygenation and (2) the effects of various substances on this control in healthy animals, (3) to test several putative preventive or therapeutic approaches for AKI and CKD in animal models, and (4) for the purpose of calibrating functional magnetic resonance imaging (MRI) including renal blood oxygenation level-dependent MRI (BOLD-MRI) that makes use of the quantitative MR parameter T_2*, which is a surrogate for blood oxygenation [18–28].

The invasive probes typically include (1) a perivascular flow probe for measurement of total renal blood flow, (2) laser-Doppler-optodes for assessment of local tissue perfusion, (3) Clark-type electrodes or fluorescence-quenching optodes for measurements of local tissue partial pressure of oxygen (pO_2), and (4) devices for invasive measurement of arterial blood pressure. These methods are considered the gold standard for the study of renal hemodynamics and oxygenation, because the methods, with the exception of the laser-Doppler fluxmetry, provide calibrated quantitative data [25, 29, 30]. Step-by-step protocols for application of these techniques in two setups, one for stand-alone experiments in laboratories for integrative physiology, and the other for experiments within small-animal MR scanners by use of a hybrid setup, are provided in the chapter by Cantow K et al. “Monitoring Renal Hemodynamics and Oxygenation by Invasive Probes: Experimental Protocol”.

As with all established modalities available in today’s experimental and translational research, these techniques have shortcomings and methodological limitations. In particular, their invasiveness, for obvious ethical reasons, precludes their use in humans. The invasiveness is, furthermore, a considerable hurdle for implementation of these methods in long-term and longitudinal studies: although invasive probes have been used in conscious, chronically instrumented animals [22, 24, 31–37], the vast majority of studies has been performed in “terminal experiments” in anesthetized animals. This is a major limitation of all invasive techniques because the measurements are by necessity potentially confounded by the effects of anesthesia (*see* the chapter by Kaucsar T et al. “Preparation and Monitoring of Small Animals in Renal MRI”).

The measurement of intrarenal tissue perfusion and tissue oxygenation is quite challenging, because of their vast spatial heterogeneity both among the renal layers (cortex, outer medulla, and inner medulla) and within the layers. In this chapter, the causes and the degree for this spatial variability are outlined first, before the basic principles of methodology to quantify renal hemodynamics and oxygenation by means of invasive probes in experimental animals are described together with a discussion of the pros and cons of the various methods.

This introduction chapter is complemented by a separate chapter describing the experimental procedure, which is part of this book.

This chapter is part of the book Pohlmann A, Niendorf T (eds) (2020) Preclinical MRI of the Kidney—Methods and Protocols. Springer, New York.

2 Heterogeneity of Intrarenal Perfusion and Oxygenation—Causes and Degree of Variability

Intrarenal local tissue pO_2 is determined by the balance between local O_2 supply and local O_2 consumption. Additionally, determinants of local O_2 diffusion play a role. Local O_2 supply depends on local blood perfusion, local vessel density, and local blood pO_2 and blood O_2 content. Local O_2 consumption is foremost determined by local metabolic demand. Blood perfusion within the kidney is much more heterogeneous than within most other organs, due to its particular vascular architecture [8, 38–40].

From the branches of the renal artery that enter the kidney at its hilus, interlobar arteries arise, which align with the medullary–cortical axis. From interlobar arteries emerge arcuate arteries that run along the boundary between the cortex and the medulla, that is, perpendicular to the medullary–cortical axis. From the latter, interlobular arteries branch off at regular intervals at angles of about 90 degrees, so that they all enter the renal cortex. For this reason, virtually all the blood flowing into the kidney perfuses the cortex first [8, 25, 38, 41–43]. The interlobular arteries are in close proximity to interlobular veins, together forming what might be called "vascular bundles" that run in parallel at regular distances from the corticomedullary boundary toward the capsule. Within the cortex, interlobular arteries branch off into afferent (preglomerular) arterioles, from which glomerular capillaries arise that, in turn, rejoin into efferent (postglomerular) arterioles. The efferent arterioles from the subcapsular and mid-cortical glomeruli branch off into networks of peritubular capillaries. The efferent arterioles of the deep cortical (juxtamedullary) glomeruli, however, branch off at about the corticomedullary boundary to form capillary-like vessels, the descending vasa recta [38–40]. These very straight and exceptionally long vessels descend toward the papilla. The descending vasa recta provide virtually all blood that perfuses the medulla. As a consequence, only 10–15% of blood that previously passes through the cortex, will reach the medulla, and the vascular density is much lower in the medulla than the cortex [8, 25, 38, 41–43]. The descending vasa recta are in close proximity with the ascending vasa recta, thus forming distinct "vascular bundles" that run in parallel at regular distances through the medulla [38–40].

These particularities of the intrarenal vascular architecture have a number of salient consequences with regard to local blood

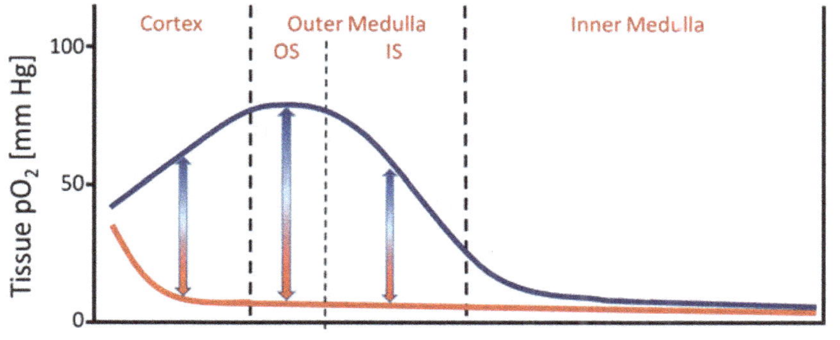

Fig. 1 Scheme depicting the range of intrarenal tissue partial pressure of oxygen (pO_2). The red curve depicts values at the greatest distance from two neighboring "vascular bundles," the blue one that directly adjacent to "vascular bundles" (for details see text); OS (outer stripe), IS (inner stripe). Original data were obtained by measurements in in anesthetized dogs and rats [43–45]

perfusion and thus the local O_2 supply. First, the striking difference in the quantity of blood perfusion between the cortex and the medulla, together with the difference in their vascular densities, is one of the major reasons for the low tissue pO_2 in the medulla. Second, the Fåhræus–Lindqvist effect that lowers the hematocrit and thereby the O_2 content of blood in the vasa recta that supply the medulla, contributes to low medullary O_2 delivery [39, 40]. Third, diffusive shunting of O_2 between the arcuate and interlobular arteries and their respective veins in the cortex as well as between the descending and ascending vasa recta in the medulla, owing to the close proximities of the respective vessels, are a further major reason behind the "physiological hypoxia" of the medulla. Thus, blood pO_2 is higher in the venous vessels than in the capillaries these venous vessels drain. Fourth, due to the particular vascular architecture with distinct "vascular bundles" that comprise arterial vessels with high pO_2 and venous vessels with relatively high pO_2 (due mainly to the low fractional O_2 extraction of the renal tissue), there are huge differences in local pO_2 even within a given renal layer under physiological conditions [25, 41, 43–47]. Fifth, plasma skimming at intrarenal vessel branches results in different hematocrit and therefore O_2 content of blood perfusing the daughter vessels, which also contributes to the local pO_2 differences [39, 48].

The schematic shown in Fig. 1 depicts the range of local pO_2 values as measured by invasive Clark-type electrodes in the kidneys of rats and dogs under physiological conditions in vivo [43–45]. These measurements reveal that local tissue pO_2 levels in the cortex vary dramatically, foremost according to the distance to the "vascular bundles" of interlobular arteries and veins: pO_2 values range from 10 mmHg at the greatest distance from two neighboring "bundles," to up to 70 mmHg around the "bundles." In addition, local cortical tissue pO_2 varies with the distance to the arcuate arteries located at the corticomedullary boundary. Also, the range of tissue pO_2 variability in the outer medulla is huge (*see* Fig. 1): whereas pO_2 is less than 10 mmHg in locations at maximum distance from the "vascular bundles" of descending and ascending vasa recta, pO_2 is up to 75 mmHg in close proximity to these "bundles." In the inner medulla, tissue pO_2 is rather homogenous: in general, it usually amounts to less than 15 mmHg.

The huge differences in tissue pO_2 among the renal layers not only reflect the differences in O_2 supply but also the different O_2 consumption of the distinct sections of the tubules located in the respective renal layers. Tubular resorption relies on active transport processes, which account for about 85% of the kidney's energy expenditure and, therefore, its O_2 consumption [8, 49]. The proximal tubule and the distal convoluted tubule, which constitute the majority of tubular segments within the cortex, consume much O_2 because a huge amount of osmolytes is resorbed by active transport in these segments. On the other hand, tubular sections such as the thin descending and the thin ascending limbs of Henle's loop and the medullary collecting duct, which are the most abundant tubular sections within the medulla, feature very low to nonexisting active transport. Yet the thick ascending limbs of Henle's loop, which are located in the outer medulla, consume much O_2, because of their active resorption of osmolytes [8, 25, 41, 43–47, 50]. The high O_2 demands of the thick ascending limbs in relation to the rather low O_2 supply of the outer medulla, consequent to its particular vascular architecture, exposes this renal layer to the greatest risk for hypoxic tissue damage [6–14, 43, 51, 52].

3 Methods: Methodologic Principles, Advantages, and Disadvantages

Techniques for invasive measurements of renal hemodynamics and oxygenation comprise readily (commercially) available methods and devices that are employed in many laboratories of integrative kidney physiology worldwide, but also techniques that are established only in one or a few laboratories. The widely used methods are described first. They include (1) perivascular flow probes for measurement of total renal blood flow, (2) laser-Doppler-optodes for assessment of local tissue perfusion, (3) Clark-type electrodes for measurements of local tissue pO_2, (4) fluorescence-quenching optodes for the same purpose, (5) devices for invasive measurement of arterial blood pressure, and (6) pimonidazole adduct immunohistochemistry for assessment of renal tissue hypoxia.

The pimonidazole technique is included here because of its widespread usage, although it is an exceptional case for two reasons. First, in contrast to the other techniques, this approach does not allow investigators to monitor a given parameter over time, but only provides a snapshot: Pimonidazole is injected at a single time point in vivo, and pimonidazole adducts formed in severely hypoxic tissue are visualized in ex vivo samples [53–55]. Second, although the technique has been used for two decades, it was subjected to close scrutiny only recently [55]. Upon this careful investigation major pitfalls were identified and detailed—which, at least in part, cast doubts on the reliability of previously published results—and methods to address and overcome these issues have been proposed [55].

In the final part of this chapter, a few selected examples of methods are discussed that are not (yet) generally available but presently established in only one or a few laboratories.

3.1 Transonic Flow Probes

Today's gold standard for whole kidney blood flow measurements is a flow probe attached to the renal artery or to the renal vein that makes use of ultrasound transit time differences. This method was established in the late 1970s and provides continuous absolute measurements of blood flow (in mL per min) independent of the actual flow velocity profile, the actual vessel diameter, and the actual hematocrit [56]. The commercially available device (Transonic™, Transonic Systems Inc.) comprises an electronic flow detection unit (flowmeter) and perivascular probes [57, 58]. The flow probe consists of two ultrasonic transducers and a fixed acoustic reflector (*see* Fig. 2a). The flow probe is positioned on the blood vessel so that the vessel lies within the acoustic sensing window defined by

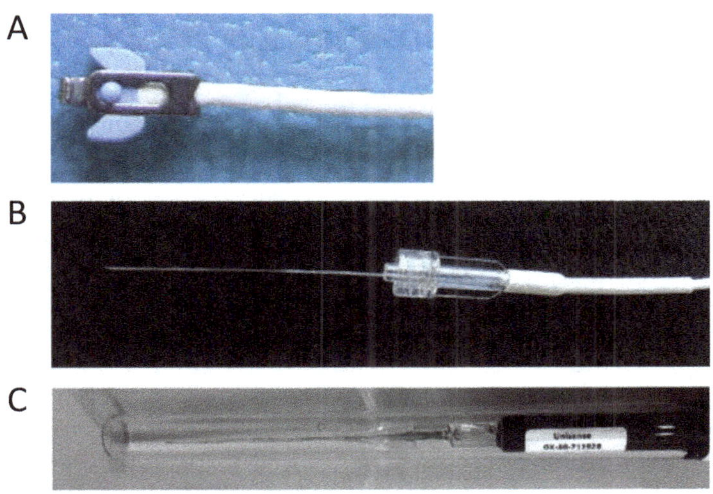

Fig. 2 Photographs of typical probes for invasive measurements. (**a**) Perivascular Transonic™ flow probe for measurement of total renal blood flow. (**b**) Combined fluorescence-quenching-laser-Doppler probe (OxyLite/OxyFlo™) for simultaneous measurements of local tissue pO_2 and assessment of local tissue perfusion in the same circumscribed area. (**c**) Clark-type electrode for measurement of local tissue pO_2

the transducers and the metallic reflector. Probes are available in various sizes to fit the dimensions of the blood vessel of interest.

The flowmeter directs the flow probe through measurement cycles [57, 58]. First, a wide beam of ultrasound is emitted by the downstream transducer. It intersects the vessel in the upstream direction, is reflected by the acoustic reflector, then intersects the vessel again before being received by the upstream transducer. The flowmeter records the transit time. Then, the transit–receive sequence is repeated, but with the transmitting and receiving functions of the transducers reversed, that is, the vessel is bisected by the beam in the downstream direction. The transit time during the upstream cycle is higher than during the downstream cycle, because the ultrasound beam travels against the blood flow in the first, and with the blood flow in the latter cycle. The difference in the transit times is directly proportional to blood volume flow. Due to the wide ultrasonic beams, all flowing blood is accounted for; thus, the transit time is sampled at all points across the vessel diameter, and the volume flow measurement is independent of the flow velocity profile [57, 58].

An accurate measure of volumetric flow is obtained by the perivascular probes even when the vessel is smaller than the acoustic window, because the parts of the ultrasonic beam that do not intersect the vessel do not contribute to the signal [57, 58]. However, air effectively blocks ultrasound transmission, and even small air bubbles compromise measurement accuracy. Therefore, all spaces between the vessel and probe must be filled with a suitable acoustic coupling agent. In case of "terminal experiments" in anesthetized animals, where the abdomen is opened, this can be achieved by simply filling the abdominal cavity with isotonic saline (at 37 °C) [27]. Acoustic coupling gels can also be used and are available from the supplier of the probes. Fatty tissue also affects the ultrasonic beam; thus, the vessel of interest must be thoroughly prepared by gently removing fatty tissue [27].

Measurements of total renal blood flow by means of Transonic™ devices have also been performed in chronically instrumented animals [22, 31, 33, 58, 59]. Here, the perivascular probe becomes encapsulated by tissue, which stabilizes its position. En route to calibration of functional MRI for the study of renal hemodynamics and oxygenation, an integrated multimodality approach was developed that enables measurements of invasive gold standard parameters and functional MR parameters simultaneously for the same kidney in an ultrahigh field small animal scanner (MR-PHYSIOL) [25–28]. For such a setup, a special Transonic™ flow probe is used: its acoustic reflector is made of Macor ceramics instead of stainless steel or brass to meet the safety and compatibility requirements of MRI (*see* the chapter by Cantow K et al. "Monitoring Renal Hemodynamics and Oxygenation by Invasive Probes: Experimental Protocol").

With the introduction of the Transonic™ technique, all other methods used for quantitative assessment of total renal blood flow in experimental animals including but not limited to electromagnetic probes and microsphere techniques were rendered obsolete.

3.2 Laser-Doppler Optodes

In the 1970s, laser-Doppler probes were developed that estimate local blood perfusion within circumscribed areas of tissue [60, 61]. For this purpose, pulsed light of a distinct wavelength (e.g., 785 nm) is guided via an optical fiber into the tissue subjacent to the tip of the fiber, where it is scattered within the tissue. A fraction of the light encounters erythrocytes, is reflected, and is fed back via the fiber to the photodetecting device of the apparatus. From the amount of reflected light the concentration of erythrocytes per tissue volume is estimated. Because erythrocytes move with the bloodstream, the reflected light becomes frequency shifted due to the Doppler effect. The photodetected signal comprises a broad spectrum of Doppler frequency shifted signals from which the average velocity of erythrocytes is derived. An estimate of microvascular blood perfusion is than calculated by the apparatus as the product of mean erythrocyte velocity and mean erythrocyte concentration in the volume of tissue under illumination from the probe [61].

The most important limitation of the laser-Doppler technique is that it can only provide arbitrary, nonabsolute, units for blood perfusion rather than an absolute value of blood flow, which is why the method is often termed laser-Doppler-fluxmetry [25]. This is due to the fact that the actual sampling volume could only be determined if it were possible to identify which erythrocytes have interacted with the light reflected from the tissue. The latter depends on the optical scattering and absorption coefficients of the tissue. Since these coefficients vary considerably with regard to the local microvasculature and its perfusion at the time of measurement, it is impossible to determine the actual sampling volume and thus the blood flow in absolute terms [61].

Estimated mean sampling depths for mammal tissues range from 0.5–1.5 mm, corresponding to "captured" volumes of roughly 1 mm^3 of tissue. However, these values must be lower in regions with large light absorption due to large amounts of erythrocytes per volume such as the renal cortex, and lower in the inner medulla with its low amount of erythrocytes per volume [38–40, 61].

Considering the rather small volume of tissue for which the laser-Doppler data are obtained versus the heterogeneity of intrarenal perfusion, extrapolation of the results of one area to other areas, even of the same renal layer, is unfeasible. Because of the impossibility to provide absolute data, laser-Doppler-fluxmetry allows investigators only to report relative changes occurring while the optode is fixed in place. Therefore, only continuous and

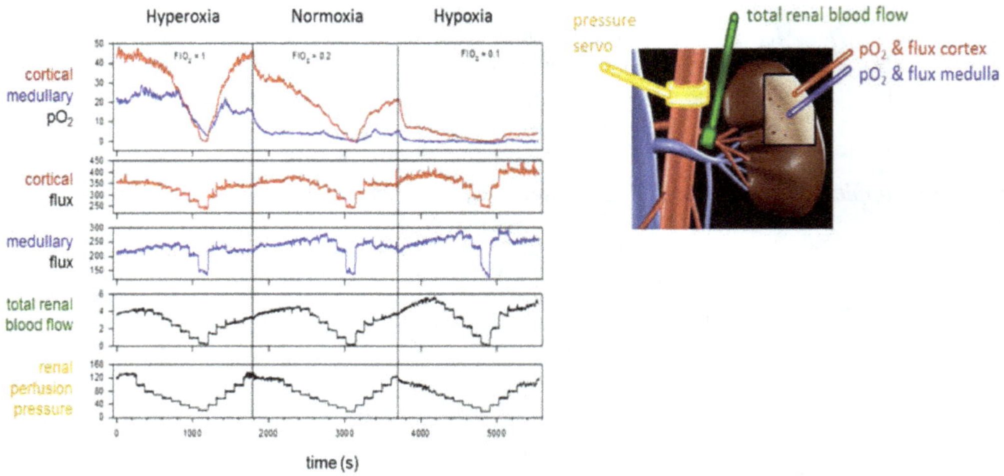

Fig. 3 Original tracings of invasively measured parameters of renal hemodynamic and oxygenation in an anesthetized rat (left panel) and sketch of the left kidney with the locations of the used probes (right panel). The rat was exposed to staircasewise reductions in renal perfusion pressure followed by staircasewise pressure restorations performed by means of a servo-controlled inflatable occluder placed around the suprarenal aorta (pressure servo) [22]. This was done under normoxic (inspiratory fraction of O_2, $FiO_2 = 0.2$), hyperoxic ($FiO_2 = 1.0$), and hypoxic ($FiO_2 = 0.1$) conditions

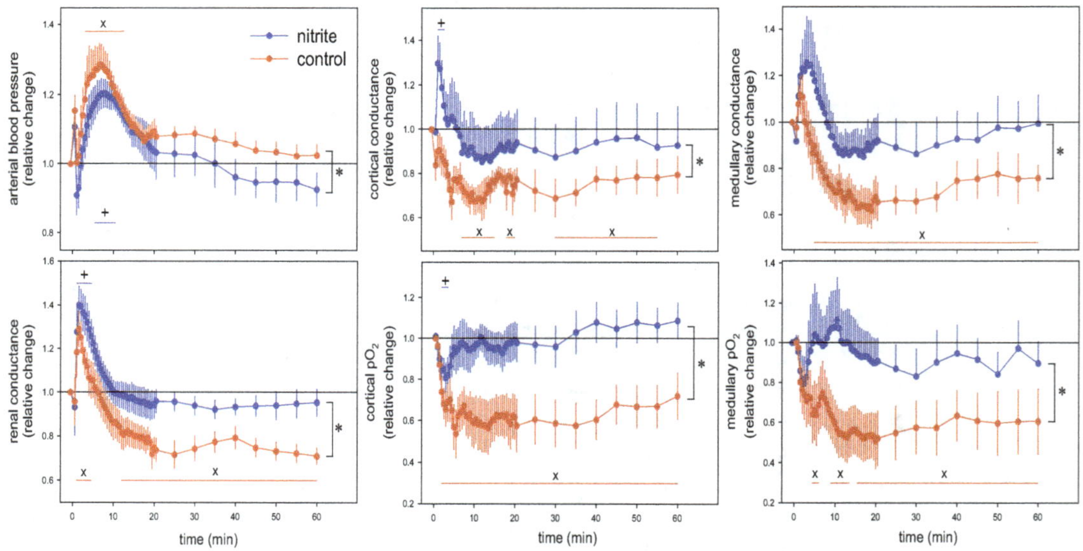

Fig. 4 Time courses of invasively measured parameters of renal hemodynamics and oxygenation in two groups of anesthetized rats that both received a 1.5 mL bolus injection of an X-ray contrast medium (iodixanol 320 mg iodine per mL) into the thoracic aorta at time 0. In the blue group, a low dose of nitrite was administered by continuous infusion, while in the red group saline was infused (control). Conductance values (the reciprocal of vascular resistance) were calculated by dividing the respective perfusion values by arterial blood pressure, in order to distinguish flow changes that result from passive circular distension/compression of vessels from those actively exerted by vascular smooth muscles. Values (mean $\pm$ SEM) are given as relative changes from baseline. Redrawn from Ref. 20

quantifiable changes relative to baseline (control) measurements are recorded, typically induced by acute interventions such as changes in renal arterial pressure or the inspiratory O_2 fraction, or by the administration of drugs (*see* Figs. 3 and 4) [18–20, 22, 23, 25, 28, 62]. Yet even interpretation of changes in laser-Doppler data recorded during such maneuvers must be done with due caution: they could rely on changes in local hematocrit, for example, due to changes in plasma skimming, rather than changes in blood flow [25, 39, 48].

In many studies on renal hemodynamics, data from two probes are recorded, one placed within the cortex and the other one in the (outer) medulla. This approach has been also employed in chronically instrumented rats [22]. It must be noted, that the potential tissue injury inflicted by the insertion of the optodes (usual tip diameters range from 50 to 300 μm) may confound the results. Laser-Doppler fluxmetry devices are supplied by various manufacturers. Oxford Optronics, Ltd., provides combined fluorescence-quenching and laser-Doppler optodes (OxyLite/OxyFlo™) that enable simultaneous recordings of local tissue pO_2 (vide infra) and of relative changes in local tissue perfusion in the same circumscribed area of renal tissue (*see* Fig. 2b).

3.3 Clark-Type Electrodes

These polarographic electrodes were developed in the 1950s by Clark and colleagues [63]. The electrodes consist of a noble metal (e.g., silver, gold, platinum) which reduces O_2 due to a negative polarizing voltage. The difference in voltage between the reference electrode (anode) and the measuring electrode (cathode) is proportional to the amount of O_2 molecules being reduced on the cathode. This enables quantification of tissue pO_2 (absolute values in mmHg). The critical technical advance was electrical insulation of the anode and cathode with a gas-permeable but liquid-impermeable membrane. This approach provided the foundation for the development of miniaturized versions (*see* Fig. 2c) with tips as small as 1–5 μm, that enable quantification of pO_2 even in specific vascular and tubular elements of the kidney [64, 65]. Using such small electrodes, Lübbers, Baumgärtl, and colleagues were the first to document the vast heterogeneity of renal tissue pO_2 among as well as within the renal layers that is depicted by Fig. 1 [43–45]. These authors generated "spatial maps" with the frequency distribution of pO_2 values ("pO_2 histograms") from the cortex to the inner medulla, by moving the electrodes through the renal tissues using a nanostepper technique (step width 50 μm).

While "pO_2 histograms" have also been obtained in a few recent studies [66, 67], the majority of studies uses fixed electrodes, making sure that the tips remain at the same location within the kidney throughout the experiment. Often, one electrode is placed within the cortex and the other one in the (outer) medulla. The tissue volume that is "captured" by the electrodes has probably about the same diameter as the tip of the electrode; thus, standard electrodes of ≤10 μm diameter obtain pO_2 values that are representative for a relatively small tissue volume only [67]. In the face of the spatial heterogeneity of intrarenal pO_2, this constitutes a major limitation of this technique. On the other hand, the potential tissue injury inflicted by the insertion of these small electrodes is less than with bigger electrodes or fluorescence quenching optodes that enable better "spatial averaging" (vide infra) [24, 35, 67]. Another drawback of Clark-type electrodes is O_2 consumption due to their electrochemical reduction, which is particularly unfavorable in areas with a fragile balance between O_2 delivery and demand such as the renal medulla [67–70].

Furthermore, it is not technically feasible to make repeated measurements in the same anesthetized animal over time-frames longer than a few hours. Yet, recently, a telemetric method using carbon paste electrodes has been developed that allows assessment of renal tissue pO_2 in conscious rats [35]. This method provides exquisite temporal resolution [24]. The major limitations of the method are (1) that it requires considerable skill and expertise to construct and implant the devices, (2) that tissue pO_2 can only be monitored at a single location in each animal, and (3) that only relative changes in tissue pO_2, rather than absolute levels are measured.

3.4 Fluorescence-Quenching Optodes

In the 1990s, a fiber-optic oxygen-sensing device was developed that measures pO_2 from the lifetime of fluorescence of a (ruthenium- or platinum-based) luminophore at the tip of an optode [70, 71]. The probe is connected to a pO_2 meter developed by Oxford Optronics, Ltd., that generates short pulses of blue LED light, which are transmitted via the fiber to the tip of the optode [70]. The resulting emission of fluorescent light is quenched by the presence of O_2 molecules. The OxyLite™ instrument measures the lifetime of each pulse of fluorescence, which is approximately inversely proportional to the pO_2 according to the Stern-Volmer equation at pO_2 values between 0 and 100 mmHg [68, 71].

Direct comparisons between Clark-type electrodes and quenching optodes reveal their respective advantages and disadvantages [67, 68, 70]. Both techniques share the disadvantage of invasiveness, and the advantage of enabling absolute quantification of pO_2 (in mmHg). Advantages of the optode include the absence of O_2 consumption and a greater accuracy at low pO_2, which is of particular importance when it comes to measurements in the renal medulla. In contrast to the electrodes that "capture" a tissue volume that is approximately equal to their tip diameter, optodes do not "capture" a proper volume. The pO_2 measured by the optodes is that within the probe-head (at the tip) of the optode itself, which covers a circular area of 230 μm diameter [67, 68, 70]. The larger diameter of the optodes as compared with that of standard pO_2 electrodes increases the risk for tissue damage. On the other hand, it facilitates a favorable "spatial averaging" of renal tissue pO_2 values in the face of their huge spatial heterogeneity. In fact, "pO_2histograms" of renal cortical pO_2 obtained in rabbits by a fluorescence optode were more tightly distributed than those provided by a Clark-type electrode, which may aid detection of (patho)-physiologically significant changes in intrarenal oxygenation [67]. Finally, the optodes have been proven to be MR compatible and MR safe [25, 26].

As mentioned earlier, combined fluorescence-quenching-laser-Doppler probes (OxyLite/OxyFlo™) enable simultaneous measurements of local tissue pO_2 and assessment of local tissue perfusion in the same circumscribed area (*see* Fig. 2b).

3.5 Monitoring of Arterial Blood Pressure

It is mandatory for in vivo studies in anesthetized experimental animals, be it studies on control of renal hemodynamics and oxygenation or on every other functional parameter, to monitor cardiovascular variables such as arterial blood pressure and heart rate throughout the experiment in order to ascertain that physiological cardiovascular control is maintained. In anesthetized animals this is best achieved by use of invasive techniques: a fluid-filled catheter inserted into a conduit artery (e.g., femoral or carotid arteries) connected to one of the various commercially available pressure transducers and quantitatively calibrated via a recording device (*see* the chapter by Cantow K et al. "Monitoring Renal Hemodynamics and Oxygenation by Invasive Probes: Experimental Protocol").

Direct intra-arterial measurements in unanesthetized animals is the most physiologically relevant means of arterial pressure determination. Telemetric pressure monitoring is the gold standard in conscious animals, and various telemetric devices are commercially available [72, 73]. A limitation of this technique is that implantation surgery and maintenance of catheters require considerable skill [72]. The tail-cuff method is a simple noninvasive plethysmographic technique to assess arterial pressure in conscious rats and mice [74, 75]. Since the conditions for tail-cuff measurements necessarily involve heating and restraint of the animal, which almost inevitably alter the measured parameter (arterial pressure), the physiological meaningfulness of the results is questionable [73].

3.6 Pimonidazole Adduct Immunohistochemistry

This method was originally developed for detection of hypoxia in tumors, but subsequently adapted for use in the kidney [53]. For this technique, pimonidazole (usually 60 mg/kg of body mass) is administered to the experimental animal in vivo [54]. Pimonidazole forms adducts within hypoxic (<approximately 10 mmHg) cells. These adducts are immunohistochemically visualized in ex vivo samples of the kidney. The advantage of this technique is that it provides good spatial resolution of renal tissue hypoxia at the

cellular level. Its major limitations include (1) that it detects severe hypoxia only, with a cutoff of about 10 mmHg, (2) that hypoxia can only be assessed postmortem, and (3) only at a single time point. Those using this technique must also be aware of two major sources of false-positive detection of hypoxia, as recently revealed [55]. Firstly, pimonidazole adducts can form postmortem in cells that were not hypoxic in the living animal. For this reason, it is recommended that kidney tissue be perfusion fixed, rather than immersion fixed. Secondly, when the standard (mouse) monoclonal antibody is used, false positive staining has been observed in damaged rat kidney tissue, presumably as a result of the anti-mouse secondary antibody binding to mouse-like antigens in the damaged tissue. This problem can be avoided by use of a newly commercially available polyclonal anti-pimonidazole antibody raised in rabbits [55].

3.7 Examples of Methods That Are Not Generally Available

3.7.1 Bladder pO_2

It is not technically feasible to measure renal tissue pO_2 in humans. It can also be technically difficult to measure renal tissue pO_2 in experimental animals unless they are deeply anesthetized. However, it is technically feasible to measure the pO_2 of urine in both experimental animals and man. There has been a long history of interest in this approach for monitoring renal medullary tissue oxygenation [76]. However, with the recent development of fiber-optic probes that can be inserted into a standard Foley bladder catheter, it has been possible to subject this method to close scrutiny [77]. Available evidence now indicates that urinary pO_2 can provide a good estimate of renal medullary pO_2 [77]. Because this technique can be deployed in humans equipped with a bladder catheter, it provides a translational pathway for development of approaches to improve renal medullary oxygenation in human patients at risk of AKI. It is also noteworthy that low urinary pO_2 during cardiac surgery requiring cardiopulmonary bypass predicts development of postoperative AKI. In light of this, urinary pO_2 measurements may provide a real-time measure of medullary oxygenation and predict the risk of AKI in critically ill patients. The major limitation of this approach is that the combination of low urine flow and high arterial pO_2 can confound the relationship between urinary pO_2 and medullary pO_2 [77].

3.7.2 Near Infrared Spectroscopy

Near infrared spectroscopy (NIRS), together with models for diffuse optical imaging affords the measurement of (1) tissue concentrations of oxygenated hemoglobin (oxyHb) and deoxygenated hemoglobin (deoxyHb), (2) oxygen saturation of Hb (StO_2) within tissues, and (3) tissue blood volume fraction in vivo. In particular, spatially resolved reflectance NIRS (SRR-NIRS), together with Monte-Carlo simulations of diffuse light propagation, has been applied to monitor these parameters within renal cortical tissue [78]. Quantification of the underlying absorption and reduced scattering coefficients of the tissue is based on analyzing the decrease of the intensity of diffusely remitted light with increasing distance from the light injection point. Recording techniques for the renal cortex of anesthetized rats have been established, with a linear fiber array placed on the ventral surface of the exposed kidney. Measurements have been done at selected near-infrared wavelengths between about 670 and 850 nm by multiplexing millisecond pulses from the different laser sources in time. In this way, quantitative measurements of renal cortex parameters have been achieved at a repetition rate of multiple Hz [78].

SRR-NIRS has been successfully combined with "classical" invasive techniques to study renal hemodynamics and oxygenation in rats [78]. Thus, SRR-NIRS-derived parameters such as the amount of Hb per tissue volume and StO_2 were obtained simultaneously with parameters including total renal blood flow, local cortical tissue perfusion and tissue pO_2 in the same kidney. Control of renal hemodynamics and oxygenation was studied by dedicated reversible test interventions including brief occlusions of the renal artery or the renal vein, short-term hypoxia, hyperoxia, and hypercapnia, and administration of adenosine. The results demonstrate that the combined approach, by providing different but complementary information, enables a more comprehensive characterization of renal hemodynamics and oxygenation [78].

The SRR-NIRS technique could also serve to help calibrate renal T_2* MRI. This MR surrogate parameter for blood oxygenation is related to the amount of deoxyHb per tissue volume. Confounders of the T_2* to tissue pO_2 relationship include the vascular volume fraction, the local hematocrit, and shifts of the oxyHb dissociation curve [25–28]. Since SRR-NIRS enables quantitative monitoring of the amount of Hb per tissue volume and of StO_2 it is an ideal candidate to unravel and quantify the contributions of confounding factors to renal T_2* MRI.

By extending the wavelength range beyond 900 nm, the tissue water content can additionally be assessed, which, together with the reduced scattering coefficients at the different wavelengths, can serve as a surrogate for other (patho)physiologically relevant parameters such as the tubular volume fraction.

Application of SRR-NIRS in reflection mode constrains measurements to the renal cortex of rats. Recently it was demonstrated that changes of rat medullary Hb parameters can also be assessed by SRR-NIRS in transmission mode using an additional fiber placed on the dorsal surface of the kidney [79].

3.7.3 Intravital Microscopy

Perhaps the "final frontier" in methods for assessing renal oxygenation are techniques that provide cellular resolution, in real time, in living animals. Hirakawa and colleagues have recently reported use of a technique they call "intravital phosphorescence lifetime imaging microscopy" [47]. This technique allows cellular pO_2 in the renal cortex of live animals to be resolved to the level of individual tubular cross-sections. It requires injection of a molecule whose phosphorescence is quenched by O_2. Thus, pO_2 can be measured by assessing the decay curve of the phosphorescence. Such probes are available that accumulate intracellularly or are retained within the vasculature. Thus, it is possible to use this approach to assess the heterogeneity of renal blood and tissue pO_2 in real time with unprecedented cellular resolution. Currently, the technique is limited for use in the superficial cortex.

Acknowledgments

This work was funded, in part (Kathleen Cantow, Thoralf Niendorf, and Erdmann Seeliger), by the German Research Foundation (Gefoerdert durch die Deutsche Forschungsgemeinschaft (DFG), Projektnummer/Project number 394046635, SFB 1365, RENOPROTECTION).

The authors wish to thank Ariane Anger and Andrea Gerhardt for expert technical assistance and Dr. Connie Ow for the image shown in Fig. 2c.

This chapter is based upon work from COST Action PARENCH IMA, supported by European Cooperation in Science and Technology (COST). COST (www.cost.eu) is a funding agency for research and innovation networks. COST Actions help connect research initiatives across Europe and enable scientists to enrich their ideas by sharing them with their peers. This boosts their research, career, and innovation.

PARENCHIMA (renalmri.org) is a community-driven Action in the COST program of the European Union, which unites more than 200 experts in renal MRI from 30 countries with the aim to improve the reproducibility and standardization of renal MRI biomarkers.

References

1. Fortrie G, de Geus HRH, Betjes MGH (2019) The aftermath of acute kidney injury: a narrative review of long-term mortality and renal function. Crit Care 23(1):24. https://doi.org/10.1186/s13054-019-2314-z
2. Selby NM, Taal MW (2019) Long-term outcomes after AKI-a major unmet clinical need. Kidney Int 95(1):21–23. https://doi.org/10.1016/j.kint.2018.09.005
3. Zuk A, Bonventre JV (2019) Recent advances in acute kidney injury and its consequences and impact on chronic kidney disease. Curr Opin Nephrol Hypertens 28(4):397–405. https://doi.org/10.1097/mnh.0000000000000504
4. Levin A, Tonelli M, Bonventre J, Coresh J, Donner JA, Fogo AB, Fox CS, Gansevoort RT, Heerspink HJL, Jardine M, Kasiske B, Kottgen A, Kretzler M, Levey AS, Luyckx VA, Mehta R, Moe O, Obrador G, Pannu N, Parikh CR, Perkovic V, Pollock C, Stenvinkel P, Tuttle KR, Wheeler DC, Eckardt KU (2017) Global kidney health 2017 and beyond: a roadmap for closing gaps in care, research, and policy. Lancet 390(10105):1888–1917. https://doi.org/10.1016/s0140-6736(17)30788-2

5. Bello AK, Levin A, Tonelli M, Okpechi IG, Feehally J, Harris D, Jindal K, Salako BL, Rateb A, Osman MA, Qarni B, Saad S, Lunney M, Wiebe N, Ye F, Johnson DW (2017) Assessment of global kidney health care status. JAMA 317(18):1864–1881. https://doi.org/10.1001/jama.2017.4046
6. Brezis M, Rosen S (1995) Hypoxia of the renal medulla--its implications for disease. N Engl J Med 332:647–655
7. Fähling M, Seeliger E, Patzak A, Persson PB (2017) Understanding and preventing contrast-induced acute kidney injury. Nat Rev Nephrol 13(3):169–180
8. Evans RG, Ince C, Joles JA, Smith DW, May CN, O'Connor PM, Gardiner BS (2013) Haemodynamic influences on kidney oxygenation: the clinical implications of integrative physiology. Clin Exp Pharmacol Physiol 40:106–122
9. Evans RG, Ow CP, Bie P (2015) The chronic hypoxia hypothesis: the search for the smoking gun goes on. Am J Physiol Renal Physiol 308 (2):F101–F102
10. Shu S, Wang Y, Zheng M, Liu Z, Cai J, Tang C, Dong Z (2019) Hypoxia and hypoxia-inducible factors in kidney injury and repair. Cell 8(3). https://doi.org/10.3390/cells8030207
11. Hultstrom M, Becirovic-Agic M, Jonsson S (2018) Comparison of acute kidney injury of different etiology reveals in-common mechanisms of tissue damage. Physiol Genomics 50 (3):127–141. https://doi.org/10.1152/physiolgenomics.00037.2017
12. Calzavacca P, Evans RG, Bailey M, Bellomo R, May CN (2015) Cortical and medullary tissue perfusion and oxygenation in experimental septic acute kidney injury. Crit Care Med 43 (10):e431–e439
13. Ma S, Evans RG, Iguchi N, Tare M, Parkington HC, Bellomo R, May CN, Lankadeva YR (2019) Sepsis-induced acute kidney injury: a disease of the microcirculation. Microcirculation 26(2):e12483. https://doi.org/10.1111/micc.12483
14. dos Santos EA, Li LP, Ji L, Prasad PV (2007) Early changes with diabetes in renal medullary hemodynamics as evaluated by fiberoptic probes and BOLD magnetic resonance imaging. Investig Radiol 42(3):157–162. https://doi.org/10.1097/01.rli.0000252492.96709.36
15. Calvin AD, Misra S, Pflueger A (2010) Contrast-induced acute kidney injury and diabetic nephropathy. Nat Rev Nephrol 6 (11):679–688
16. Hansell P, Welch WJ, Blantz RC, Palm F (2013) Determinants of kidney oxygen consumption and their relationship to tissue oxygen tension in diabetes and hypertension. Clin Exp Pharmacol Physiol 40(2):123–137
17. Seeliger E, Flemming B, Wronski T, Ladwig M, Arakelyan K, Godes M, Mockel M, Persson PB (2007) Viscosity of contrast media perturbs renal hemodynamics. J Am Soc Nephrol 18 (11):2912–2920
18. Hoff U, Lukitsch I, Chaykovska L, Ladwig M, Arnold C, Manthati VL, Fuller TF, Schneider W, Gollasch M, Muller DN, Flemming B, Seeliger E, Luft FC, Falck JR, Dragun D, Schunck WH (2011) Inhibition of 20-HETE synthesis and action protects the kidney from ischemia/reperfusion injury. Kidney Int 79(1):57–65
19. Cantow K, Flemming B, Ladwig-Wiegard M, Persson PB, Seeliger E (2017) Low dose nitrite improves reoxygenation following renal ischemia in rats. Sci Rep 7(1):14597–15058
20. Seeliger E, Cantow K, Arakelyan K, Ladwig M, Persson PB, Flemming B (2014) Low-dose nitrite alleviates early effects of an X-ray contrast medium on renal hemodynamics and oxygenation in rats. Investig Radiol 49(2):70–77
21. Seeliger E, Wronski T, Ladwig M, Dobrowolski L, Vogel T, Godes M, Persson PB, Flemming B (2009) The renin-angiotensin system and the third mechanism of renal blood flow autoregulation. Am J Physiol Renal Physiol 296(6):F1334–F1345
22. Flemming B, Seeliger E, Wronski T, Steer K, Arenz N, Persson PB (2000) Oxygen and renal hemodynamics in the conscious rat. J Am Soc Nephrol 11(1):18–24
23. Cantow K, Pohlmann A, Flemming B, Ferrara F, Waiczies S, Grosenick D, Niendorf T, Seeliger E (2016) Acute effects of ferumoxytol on regulation of renal hemodynamics and oxygenation. Sci Rep 6:29965. https://doi.org/10.1038/srep29965
24. Emans TW, Janssen BJ, Pinkham MI, Ow CP, Evans RG, Joles JA, Malpas SC, Krediet CT, Koeners MP (2016) Exogenous and endogenous angiotensin-II decrease renal cortical oxygen tension in conscious rats by limiting renal blood flow. J Physiol 594(21):6287–6300. https://doi.org/10.1113/jp270731
25. Pohlmann A, Cantow K, Hentschel J, Arakelyan K, Ladwig M, Flemming B, Hoff U, Persson PB, Seeliger E, Niendorf T (2013) Linking non-invasive parametric MRI with invasive physiological measurements (MR-PHYSIOL): towards a hybrid and integrated approach for investigation of acute

kidney injury in rats. Acta Physiol (Oxf) 207 (4):673–689

26. Niendorf T, Pohlmann A, Arakelyan K, Flemming B, Cantow K, Hentschel J, Grosenick D, Ladwig M, Reimann H, Klix S, Waiczies S, Seeliger E (2015) How BOLD is blood oxygenation level-dependent (BOLD) magnetic resonance imaging of the kidney? Opportunities, challenges and future directions. Acta Physiol (Oxf) 213(1):19–38
27. Cantow K, Arakelyan K, Seeliger E, Niendorf T, Pohlmann A (2016) Assessment of renal hemodynamics and oxygenation by simultaneous magnetic resonance imaging (MRI) and quantitative invasive physiological measurements. Methods Mol Biol 1397:129–154. https://doi.org/10.1007/978-1-4939-3353-2_11
28. Pohlmann A, Arakelyan K, Hentschel J, Cantow K, Flemming B, Ladwig M, Waiczies S, Seeliger E, Niendorf T (2014) Detailing the relation between renal T2* and renal tissue pO_2 using an integrated approach of parametric magnetic resonance imaging and invasive physiological measurements. Investig Radiol 49(8):547–560
29. Evans RG, Gardiner BS, Smith DW, O'Connor PM (2008) Methods for studying the physiology of kidney oxygenation. Clin Exp Pharmacol Physiol 35(12):1405–1412
30. Hirakawa Y, Tanaka T, Nangaku M (2017) Renal hypoxia in CKD; pathophysiology and detecting methods. Front Physiol 8:99. https://doi.org/10.3389/fphys.2017.00099
31. Flemming B, Arenz N, Seeliger E, Wronski T, Steer K, Persson PB (2001) Time-dependent autoregulation of renal blood flow in conscious rats. J Am Soc Nephrol 12(11):2253–2262
32. Calzavacca P, Evans RG, Bailey M, Bellomo R, May CN (2015) Variable responses of regional renal oxygenation and perfusion to vasoactive agents in awake sheep. Am J Physiol Regul Integr Comp Physiol 309(10):R1226–R1233
33. Calzavacca P, Evans RG, Bailey M, Lankadeva YR, Bellomo R, May CN (2015) Long-term measurement of renal cortical and medullary tissue oxygenation and perfusion in unanesthetized sheep. Am J Physiol Regul Integr Comp Physiol 308(10):R832–R839
34. Evans RG, Madden AC, Denton KM (2000) Diversity of responses of renal cortical and medullary blood flow to vasoconstrictors in conscious rabbits. Acta Physiol Scand 169 (4):297–308
35. Koeners MP, Ow CP, Russell DM, Abdelkader A, Eppel GA, Ludbrook J, Malpas SC, Evans RG (2013) Telemetry-based oxygen sensor for continuous monitoring of kidney oxygenation in conscious rats. Am J Physiol Renal Physiol 304(12):F1471–F1480
36. Koeners MP, Ow CPC, Russell DM, Evans RG, Malpas SC (2016) Prolonged and continuous measurement of kidney oxygenation in conscious rats. Methods Mol Biol 1397:93–111. https://doi.org/10.1007/978-1-4939-3353-2_9.:93-111
37. Lankadeva YR, Kosaka J, Evans RG, Bailey SR, Bellomo R, May CN (2016) Intrarenal and urinary oxygenation during norepinephrine resuscitation in ovine septic acute kidney injury. Kidney Int 90(1):100–108
38. Pitts RF (1974) Anatomy of the kidney. In: Pitts RF (ed) Physiology of the kidney and body fluids. Year Book Medical Publishers, Inc., Chicago
39. Edwards A, Silldforff EP, Pallone TL (2000) The renal medullary microcirculation. Front Biosci 5:E36–E52
40. Zimmerhackl BL, Robertson CR, Jamison RL (1987) The medullary microcirculation. Kidney Int 31(2):641–647
41. Evans RG, Gardiner BS, Smith DW, O'Connor PM (2008) Intrarenal oxygenation: unique challenges and the biophysical basis of homeostasis. Am J Physiol Renal Physiol 295 (5):1259–1270
42. Niendorf T, Pohlmann A, Arakelyan K, Flemming B, Cantow K, Hentschel J, Grosenick D, Ladwig M, Reimann H, Klix S, Waiczies S, Seeliger E (2015) How BOLD is blood oxygenation-dependent (BOLD) magnetic resonance imaging of the kidney? Opportunities, challenges and future directions. Acta Physiol (Oxf) 213(1):19–38
43. Schurek HJ (1988) Kidney medullary hypoxia: a key to understanding acute renal failure? Klin Wochenschr 66(18):828–835
44. Baumgartl H, Leichtweiss HP, Lubbers DW, Weiss C, Huland H (1972) The oxygen supply of the dog kidney: measurements of intrarenal pO_2. Microvasc Res 4(3):247–257
45. Lubbers DW, Baumgartl H (1997) Heterogeneities and profiles of oxygen pressure in brain and kidney as examples of the pO_2 distribution in the living tissue. Kidney Int 51(2):372–380
46. Evans RG, Ow CPC (2018) Heterogeneity of renal cortical oxygenation: seeing is believing. Kidney Int 93(6):1278–1280. https://doi.org/10.1016/j.kint.2018.01.039
47. Hirakawa Y, Mizukami K, Yoshihara T, Takahashi I, Khulan P, Honda T, Mimura I, Tanaka T, Tobita S, Nangaku M (2018) Intravital phosphorescence lifetime imaging of the renal cortex accurately measures renal hypoxia.

Kidney Int 93(6):1483–1489. https://doi.org/10.1016/j.kint.2018.01.015

48. Pappenheimer JR, Kinter WB (1956) Hematocrit ratio of blood within mammalian kidney and its significance for renal hemodynamics. Am J Physiol 185:377
49. Evans RG, Harrop GK, Ngo JP, Ow CP, O'Connor PM (2014) Basal renal O_2 consumption and the efficiency of O_2 utilization for Na^+ reabsorption. Am J Physiol Renal Physiol 306(5):F551–F560
50. Pitts RF (1974) Mechanisms of reabsorption and excretion of salt and water. In: Pitts RF (ed) Physiology of the kidney and body fluids. Year Book Medical Publishers, Inc., Chicago
51. Palm F, Carlsson PO, Hansell P, Hellberg O, Nygren A, Liss P (2003) Altered response in renal blood flow and oxygen tension to contrast media in diabetic rats. Acta Radiol 44 (3):347–353
52. Palm F, Cederberg J, Hansell P, Liss P, Carlsson PO (2003) Reactive oxygen species cause diabetes-induced decrease in renal oxygen tension. Diabetologia 46(8):1153–1160
53. Zhong Z, Arteel GE, Connor HD, Yin M, Frankenberg MV, Stachlewitz RF, Raleigh JA, Mason RP, Thurman RG (1998) Cyclosporin a increases hypoxia and free radical production in rat kidneys: prevention by dietary glycine. Am J Physiol 275(4):F595–F604. https://doi.org/10.1152/ajprenal.1998.275.4.F595
54. Rosenberger C, Rosen S, Paliege A, Heyman SN (2009) Pimonidazole adduct immunohistochemistry in the rat kidney: detection of tissue hypoxia. Methods Mol Biol 466:161–174. https://doi.org/10.1007/978-1-59745-352-3_12
55. Ow CPC, Ullah MM, Ngo JP, Sayakkarage A, Evans RG (2019) Detection of cellular hypoxia by pimonidazole adduct immunohistochemistry in kidney disease: methodological pitfalls and their solution. Am J Physiol Renal Physiol 317(2):F322. https://doi.org/10.1152/ajprenal.00219.2019
56. Drost CJ (1978) Vessel diameter-independent volume flow measurements using ultrasound. In: Proceedings of San Diego Biomedical Symposium, vol 17. San Diego Biomedical Society, San Diego, CA, pp 299–302
57. Dean DA, Jia CX, Cabreriza SE, D'Alessandro DA, Dickstein ML, Sardo MJ, Chalik N, Spotnitz HM (1996) Validation study of a new transit time ultrasonic flow probe for continuous great vessel measurements. ASAIO J 42(5): M671–M676
58. Charbel FT, Hoffman WE, Misra M, Ostergren L (1998) Ultrasonic perivascular flow probe: technique and application in neurosurgery. Neurol Res 20(5):439–442
59. Lankadeva YR, Cochrane AD, Marino B, Iguchi N, Hood SG, Bellomo R, May CN, Evans RG (2019) Strategies that improve renal medullary oxygenation during experimental cardiopulmonary bypass may mitigate postoperative acute kidney injury. Kidney Int 95(6):1338–1346. https://doi.org/10.1016/j.kint.2019.01.032
60. Stern MD, Bowen PD, Parma R, Osgood RW, Bowman RL, Stein JH (1979) Measurement of renal cortical and medullary blood flow by laser-Doppler spectroscopy in the rat. Am J Physiol 236(1):F80–F87. https://doi.org/10.1152/ajprenal.1979.236.1.F80
61. Obeid AN, Barnett NJ, Dougherty G, Ward G (1990) A critical review of laser Doppler flowmetry. J Med Eng Technol 14(5):178–181
62. Ferrara F, Cantow K, Flemming B, Skalweit A, Ladwig M, Fähling M, Seeliger E (2017) Effects of liraglutide on control of renal hemodynamics and oxygenation in diabetic rats. Acta Physiol (Oxf) 219(Suppl. 711):38
63. Clark LC Jr, Misrahy G, Fox RP (1958) Chronically implanted polarographic electrodes. J Appl Physiol 13(1):85–91. https://doi.org/10.1152/jappl.1958.13.1.85
64. Whalen WJ, Riley J, Nair P (1967) A microelectrode for measuring intracellular PO2. J Appl Physiol 23(5):798–801. https://doi.org/10.1152/jappl.1967.23.5.798
65. Welch WJ, Baumgartl H, Lubbers D, Wilcox CS (2001) Nephron pO_2 and renal oxygen usage in the hypertensive rat kidney. Kidney Int 59(1):230–237. https://doi.org/10.1046/j.1523-1755.2001.00483.x
66. Ow CPC, Ngo JP, Ullah MM, Barsha G, Meex RC, Watt MJ, Hilliard LM, Koeners MP, Evans RG (2018) Absence of renal hypoxia in the subacute phase of severe renal ischemia-reperfusion injury. Am J Physiol Renal Physiol 315(5):F1358–f1369. https://doi.org/10.1152/ajprenal.00249.2018
67. Leong CL, O'Connor PM, Eppel GA, Anderson WP, Evans RG (2008) Measurement of renal tissue oxygen tension: systematic differences between fluorescence optode and microelectrode recordings in anaesthetized rabbits. Nephron Physiol 108(2):11–17
68. Shaw AD, Li Z, Thomas Z, Stevens CW (2002) Assessment of tissue oxygen tension: comparison of dynamic fluorescence quenching and polarographic electrode technique. Crit Care 6(1):76–80
69. Carreau A, El Hafny-Rahbi B, Matejuk A, Grillon C, Kieda C (2011) Why is the partial

oxygen pressure of human tissues a crucial parameter? Small molecules and hypoxia. J Cell Mol Med 15(6):1239–1253. https://doi.org/10.1111/j.1582-4934.2011.01258.x

70. Griffiths JR, Robinson SP (1999) The OxyLite: a fibre-optic oxygen sensor. Br J Radiol 72 (859):627–630. https://doi.org/10.1259/bjr.72.859.10624317
71. Young WK, Vojnovic B, Wardman P (1996) Measurement of oxygen tension in tumours by time-resolved fluorescence. British J Cancer Suppl 27:S256–S259
72. Sponer G, Müller-Beckmann B, Martin U (1993) Blood pressure recording in rats: pitfalls and problems. In: Gretz N, Strauch M (eds) Experimental and genetic rat models of chronic renal failure. Karger, Basel, pp 319–330
73. Nalivaiko E (2011) Animal models of psychogenic cardiovascular disorders: what we can learn from them and what we cannot. Clin Exp Pharmacol Physiol 38(2):115–125. https://doi.org/10.1111/j.1440-1681.2010.05465.x
74. Byrom FB, Wilson C (1938) A plethysmographic method for measuring systolic blood pressure in the intact rat. J Physiol 93 (3):301–304. https://doi.org/10.1113/jphysiol.1938.sp003641
75. Krege JH, Hodgin JB, Hagaman JR, Smithies O (1995) A noninvasive computerized tail-cuff system for measuring blood pressure in mice. Hypertension 25(5):1111–1115. https://doi.org/10.1161/01.hyp.25.5.1111
76. Aperia AC, Liebow AA (1964) Implications of urinary pO2 for renal medullary blood flow. Am J Physiol 206:499–504
77. Ngo JP, Lankadeva YR, Zhu MZL, Martin A, Kanki M, Cochrane AD, Smith JA, Thrift AG, May CN, Evans RG (2019) Factors that confound the prediction of renal medullary oxygenation and risk of acute kidney injury from measurement of bladder urine oxygen tension. Acta Physiol (Oxf) 227(1):e13294. https://doi.org/10.1111/apha.13294
78. Grosenick D, Cantow K, Arakelyan K, Wabnitz H, Flemming B, Skalweit A, Ladwig M, Macdonald R, Niendorf T, Seeliger E (2015) Detailing renal hemodynamics and oxygenation in rats by a combined near-infrared spectroscopy and invasive probe approach. Biomed Opt Express 6(2):309–323
79. Gladytz T, Cantow K, Flemming B, Pohlmann A, Niendorf T, Seeliger E, Grosenick D Towards depth-resolved characterization of hemodynamics and oxygenation in the rat kidney. In Proc SPIE, 2019. vol 11074, pp 1107415-1107411-1107415–1107413

Permissions

All chapters in this book were first published in PMRITKMP, by Springer; hereby published with permission under the Creative Commons Attribution License or equivalent. Every chapter published in this book has been scrutinized by our experts. Their significance has been extensively debated. The topics covered herein carry significant findings which will fuel the growth of the discipline. They may even be implemented as practical applications or may be referred to as a beginning point for another development.

The contributors of this book come from diverse backgrounds, making this book a truly international effort. This book will bring forth new frontiers with its revolutionizing research information and detailed analysis of the nascent developments around the world.

We would like to thank all the contributing authors for lending their expertise to make the book truly unique. They have played a crucial role in the development of this book. Without their invaluable contributions this book wouldn't have been possible. They have made vital efforts to compile up to date information on the varied aspects of this subject to make this book a valuable addition to the collection of many professionals and students.

This book was conceptualized with the vision of imparting up-to-date information and advanced data in this field. To ensure the same, a matchless editorial board was set up. Every individual on the board went through rigorous rounds of assessment to prove their worth. After which they invested a large part of their time researching and compiling the most relevant data for our readers.

The editorial board has been involved in producing this book since its inception. They have spent rigorous hours researching and exploring the diverse topics which have resulted in the successful publishing of this book. They have passed on their knowledge of decades through this book. To expedite this challenging task, the publisher supported the team at every step. A small team of assistant editors was also appointed to further simplify the editing procedure and attain best results for the readers.

Apart from the editorial board, the designing team has also invested a significant amount of their time in understanding the subject and creating the most relevant covers. They scrutinized every image to scout for the most suitable representation of the subject and create an appropriate cover for the book.

The publishing team has been an ardent support to the editorial, designing and production team. Their endless efforts to recruit the best for this project, has resulted in the accomplishment of this book. They are a veteran in the field of academics and their pool of knowledge is as vast as their experience in printing. Their expertise and guidance has proved useful at every step. Their uncompromising quality standards have made this book an exceptional effort. Their encouragement from time to time has been an inspiration for everyone.

The publisher and the editorial board hope that this book will prove to be a valuable piece of knowledge for researchers, students, practitioners and scholars across the globe.

List of Contributors

Pietro Irrera, Lorena Consolino, Phillip Zhe Sun and Michael T. McMahon

Tamas Kaucsar, Adam Hosszu and Henning M. Reimann

Michael Pedersen, Walter Dastrù, Frank G. Zöllner, Kevin M. Bennett, Scott C. Beeman, G. Larry Bretthorst, Joel R. Garbow and Dario Livio Longo

Jason M. Millward, João S. Periquito, Paula Ramos Delgado, Christian Prinz and Sonia Waiczies

Stefanie J. Hectors, Philippe Garteiser, Sabrina Doblas, Gwenaë Page, Bernard E. Van Beers, John C. Waterton and Octavia Bane

Min-Chi Ku, Mariá A. Fernández-Seara, Frank Kober and Thoralf Niendorf

Delgado, Ekkehard Kü stermann, André Kü hne, Andreas Pohlmann and Martin Meier

Susan J. Back, Iris Friedli, Stefanie Hectors, Periquito, Suraj D. Serai, Steven Sourbron and Christoffer Laustsen

Tamas Kaucsar and Andrea Fekete

Sandra Meyer and Dieter Fuchs

Lu-Ping Li, Bradley Hack and Pottumarthi V. Prasad

Kathleen Cantow, Mechthild Ladwig-Wiegard and Erdmann Seeliger

Neil Peter Jerome, Anna Caroli and Alexandra Ljimani

Roger G. Evans, Dirk Grosenick, Thomas Gladytz and Bert Flemming

Index

A

Acute Kidney Injury, 1, 9-10, 12, 16, 18, 25, 43, 45, 49, 69-70, 72-73, 77, 82, 84-85, 110-111, 133, 146-148, 156, 171, 174, 182, 184, 186-187, 200-201, 220, 222, 236-240

Analgesia, 23, 25, 27, 162

Anesthesia, 17-27, 44, 53-54, 110, 123, 139, 152, 162-163, 165-167, 180, 185, 223

Anisotropy, 204, 208, 213-215

Antibiotics, 24

Antidiabetic Liraglutide, 195-196

Apparent Diffusion Coefficient (adc), 125, 127, 204, 207, 210, 212, 217

Arbitrary, 118, 122, 229

Arterial Blood Pressure, 76, 223, 226, 230, 233

Arterial Spin Labeling (asl), 43, 69, 75-77, 80, 83, 87, 101, 120, 125-126

B

Blood Oxygenation Level Dependent (bold), 120, 172

Body Temperature, 17-18, 22-23, 27, 105, 139, 163

C

Cardiovascular Disease, 156-157

Chronic Kidney Disease, 17, 24, 45, 72, 111, 141, 145-146, 156-157, 171, 183, 186-187, 200, 215, 219, 222, 236

Clark-type Electrodes, 188, 223, 225-226, 232

Contrast Agent, 5, 11, 14, 16, 28-30, 33, 35, 37-38, 42, 44, 48-49, 60, 82, 141, 152, 156, 160-162, 165-166, 169-170, 179 188, 220

Cortex, 3, 6, 10, 21, 26, 28-29, 37, 39, 43-44, 69-71, 75-76, 85, 152, 157, 161, 169, 173, 175, 177-178, 181, 183, 189-190, 192, 202-203, 212, 223-226, 229, 231, 235-236, 238

D

Deoxygenated Hemoglobin, 172, 234

Diffusion-weighted Imaging (dwi), 87, 204, 210, 212

Disarticulation, 55-56

Dissection, 53

Doppler, 77, 150, 155-160, 164-166, 169, 171, 188, 223, 226-227, 229, 231, 239

E

Echo Time, 9, 65, 81, 91, 104, 109, 176, 194, 210

Ex Vivo Methods, 51

F

Fixation, 52-54, 60-61

Fluorescence-quenchingOptodes, 188, 223, 226

G

Gadolinium, 28-30, 33, 35-36, 43-44, 46-47, 49, 60, 69, 205, 218

Glomerular Filtration Rate (gfr), 28, 75, 189

Glycerol, 10, 141

Gradient Systems, 91, 106

H

Hematocrit, 173, 177-179, 190, 225, 227, 231, 235

Hemoglobin, 160, 169, 172, 175-176, 178-179, 191, 234

Heterogeneity, 37, 137, 173, 179, 195, 202, 222-224, 229, 231-233, 236, 238

Hydration, 17-19, 140

Hydronephrosis, 141, 155-157, 170

Hypoxia, 19, 73, 83, 95, 108, 140, 147, 172, 174-175, 179-187, 190, 192, 195-197, 200-202, 219, 222, 225-226, 233-235, 237-240

I

Image Distortion, 88, 177

Inhomogeneities, 9, 35, 82, 88, 104

Intravoxel Incoherent Motion (ivim), 125, 127, 204, 210-212, 217, 219

Ischemia, 1, 10-13, 16, 19-20, 22-23, 25-27, 45, 50, 69-70, 72, 77, 82-83, 133, 135-136, 138-139, 141, 145-147, 156, 171, 174, 182, 186, 202, 237

L

Laser-doppler Optodes, 231

Latex Covering, 53

M

Magnetic Resonance Imaging (mri), 1-2, 17, 28, 51, 62-63, 75, 86, 111-112, 132, 150, 172, 187, 204, 223

Medulla, 3, 6, 10, 28-29, 69-71, 75-76, 84, 157, 161-162, 169, 173, 175, 177-178, 181-183, 185, 189-190, 192, 195, 212, 223-226, 229, 231-232, 237

Multimodality, 150, 228

Multinuclear Imaging, 99

N

Near Infrared Spectroscopy, 192, 234

O

Oxygenation, 1-2, 12-13, 17-20, 25-26, 50, 58, 69, 82, 87-88, 101, 107, 114, 120, 125-127, 132-133, 160, 170, 172-174, 176-177, 179-191, 193, 195-203, 219, 222-224, 226, 228, 230, 233-235, 237-240

P

Parametric Imaging, 62

Parenchima, 1, 12, 17, 24, 28, 46, 51, 60-62, 72, 75, 81, 83, 86, 107, 111, 115, 119-120, 123, 129-130, 132, 144-145, 150, 170, 172, 184, 187, 200, 204, 215, 218, 222, 236

Perfusion, 2, 12, 17, 25-26, 28, 33, 39, 43, 53, 70, 75, 81, 87, 95, 101, 109, 114, 120, 125, 132, 140, 146, 152, 156, 160-161, 165-166, 169, 171, 173, 179, 188, 195-196, 200-201, 203, 208, 211, 218-219, 222-227, 229, 233-235, 237

Phantom, 8, 51-53, 55-60, 109

Pharmacokinetic, 37-38, 40, 45, 48, 73

Photoacoustic Imaging (pa), 150

Physiological Monitoring, 22, 25, 101-103, 105, 121, 123, 152-153

Pimonidazole, 174-175, 180-181, 184, 226-227, 233 234, 239

Pseudodiffusion, 207-209, 211-213

Pulsed Asl (pasl, 78-79

Q

Quantitative Invasive Probes, 222

R

Radio Frequency (rf) Coils, 94

Radiologists, 113-114

Renal Blood Flow (rbf), 29, 43, 75, 189

Renal Hemodynamics, 26, 82, 126, 147, 172, 179, 185-189, 191, 193, 195-199, 201-202, 222-223, 226, 228, 230-231, 233, 235, 237-240

Renal Transplantation, 50, 138-139

Respiration, 23, 94, 102-103, 105-106, 153, 164-165, 180

Rodents, 2, 18, 22-23, 25, 29, 77, 79, 86, 96-97, 101, 108, 132, 135-137, 139, 141-142, 174, 177-178

S

Scintigraphy, 77

Sepsis, 139-140, 174, 200, 237

Sodium Reabsorption, 173-174

Sonography, 77

Spatial Resolution, 2, 34, 68, 86-87, 89, 103, 106, 108, 119, 152, 174-175, 177, 194, 205, 208, 210, 216, 233

Suprarenal Aortic Occlusion, 179, 182, 191, 193

T

Tomography, 49, 77, 86, 140, 150, 185, 203

U

Ultrasound Imaging (us), 150

Unilateral Ureteral Obstruction (uuo), 182

V

Vascular Bundles, 224-226

X

X-nuclei, 95, 101, 105, 109